# *Bennett's* Ophthalmic Prescription Work

*Acquisitions editor*: Caroline Makepeace
*Development editor*: Zoë Youd
*Production controller*: Chris Jarvis
*Desk editor*: Claire Hutchins
*Cover Designer*: Fred Rose

# *Bennett's* Ophthalmic Prescription Work

Fourth edition

Kelvin G. Wakefield SMC(Tech)

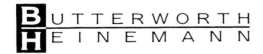

OXFORD  AUCKLAND  BOSTON  JOHANNESBURG  MELBOURNE  NEW DELHI

Butterworth-Heinemann
Linacre House, Jordan Hill, Oxford OX2 8DP
225 Wildwood Avenue, Woburn, MA 01801-2041
A division of Reed Educational and Professional Publishing Ltd

℞ A member of the Reed Elsevier plc group

First published 1963
Second edition 1983
Third edition 1994
Reprinted 1995
Fourth edition 2000

**British Library Cataloguing in Publication Data**
A catalogue record for this book is available from the British Library

**Library of Congress Cataloging in Publication Data**
A catalogue record for this book is available from the Library of Congress

ISBN 0 7506 4669 1

Printed and bound by Antony Rowe Ltd, Eastbourne

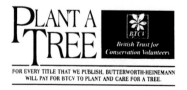

# Contents

*Preface*                                                              vii
*Acknowledgements*                                                      ix

**Part One**

 1  General introduction                                                 3
 2  The ophthalmic lens industry and materials                          13
 3  The spectacle frame industry and materials                          22
 4  Spectacle frame nomenclature                                        39
 5  Spectacle frame dimensions                                          53
 6  Lens shapes and sizes                                               60
 7  The prescription order form                                         69
 8  Spherical lenses                                                     75
 9  Astigmatic lenses                                                   102
10  Toric lenses                                                        111
11  Chapter revision                                                    123

**Part Two**

12  Optical centration                                                  129
13  Ophthalmic prisms                                                   144
14  Neutralisation                                                      161
15  The focimeter (lens analyser or lensmeter)                          167
16  Glazing                                                             180
17  Inspection/final verification                                       205
18  Chapter revision                                                    212

**Part Three**

19  Fused multifocals                                                   219
20  Glass solid multifocals                                             236
21  Resin multifocals                                                   244
22  Progressive lenses (PALs – progressive addition lenses)            248

23   Franklin (split) and 'bonded' lenses                     263
24   High powered and lenticular lenses                       268
25   Aspheric lenses                                          280
26   Anti-reflection, tinted and protective lenses            290
27   Lens surfacing/manufacturing                             320

## Part Four   Appendices

1   Vertex power allowances                                    337
2   Sags of lens surfaces                                      345
3   Powers of cylinders at oblique meridians                   352
4   Decentrations and prismatic effects                        354
5   Compensation for change in vertex distance                 358
6   Flow chart for a prescription house                        360

Index                                                          361

# Preface

In 1993 a great honour was bestowed upon me when Arthur Bennett gave me permission to update his book, which resulted in the third edition being published in 1994. I soon discovered that a lot had changed since Arthur produced the first edition back in 1963.

With the help of Simon Blumlein, Arthur produced a second edition in 1983.

Arthur died on 23rd March, 1994, aged 83, so he never saw the third edition, but I hoped he would have approved of my 'updating' of his original publication. 'Updating' is probably not the correct terminology, after 31 years it was probably more of a 're-write'. He possessed the rare ability of taking the complex and rendering it comprehensible. I trust you agree that I have continued that theme.

It is therefore an even greater honour to be asked by the publishers to produce this fourth edition. As I read through my original notes I realise how quickly manufacturing optics is changing. This can be appreciated by the fact that there was a gap of 20 years between the first and second editions of this book. The gap narrowed to 11 years between the second and third edition, and now a mere 6 years between the third and fourth. Many things have changed and I have therefore tried to incorporate as many as possible within this new edition.

Who is this book for? Anyone and everyone who has an interest or connection with optics. Be it the ophthalmic optician who wants to update his/her knowledge of modern manufacturing methods, be it the student or technician embarking on a career in optics or be it a receptionist or optical assistant, this book is for you – ENJOY.

Kelvin G. Wakefield SMC(Tech)

# Acknowledgements

The author gratefully acknowledges the help and assistance gained from articles written and diagrams supplied by the following.

M. Jalie SMSA, FBDO (Hons), MIMgt, Hon FCGI
A. J. Jarratt FBDO
G. Walsh
P. O'Neill
L. Sasieni FBDA, FSMC, DOrth, DCLP
F. Blackwood
B. Such
S. Johnson SMC(Tech)
Dr R. Barth
J. Bruneni
G. Walsh
M. Emes
Dr P. Wilkinson

*Younger Optics*
*The Optician*
*Optical World*
*Dispensing Optician*
BSI

Without reference to these articles this book would never have been possible.

Special thanks to Dr C. Fowler BSc, PhD, FBCO for his valuable contributions and advice.

A special mention also to Professor Mo Jalie who very kindly reviewed the manuscript prior to publication, providing the author with some very valuable 'fine tuning'.

And last but not least, a very special thanks to Imelda Walden for patiently working through the updated manuscript allowing yours truly to submit to the publishers on time.

# Part One

# Chapter 1

# General introduction

The wearing of spectacles has now become a common everyday need for millions of people around the world. Without spectacles their perception of life would be very different. Distance or near objects would not be seen clearly and participation in sport and leisure activities would be affected – but it has not always been like this.

Who invented spectacles? Whether it was Roger Bacon (1216–1294) or Salvino d'Amarti or somebody else, or whether they were first used by the Chinese, Greeks or Druids is not clearly determinable. There is a suggestion that spectacle making became more common with the advent of printing (Caxton produced the earliest printed book in England in 1476). References to spectacles certainly became more frequent after that date!

The earliest spectacles were comparatively crude affairs but were found to be such a boon that they came into common use long before the optical system of the eye was properly understood.

In Great Britain the Worshipful Company of Spectacle Makers, a City of London Livery Company, is predominant whenever mention is made of both past and present optical history. Founded by Royal Charter in 1629, its function is to ensure high standards of quality and service in optics. In fact, with time, the activities of the Company have extended across the whole field of optics, covering education and training. The Great Fire of London in 1666 destroyed all of the Company's documents with the exception of its Charter and Ordinances. The Court Minutes are therefore complete from 1666 until the present day.

The great Samuel Pepys had spectacles made for him by John Turlington who was Master of the Company from 1665 until 1668. He was a well-known spectacle maker in his day and was described by Samuel Pepys in his Diary as 'The Great Spectacle Maker'.

For many centuries spectacles could only have been provided on a basis of trial and error, and were incapable of providing any proper relief for astigmatism. Indeed, it was not until the nineteenth century that the prescribing of spectacles began to be put on to a scientific basis.

The existence of ocular astigmatism was first demonstrated by the English scientist Thomas Young in 1801. In 1825, Sir George Airy, afterwards Astronomer Royal, measured his own astigmatism and was the first to specify and wear the proper type of lens for its correction.

Perhaps the greatest single contributor to the science of refraction was the Dutch ophthalmologist Donders, whose classic work *Accommodation and Refraction of the Eye*, published in English in 1864, cleared away many of the previously confused ideas. The latter half of the nineteenth century also saw the introduction of the trial case, the retinoscope, and the ophthalmoscope, which now form the basic equipment of the optical practitioner. Over the years, spectacle lenses have become more accurate and considerably more complex. As a result, good prescription work demands a wider range of knowledge than ever before.

A similar development has taken place with regard to frames. The greater accuracy of lenses requires a corresponding accuracy in frame fitting and measurement so that the lenses are held in the correct position with respect to the eyes. Much greater attention is now paid to the cosmetic aspect, that is, the appearance of the spectacles on the wearer's face. Spectacle frames and mounts are now made in a bewildering variety of styles and lens shapes and in many different materials, obtainable in an enormous range of colours.

Besides prescription lenses mounted in frames, ocular corrections can also be achieved by the use of contact lenses. Advancements in technology have allowed the development of materials that enable the eye to 'breathe', by permitting oxygen to pass through them thereby making them more comfortable to wear. A recent development has been *photorefractive keratectomy* (PRK). By use of a low energy excimer laser, corneal tissue is selectively removed to have the desired corrective effect on the eye's system, thereby restoring good vision. Whilst both contact lenses and PRK represent important advancements in the treatment of sight defects it is not the intention of this book to explore these particular aspects.

## Some terms explained

The term *optics* is derived from a Greek root meaning 'pertaining to the eyes or sight'. It denotes a science, divided into many branches, covering a vast range of phenomena connected with light and sight. *Geometrical optics*, the oldest branch of the subject, is mainly concerned with lenses, mirrors and prisms, together with the optical instruments that can be made from them. Therefore, as expected, geometrical optics provides the basis for the theoretical study of spectacle lenses.

*Ophthalmic optics* – rather a broad term – is that branch of the subject dealing with vision, the word 'ophthalmic' having been derived from another Greek root meaning 'the eye'. *Ophthalmology* is that branch of medicine and surgery dealing with the eye, and its practitioners are called *ophthalmic surgeons* or *ophthalmologists*. *Ocular*, pertaining to the eye, is derived from the Latin word 'oculus'. *Oculist* is the popular name frequently used by laymen when referring to an ophthalmic surgeon.

The action of a lens or prism, i.e. its effects on light passing through it, is described by the general term *refraction*, and the defects of vision briefly outlined below are termed *refractive errors*. The term *refraction* is also used to denote the process of detecting and estimating such errors, commonly known as *sight-testing*. A *refractionist* is an optician or other practitioner carrying out refraction.

Over the years, the term 'optician' has had several meanings. It originally denoted someone versed in optical science and was later applied to a maker of (or dealer in) optical instruments including spectacles.

It may be useful at this point to clarify the names and roles of the various 'professionals' involved in the important task of eye care. There are four types of practitioner who are registered and qualified within the UK:

*Ophthalmic medical practitioners (OMPs)* are fully qualified doctors who specialise in eyes and eye care. In addition to their medical skills in detecting abnormalities and diseases of the eye, they are also qualified to test sight and prescribe spectacles and other appliances. They are registered with the General Medical Council and work either in Medical Eye Centres, which are operated by firms of opticians, or from their own consulting rooms.

*Hospital Eye Service consultant ophthalmologists*, otherwise known as ophthalmic surgeons, work in the Hospital Eye Service, as do some opticians. In their treatment of eye disorders they sometimes provide corrective lenses. They do not dispense or fit spectacles, although a dispensing service is available at some eye hospitals.

*Ophthalmic opticians (OOs)*, also known as optometrists, are qualified to test sight and both to prescribe and dispense spectacles and other optical appliances. They are trained to recognise abnormalities and diseases which are revealed in the eyes.

*Dispensing opticians (DOs)* are qualified to dispense, fit and supply spectacles. The main function of the DO is the interpretation of a patient's individual visual and fitting requirements and the translation of the prescription into specifications and instructions to which the optical manufacturer will work.

A vast array of different lens types and forms are available and it is the responsibility of the dispenser to ascertain, in conjunction with the patient with regard to their occupation and lifestyle, which lens type or form would be most suitable. Measurements then have to be taken to position the lenses accurately before the eye. Therefore linked to this is the function of helping the patient to select a frame that is suitable for their particular prescription and facial contours.

When the prescribed spectacles have been fabricated the dispenser will make the minor adjustments necessary to ensure the correct fit. A recent change in the law means that DOs must now be specially certified to fit contact lenses.

The titles and roles may vary in different countries whose health regulations and practices are different.

The supply of finished spectacles to the public also relies on the skills of optical receptionists, assistants and technicians.

The *'prescription'* ('Rx' for short) is a specification of the lenses needed by the patient. The same term is sometimes used in connection with a spectacle frame or mounting, in which case it means a concise description covering material, style and measurements.

The concept of a *lens* is developed throughout this book but a definition of a lens may be considered as 'an optical medium, bounded by two polished surfaces, one of which must be curved'.

## Why spectacles?

It is natural for anyone engaged in making or supplying spectacles to wonder how and why they work. A brief explanation is given in this section. It should be borne in mind that it represents only the merest outline of the subject, which constitutes an entire field of study in itself.

Spectacles can be used to correct sight defects, protect against impact, and protect against certain radiation. One must also not forget the cosmetic function that they perform in providing a fashion accessory as well as the more serious roles mentioned above.

A good idea of the structure of the human eye can be obtained from an elementary textbook of anatomy and physiology, which the interested reader should consult. From an optical point of view, the eye can be compared to a camera.

The most important part of a camera is the lens or lens combination, the function of which is to throw a picture or image of the scene in front of it on to a sensitive film or plate. In the same way, the optical system of the eye forms an image on the retina, a sensitive screen connected to the brain by means of the optic nerve.

When the camera is properly adjusted, the film is at the correct distance from the lens and receives a sharply focused image. If the film is too near or too far from the lens, the image becomes 'out of focus' or blurred. In this event, sharp focusing could be restored by one of two methods: (1) by adjusting the distance between lens and film or (2) by mounting an additional lens of the correct power in front of the camera. The wearing of spectacles corresponds to this latter method.

Suppose a camera that is properly adjusted for distant objects is used to take a close-up portrait. It will be found that the picture is blurred because, according to a well-known law of geometrical optics, the image of a near object is formed at a different distance from the lens than the image of a more distant object (*Figure 1.1*). Again, to bring the image into focus, either of the methods already mentioned could be adopted. That is, move the lens away from the film, or use a supplementary lens. Modern cameras allow adjustment of the lens position relative to the film. However, supplementary or 'portrait attachments' can be fitted.

A method more subtle than either of these two is used by the human eye (*Figure 1.2*). The crystalline lens *changes shape* to accommodate different distances.

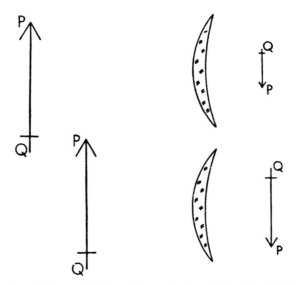

**Figure 1.1** The inverted image QP formed by a plus lens of the object PQ. If the object is brought nearer to the lens, the image moves further away and increases in size.

Listed below are some of the components that make up the human eye.

*Cornea.* The outer coat, the window of the eye, which carries out most of the focusing of light to form a sharp image within the eye. The eyelids protect the cornea by reacting very quickly if anything tries to come into contact with it.

*Pupil.* Actually a hole, behind the cornea, through which light passes. From an observer's point of view, it is the black circular part of the eye.

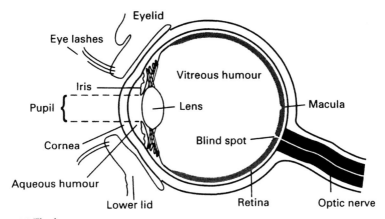

**Figure 1.2** The human eye.

*Iris.* In contrast to the pupil, this is the coloured part of the eye. At birth, the colour varies from light grey to blue. The true colour, usually inherited, forms when the pigment cells begin to grow. The iris contains muscle which controls the size of the pupil aperture. At night or in conditions of low illumination the iris dilates allowing the pupil to be larger, thus permitting more light to reach the eye.

*Lens.* Full name is 'crystalline lens', and it has the ability to change shape, which enables the eye to focus at different distances. For example, when looking at a near object, the lens becomes bulbous but when looking into the distance, it is relaxed and thinner.

*Retina.* The inside surface at the back of the eye, made up from 10 layers of nerve fibres and cells. Some of the cells are sensitive to light but the nerve fibres are not, their job being to conduct the light impulses given out by the cells. The cells can be divided into two groups, rods and cones. There are some 120 million rods and 6 million cones in a human eye. The rods are insensitive to colour but react to the light. The cones, on the other hand, distinguish colours but only in daylight or conditions of high illumination. This is why at night trees and fields are seen as a tone of grey rather than green. Cones are located at the macula, and are used for tasks requiring good visual acuity. Rods are found in other areas of the retina.

*Macula.* It is only 1.5 mm in diameter and is at the centre of the retina. The parts surrounding the macula give us visual awareness – peripheral vision.

*Optic nerve.* This provides the link between the images received by the retina and the brain. It transmits the images to the brain.

*Blind spot.* The name given to the place where all retinal nerve fibres come together to enter the optic nerve. It covers an area of 2 mm diameter and contains no receptor cells, hence it is a blind spot. This tends not to be noticed as the blind spots are positioned in the nasal area of the retina in each eye and each eye makes up for the other.

*Sclera.* The white part of the eye. A very tough external coat, continuous with the transparent cornea.

*Vitreous humour and aqueous humour.* The vitreous humour fills most of the eyeball, maintaining its basic shape, and is jelly-like in substance. Aqueous humour is liquid-like, providing the metabolism of the lens and cornea and controlling the intra-ocular pressure.

The transparent outer portion, the cornea, acts in the same way as a lens but is supplemented by another one – the crystalline lens – hidden from view behind the iris. In the perfect eye the two combine to form a sharply focused image of distance objects on the retina (*Figure 1.3*). When a near object is viewed, the crystalline lens alters its shape and curvature

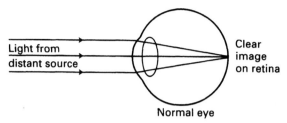

**Figure 1.3** The 'perfect' eye.

as the result of an unconscious muscular effort, making the eye as a whole more powerful, and once again sharp focusing is obtained. This ability of the eye to focus at different distances is known as 'accommodation'.

The optical defects which can be corrected by spectacles fall into five main categories.

## Hypermetropia (long-sightedness)

In hypermetropia the eye is too short to suit its optical system and additional focusing power is required (*Figure 1.4*). If the deficiency is not too great, the additional power can be supplied by exerting an effort of accommodation, in which case clear vision of distant objects can be obtained. However, this means that less than the normal amount of accommodation is available for use in near vision, which may prove to be an inconvenience. The remedy is to wear a supplementary lens of such power that clear distance vision is enjoyed without any effort of accommodation (*Figure 1.5*).

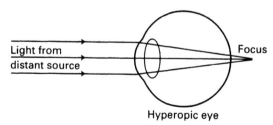

**Figure 1.4** The hyperopic eye.

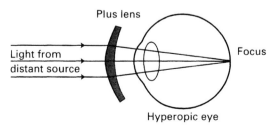

**Figure 1.5** The action of a plus lens on a hyperopic eye.

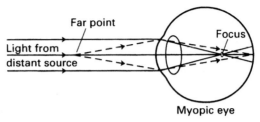

**Figure 1.6** The myopic eye.

## Myopia (short-sightedness)

Myopia is the reverse condition: the eye is too long to suit its optical system (*Figure 1.6*). As a result, only near objects can be seen distinctly for these are imaged at a greater distance from the lens. Since the focusing power of a myopic eye is too great to suit its length, the remedy consists of wearing a minus lens to reduce it to the required amount. Unlike the plus lens that is capable of focusing light on to a screen or film, a minus lens spreads it out more. Hence, when used in conjunction with a strong plus lens it reduces the power of the latter (*Figure 1.7*).

In extreme cases of myopia, surgical techniques may be employed.

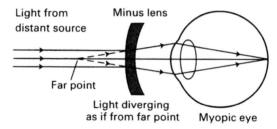

**Figure 1.7** The action of a minus lens on a myopic eye.

## Presbyopia

As already mentioned, the ability of the eye to accommodate for different distances depends on the crystalline lens. As the result of biological processes which cannot at present be controlled, the crystalline lens gradually hardens with the passage of time and so the amount of accommodation that can be brought into play slowly declines. Consequently, even though perfect distance vision is enjoyed with or without glasses, a time is reached when viewing at a normal reading or working distance becomes difficult. This condition is known as presbyopia and as a rule makes itself felt at an age in the early or middle forties. The remedy is to wear either bifocals, trifocals or progressives to provide the additional power hitherto supplied by accommodation. A less common solution today is to provide separate distance and reading spectacles.

## Aphakia

Aphakia is the term applied to the eye when the crystalline lens has been removed. In cases of cataract, the lens becomes opaque and blindness results but vision can often be restored by the operation of removing the lens. Unfortunately, the focusing power of the eye is then greatly reduced and so a high-powered lens is required to make up the deficiency. The power of accommodation is also lacking in the aphakic eye and so a still more powerful lens is needed for reading. Most patients operated on for removal of the crystalline lens will be suitable to have an IOL (intra-ocular lens) or implant positioned within the eye to replace what the eye surgeon has just removed. This means the need for bulbous high powered lenses to be worn in front of the patient's eyes in the form of spectacles is eliminated. They will probably still need some form of correction, especially for reading purposes but not the very high powered lenses that used to be associated with this condition.

## Astigmatism

Astigmatism is a defect which may be found in conjunction with any of the other defects already mentioned. It is usually due to one of the eye's optical surfaces, often the front surface of the cornea, not being perfectly spherical but shaped, for example, like a portion of the surface of a pumpkin or a motor tyre, which is differently curved in different directions. A surface of this kind is termed 'astigmatic' (from the Greek, meaning 'without a point') because, unlike a spherical surface, it is incapable of bringing all the rays of light emanating from a point on the object to a corresponding point on the image. In other words, by itself it is incapable of forming a well-focused image. A non-astigmatic person, on looking at a diagram such as *Figure 1.8* will see all the radiating lines equally clearly; if astigmatism is present the lines may not appear to be equally distinct, some being apparently blacker or more sharply defined than the rest.

The remedy is to wear a lens having one surface unequally curved in different directions so as to counteract or neutralise the defect in the eye itself.

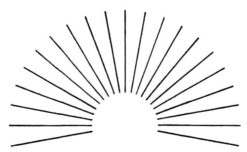

**Figure 1.8** The 'astigmatic fan'. Some of these lines may appear blacker than others to an astigmatic eye.

## Some practical experiments

The best way to understand what has been described in this chapter is to experiment with a few lenses. For example, with a meniscus lens about +6.00 DS it will be seen that an image of a window can be formed on a screen such as a sheet of white paper or cardboard by holding the lens at the correct distance from it. If the lens is moved too near or too far away from the screen, the image becomes blurred. It can also be verified that if the lens is brought much nearer to the window the screen has to be placed further from the lens than before to bring the image into focus. The image on the screen will be seen to be inverted, that is to say turned through 180 degrees. The image formed on the retina is also inverted despite which we still see things the right way up.

A good idea of the effect of astigmatism can be obtained by repeating the experiments with a spherocylindrical or toric lens about +6.00 DS + 4.00 DC, held with its axis horizontal or vertical. It will be found that at a certain distance of the lens from the screen the horizontal window bars are sharply imaged and that the vertical bars seem clearer at another distance, but in no position can a really sharp and satisfactory image of the whole window be obtained. In view of the peculiar nature of this defect it is not surprising that it escaped analysis for so long.

# Chapter 2

# The ophthalmic lens industry and materials

Even when ignoring ophthalmic instruments, equipment and contact lenses, the ophthalmic lens industry covers many different skills which have little in common from the standpoint of manufacturing techniques.

Firstly, there are the international companies such as Pilkington, Corning, Schott, PPG and Toray who supply the basic raw materials from which others will produce lenses. This again is a very much 'across the world' operation with ophthalmic lenses being made in the USA, Mexico, Australia, Japan, Philippines, Singapore and Taiwan, to name but a few. These are locations that convert the raw materials into the semi-finished and finished lens products which are further processed by national and regional prescription laboratories.

Prescription laboratories, sometimes referred to as prescription houses, deal with individual orders for single spectacles or lenses to prescription. A modern prescription house will have in stock both finished and semi-finished blanks, the latter being used for all but the simplest of prescriptions. The term *semi-finished* is used because the prescription house has probably purchased-in these blanks with one surface, normally the front, completely finished, with the 'other' surface yet to be processed. The blank has no dioptric power until the prescription house works specific curves on the unfinished side. For this reason the prescription house has to operate a surfacing shop to make such lenses singly, as and when required. These lenses can then be supplied to the customer, the customer being the optician or another prescription house, in either what is termed 'uncut' form, where the finished lens is sent out unfitted to any frame or, in 'glazed' form, where the lenses have been cut to the shape of the frame and glazed.

The prescription house will have a large stockroom to store its supplies of finished and semi-finished lenses, its frames and other related items and may also perform the useful function of acting as a wholesaler and distributor of ophthalmic products in general, including instruments and equipment used in the ophthalmic practice.

There are also small 'workshops' attached to opticians' premises often referred to as CEF (cut, edge and fit) establishments. In this instance the optician obtains the lenses from a prescription house, then cuts and glazes them to the frame 'in-house', most likely holding a stock of finished single vision lenses to allow 'easier' prescriptions to be fabricated very quickly. The system is very common in Europe and is gaining acceptance in the UK.

A natural follow-on to this has been the emergence of what is termed 'superopticals' from the USA where refraction, dispensing and manufacture, including lenses, are combined in one retail site.

## Glass lenses

The modern techniques employed for the manufacture of spectacle glass is both highly controlled and automated, normally as a continuous process.

First stage is batch preparation where the raw materials such as silica, alumina, calcium carbonate, magnesium oxide, sodium carbonate, sodium sulphate, potassium carbonate, barium carbonate and borax are carefully checked against specifications, weighed and blended together before transfer to the furnace. The procedure is very much the same for higher index or photochromic-type glass, with different chemicals being added or, indeed, omitted.

The 'ingredients' are then mixed with cullet (rejected glass from a previous similar mix) which facilitates the mixing/melting, and heated in the furnace to between 1000 and 1500°C which in turn converts the mix into a viscous mass.

The refining stage involves the temperature being raised to 1600°C to eliminate all gases still present and to purify the composition. To prevent the risk of contamination the chamber can be lined with platinum.

The conditioning stage follows. The glass is too liquid from the previous process and now has to be brought down in temperature to make it more homogeneous for moulding. The mixture is constantly stirred during conditioning. When the correct consistency is reached (similar to that of treacle) the glass is moulded to shape.

The final stage is annealing where the lens is slowly cooled to room temperature to avoid internal stresses.

Glass is available in a whole range of different indices (refractive index) but for ophthalmic use the following are typically used: $n = 1.523, n = 1.60, n = 1.70, n = 1.80$ and $n = 1.90$ ($n$ is an abbreviation for refractive index).

The refractive index of a lens is obtained by:

$$n = \frac{\text{Speed of light in air}}{\text{Speed of light in medium}}$$

the medium in this instance being the lens.

The indices quoted have, in the main, been rounded for simplicity. Besides being available in 'white glass', photochromics are also available in the 1.523 and 1.60 categories.

Traditionally, 1.523 spectacle crown was the most popular. This material has many excellent properties; it is highly transparent, colourless and odourless; it is resistant to heat and atmospheric attack; it does not easily tarnish nor become scratched as easily as some other types of glass. With the introduction of resin lenses its use has drastically declined over the years.

Although there has been a decline in the use of spectacle crown, an increase has occurred in the higher index materials such as 1.70, 1.80 and 1.90 (available under various trade names). These may have a weight disadvantage compared to resin lens materials but they do have the advantage of being thinner.

Photochromic glass is another interesting development. These lenses darken on exposure to bright light and clear again once removed from the light. This is achieved through silver halide crystals contained within the glass. When subjected to UV radiation between 320 and 420 nm a metallic silver deposit forms on the surface of the crystals within the lens. This causes the lens to effectively darken. Removal from the activating light causes the reconversion into silver halide, thus the lens clears. The silver halide crystals are generally between 0.008 and 0.0015 µm in size.

Overall, in the UK, glass lenses form about 10% of the ophthalmic lens market, resin taking up the remaining 90%. However, these figures will vary in different parts of the world, with less developed countries using a greater proportion of glass lenses. Optical surfaces on glass are produced by the processes of generating, smoothing and polishing. The first stage, generating, is where the lens has the curve or curves machined or cut into it and at the same time is reduced to the correct substance (although there is a small allowance for material removed in subsequent processes). This is normally done by a diamond-bonded disc or cutter.

Smoothing is the name given to the process that improves the finish on the generated surface. To facilitate this a tool representing the same but opposite curvature to that of the lens is used, a compensation having been made to the tool radius to allow for the thickness of the pads applied for smoothing and polishing (see Chapter 27). Normally a smoothing pad will be placed on the tool surface. Lens, tool and pad are then mounted into a machine that will, with the aid of smoothing powder mixed with water, improve the surface of the generated lens. The curvature is kept true by the fact that the pad is resting on an appropriate tool, machined with the correct curvature.

The polishing procedure is very similar to that of smoothing but this time a polishing pad is placed on the tool and the abrasive is so fine it can be considered a polish.

Mention should also be made of a process called *trepanning* or *cribbing*, which is normally performed before generating. It involves reducing the lens blank down to a more suitable diameter taking into account the frame size and the lens setting details. For example, some lens types are available from the semi-finished manufacturers with a minimum blank size of, say, 70 mm. This is fine on a large frame but why surface a lens as large as 70 mm when, for a small frame, the glazing department is going to cut most of it away? Surely, it is much better to reduce it to a diameter more compatible with that of the frame being glazed. Besides this, the smaller the lens the thinner it can be made and the easier it is to process.

## Resin lenses

Resin lenses have two great advantages over glass. They are only about half the weight and are far less easily broken.

The first range of resin ophthalmic lenses ever produced was made in England by a patented process whereby 'preforms' cut from solid polymethyl methacrylate – an acrylic resin – were compression moulded between highly polished stainless steel dyes. The lenses were marketed under the trade name 'Igardi', subsequently shortened to 'Igard'. An additional process was later introduced whereby the lenses were coated with another and harder material giving them a greatly increased scratch resistance. Lenses made by this method are sometimes referred to as 'thermoplastic'.

Although Igard lenses are still available today, by far the most popular resin material is CR39 developed in America by the Columbia Southern Chemical Corporation in the 1940s (the 'C' indicating Columbia, from the company that developed it, the 'R' for resin and '39' because the 39th attempt was the most promising as it offered some unique character-istics). The first commercial use of this new monomer involved combining with fibre glass to form moulded fuel tanks for American B17 bombers!

The scientific name for CR39 is Allyl Diglycol Carbonate and it has a refractive index of 1.498. The appearance is of a limpid liquid possessing a viscosity identical to glycerine oil. It is a thermosetting material that will withstand temperatures up to 100°C without deformation.

Development of today's CR39 lenses came primarily from the efforts of companies such as Univis, Armorlite (later to become Signet Armorlite), Sola and Essilor.

Initially there were two main production problems, that of shrinkage and that of scratching. During the curing process there can be up to a 14% shrinkage, the greater the difference between the front and back surface curvatures, the greater the shrinkage. The problem was overcome by the use of a different glass for the moulds and the inclusion of a release agent in the monomer.

The problem of CR39 lenses scratching was conquered in the 1970s when Minnesota Mining and Manufacturing (3M) developed a coating (to be marketed by Armorlite as 'RLX') that could be applied to give greater scratch resistance. Most CR39 lens manufacturers now have their own brand hardcoating (see Chapter 26).

The process of resin lens manufacture involves injecting the liquid monomer between two glass-toughened moulds. Sometimes a harder metallic coating will also be applied to the surface of the mould. Utmost skill and care is required since the lens faces automatically reproduce all the qualities or defects of these moulds.

The moulds are separated by a type of ring, often referred to as a gasket. It has two functions: to hold the monomer liquid between the two faces of the moulds and to give the lens its centre and edge thickness. The material chosen for the gasket has to be able to withstand the temperatures incurred during the polymerisation process and cope with the average 14% shrinkage factor. A metal clip is used to hold the whole assembly together. Very carefully the monomer is injected between the moulds where the formation of air bubbles must be avoided. The filled moulds are then subjected to heat by either oven or immersion in hot water. Alone it cannot grow harder, so to harden it a catalyst such as benzoyl peroxide is added in suitable proportions which initiates the polymerisation process under the combined action of heat and transforms the monomer liquid into polymer (a solid). A diagrammatic representation is shown in *Figure 2.1*.

The cast lens can either be finished, in the case of stock single vision, or semi-finished, which will require further processing in a prescription house. This further processing is similar to that described for glass surfacing, namely, generating, smoothing and polishing, except to say that smoothing is often referred to as *fining* and that the smoothing and polishing pads along with the abrasives used are of different grades. CR39, unlike Igard, is a 'thermosetting' material.

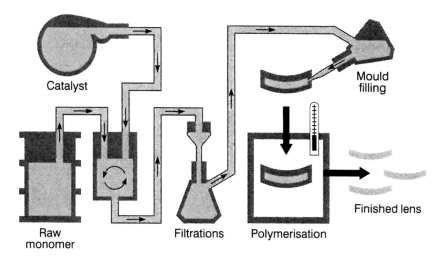

**Figure 2.1** Resin lens manufacture.

Recent development work has brought about the availability of high index resins such as 1.586, 1.60, 1.66 and even 1.70, – all marketed under various trade names.

Another high index resin material is polycarbonate. Originally developed and manufactured in 1957 by the General Electric Company and known by the name of *Lexan*. In 1978, 21 years after its introduction, the first ophthalmic lens, commercially available, came on to the market. Its initial manufacture is by injection moulding between steel dyes. The foremost differentiation is that it is a thermoplastic as opposed to thermosetting.

A thermoplastic softens when heated. Polycarbonate begins as a solid, is melted, then injected into moulds under temperatures of approximately 320°C. The moulding machines apply considerable pressure and, in roughly 2–5 minutes the lenses are ready to be removed from the moulds.

Because it is thermoplastic, polycarbonate must be guarded against excessive heat during all laboratory processing procedures. The physical properties which give it outstanding impact resistance also leave it susceptible to scratching and therefore it is essential to supply the lens to the patient with some form of hardcoat/scratch resistant coating. It has a strength-to-weight ratio equal to aluminium. Its impact strength is four times higher than aluminium or zinc. For this reason it is sometimes referred to as a thermoplastic 'metal'. Traditionally, polycarbonate has always been used in the field of industrial eye safety because of its strength. However, because of its index (1.586) it is also thinner than ordinary CR39, so its cosmetic advantages are gradually being appreciated. This coupled with the availability of aspheric, photochromic and polarised lenses in polycarbonate material has further increased its popularity.

The special contribution that antireflection coatings have made to enhancing the appearance of both resin and glass lenses must not be forgotten.

## Standards

The entire field of spectacle manufacturing and in particular prescription lens production depends on consistent adherence to standards. Quality starts with standards. Standards lay down the criteria for products, processes and systems, to ensure that they will do the job properly. They influence every aspect of production from design to after-sales service. They apply from the time a product is conceived, through design development and manufacture, to testing for fitness of purpose and durability. Standards help improve safety and cost-effectiveness and save our precious resources.

The first official British standard dates back to 1901 when the forerunner to the British Standards Institute (BSI), the Engineering Standards Committee, started work on a standard for the sizes of tramway rails. Now there are approximately 80 000 standards covering everything from abrasives to zip fasteners. When a new standard is needed, BSI calls together everyone who has an interest – manufacturers, consumers, major purchasers, safety experts, trade bodies – to ensure that standards are fair and accepted by everyone.

BSI is Britain's voice in European and world standardisation, putting industry and consumers' points of view and bringing back information on changes that will affect them. BSI represents the UK through two organisations: the European Committee for Standardization (CEN) and the European Committee for Electrotechnical Standardization (CEN-ELEC), CEN and CENELEC aim to harmonise their members' national standards on the basis of the work of their corresponding international bodies, the International Organization for Standardization (ISO) and the International Electrotechnical Commission (IEC). Although CEN and CENELEC cannot compel anyone to use their standards, BSI, as members, are obliged to implement European standards known as BSENs in the UK, by giving them the status of national standards and by ceasing work on any conflicting proposal or existing national standards while the EN is developed.

Under the current approach, the harmonisation of legislation is limited to setting the essential requirement for health, safety, consumer protection and the environment while the technical details of how the directives can be met will be worked out by CEN and CENELEC. All products which comply with these requirements will necessarily carry a CE mark – the EC stamp of approval – which will allow them to be circulated freely in the rest of the European Community.

Standards have always been an important element for optical producers. UK optical trade and professional organisations have worked with BSI, CEN and ISO to rationalise existing and new optical standards for semi-finished, uncut and glazed spectacles.

Many companies operating in the optical field have been accredited to ISO 9000 an international standard that requires organizations to have an agreed quality policy and control system. Companies are assessed several times each year to ensure they are complying with the standards set out in their policy procedures within their quality manuals. This is a stepping stone for Total Quality Management (TQM) benchmarking disciplines.

The following list demonstrates to the reader the scope and variety of standards within the optical community:

BS EN 1836 (1997)   *Sunglass and Sunglare Filters*
BS 2738 Part 1 (1998)   *Mounted Spectacle Lenses*
BS 2738 Part 3 (1991)   *Presentation of Rx Orders*
BS EN ISO 10322–1 (1997) (BS 2738 Part 4)   *Specification for Semi-Finished SV and Multifocal Blanks*
BS EN ISO 10322–2 (1997) (BS 2738 Part 5)   *Specification for Semi-Finished Progressives*
BS EN ISO 8980 Part 1 (1997) (BS 2738 Part 6)   *Uncut Finished Spectacle Lenses – Single Vision and Multifocals*
BS EN 8980 Part 2 (1997) (BS 2738 Part 7)   *Uncut Finished Spectacle Lenses – Progressives*
BS EN ISO 14889 (1997) (BS 2738 Part 8)   *Fundamental Requirements for Uncut Finished Lenses*
BS 3199 (1992) (ISO 8624: 1997)   *Measurements for Spectacle Frames*
BS 7930–1 (1998)   *Eye Protectors for Racket Sports – Part 1 Squash*
BS EN 166 (1996)   *Personal Eye Protection Specifications*
BS EN 167 (1995)   *Personal Eye Protection Optical Test Methods*
BS EN 168 (1995)   *Personal Eye Protection. Non Optical Test Methods*
BS 7394 Part 2 (1994)   *Specification for Complete Spectacles to Rx*
BS EN ISO 12870 (1998) (BS 6625: 1998)   *Spectacle Frames – General Requirements and Test Methods*
BS 6625 Part 2 (1992) (ISO 9456: 1991)   *Spectacle Frame Specification for Marking*
BS 7394 Part 1 (1996)   *Ready to Wear Near Vision Spectacles*
BS 6001 Part 1 (1991) (ISO 2859–11: 1994)   *Sampling Methods*
BS EN ISO 9002 (1994)   *Quality Systems*
ISO 13666 (1998)   *Ophthalmic Optics – Spectacle Lenses – Vocabulary*
BS EN 165 (1996)   *Eye Protection Vocabulary*
BS EN 172 (1995)   *Specification for Sunglare Filters used in Personal Eye Protectors for Industrial Use*
BS EN ISO 8624 (1997)   *Measuring System for Spectacle Frames*
BS 3521:2 (1991)   *Glossary of Terms Relating to Spectacle Frames*

BS EN ISO 7998 (1996)   *Spectacle Frames – Vocabulary and Lists of Equivalent Terms*
BS EN 11380 (1997)   *Ophthalmic Optics – Formers*
BS EN ISO 8429: 1007   *Optics and Optical Instruments Ophthalmology – Graduated Dial Scale*
BS ISO 8598 (1996)   *Optics and Optical Instruments – Focimeters*
BS ISO 9342 (1996)   *Optics and Optical Instruments – Test Lenses For Calibration of Focimeters*
BS EN ISO 13230 (1999)   *Ophthalmic Optics – Bar Code Specifications*
BS EN ISO 8980 Part 3   *Uncut Finished Spectacle Lenses – Transmittance Specifications and Test Methods*

The list above does not pretend to be a totally comprehensive representation of all standards applicable to optics, but it provides the reader with details of the 'main' ones. Standards are constantly being changed and supplemented in line with current thinking and technology. Always ensure you are using the latest version.

Whilst on the subject of standards, earlier in the chapter mention was made of refractive index. BS 7394 Part 2 (1994) advises of the various categories into which refractive indices can be classified. Any material with an index of 1.48 but below 1.54 is classed as 'normal index'. Material of 1.54 but less than 1.64 is 'mid index'. Material of 1.64 but below 1.74 is 'high index' and any material 1.74 and above is classified as 'very high index'.

In concluding this section of the chapter it would be of use to the reader to consider one other element or characteristic of lens material, that is its constringence (also referred to as v-value or Abbe number). Constringence is the reciprocal of the dispersive power of the material and indicates the degree of transverse chromatic aberration.

The effect is to cause colour fringing around items viewed through different materials. Standard Crown glass and CR39 material have v-values in the region of 59. These low dispersion materials rarely give rise to complaints of colour fringing. However, as a general statement higher index materials whilst being thinner than 'standard' materials, do have a problem that the chemical/ingredients used to give the lens its higher index do have a tendency to bring the v value down, which in turn causes colour fringing. Lenses with higher v-values have less chromatic aberration than those with low v-values.

BS 7394 Part 2 1994 classifies lenses with v-values of 45 and above as being 'low dispersion', between 39 but less than 45 as 'medium dispersion' and less than 39 'as high dispersion'.

Hopefully the reader can appreciate the important role that standards have to play. They provide an accepted benchmark and the correct terminology which any dialogue or written material can be based around.

## Quality

Standards go a long way to help ensure that optical products are of an acceptable quality. They provide the consumer the assurance and benefits linked to working from a nationally or internationally accepted standard.

EEC Regulations also have an impact on 'Quality Assurance' in as much that many of the requirements go 'hand in hand' with certification to, for example, a BSI scheme.

CE marking means that a manufacturer claims his product satisfies the requirements essential for it to be considered safe and fit for the intended purpose. It also means that the product can be marketed anywhere in the European Community without further controls.

With regard to CE marking, there are two Directives to consider: the Personal Protective Equipment (PPE) and Medical Devices (MD).

Taking PPE first. Can we dispel a popular myth – the CE mark replaces the Kitemark – IT DOES NOT! One cannot replace the other but they can co-exist. The CE mark is a legal requirement, the Kitemark is a quality mark. Since the first of July 1995, it has been a requirement that the CE mark be displayed on safety eyewear.

Many companies will, however, also continue using the Kitemark as it represents a more rigorous scheme than the CE mark, which once awarded does not have to be independently verified, whilst the Kitemark gives independent third party assurance of continuing product conformity through audits, factory surveillance and test records.

Now to the MD Directive. A medical device can be described as any instrument, apparatus, appliance, material or article, whether used alone or in combination, including the software necessary for its proper application, intended by the manufacturer to be used for human beings for the purpose of diagnosis, prevention, monitoring, treatment or alleviation of disease.

The MD regulations came into effect on 14th June 1998.

The directive states that all frames sent for glazing should carry the CE label on the frame itself unless it is too small. Frames should be checked for compatibility with the lens type being prescribed. In conclusion, with the components that go towards making a pair of spectacles now having to be CE marked, it is important that a traceability route be established. For example, under the Consumers Protection Act of 1987, you would need to provide proof to Trading Standards that the components were considered safe and fit for the intended purpose. The CE mark helps ensure compliance with consumer legislation.

# Chapter 3

# The spectacle frame industry and materials

One of the earliest references to 'eyeglasses' was by Meissener, a priest who in 1270 makes reference in his sermon to the fact that old people derived much benefit from wearing them. Archives of 1282 reveal that Michael Bullet, a priest of the Abbey of Saint Bavon-le-Grande used his eyeglasses to help him sign a document.

Very early designs of eyeglasses were fashioned from leather. Why leather you may say? During these times the leather working trade employed the second greatest labour force after agriculture, so it was natural to use a material that craftsmen had grown used to working with.

Other materials such as bone, tortoiseshell and horn were used especially for those requiring, and who could afford more ornate designs. In the 14th century the possession of a pair of spectacles was as much a statement of the owners wealth and standing in the community as it was an aid to reading.

Today the mass production of ophthalmic spectacle frames is another separate facet to manufacturing optics. Production has been mechanised to a considerable degree by breaking it down into a number of regular engineering processes such as cutting, forming, stamping, cropping, milling, slotting, shaping and so on.

As with lenses, manufacture of spectacle frames is an international industry. Increasingly, frame manufacturing is moving from the traditional centres in France and Italy and springing up in areas of the Far East. Notwithstanding, Europe remains the originators for new fashion and styling trends with often long lead times for special frame materials, factory tooling and jigs and in preparation of promotional literature. It can be 12–18 months before the product finally reaches the market. One could dub spectacles frames the 'risk element of ophthalmic manufacturing'.

The advent of fashion frames has had its effect on spectacle case designs and thus their original purely protective role has been combined with styling to complement the frame. In response to increasing consumer interest in thinner and lighter eyewear, frame companies have developed a variety of innovative new materials. Each new material has distinctive properties, and requires special techniques and care when inserting lenses or adjusting the frames. Some materials possess no ability to shrink. If lenses are not edged exactly on size or slightly undersize, new lenses may be required. Other materials require only minimum heat when inserting lenses. Overheating, even slightly, will cause some materials to shrink beyond repair. Some materials withstand almost any amount of heat, others want no heat at all and must be glazed 'cold'. Those in the optical world and especially technicians, need to have an exact knowledge of these materials. When new materials are developed it is often the technician who through 'trial and error', has to develop procedures and precautions required.

What follows will hopefully prove useful.

## Desirable properties

The term spectacle is used for brevity to include any of the devices employed for holding spectacle lenses before the eyes.

Many different materials have been used at various times for spectacle frames. Among the properties which any such materials should possess we may name the following: freedom from injurious effects, pleasing appearance, resistance to corrosion, non-flammability, cost-effective manufacture, durability, ease of working, rigidity, adjustability. Some of these properties are clearly essential. Others, though highly desirable, may have to be sacrificed to a greater or lesser extent for the sake of compensating advantages. Others, again, are hard to reconcile – for example, rigidity and adjustability.

The choice of materials for any manufactured article is dictated by a number of factors, principally economic. Because of scarcity and inherent drawbacks, natural materials tend to be replaced by synthetic or manufactured ones. Also, the whole trend of industrial development has been towards mass production and the use of materials which lend themselves most readily to this system of manufacture. Whereas, for example, spectacle frames in carbon steel were still fairly common over 70 years ago, they have now all but disappeared together with the highly skilled craftsmen who could make them from wire with the simplest of tools.

## Precious metals

Silver and gold, the most common of the precious metals, have both been popular materials for hand-made spectacles. In fact, the latter is still widely used in the form of rolled gold (sometimes mistakenly called 'gold filled', a term now illegal in the UK, but still in use in the USA).

Gold has probably been valued by human society as a personal adornment for longer than any other metal. Its rarity, ability to resist corrosion and stability in contact with skin have ensured its continued use and value throughout history. Since a special system of weights and measures is in force for precious metals and jewels, a few words of explanation may not be out of place.

Gold and silver are still legally weighed according to the 'Troy system' in which

24 grains = 1 pennyweight (dwt)

20 dwt = 1 ounce Troy

There are thus 480 grains in the Troy ounce as against 437.5 grains in the ounce avoirdupois. The name Troy, incidentally, does not refer to the site of the Trojan war but to the French cathedral of Troyes, capital of the old province of Champagne and the scene of many historical events.

Apart from its noble appearance gold has the great merit of being highly resistant to tarnishing and corrosion. Unlike base metals it is impervious to the more common acids even in their concentrated form. Another well-known property of gold is the ease with which it can be shaped; for example, it can be drawn into the finest wire and beaten into gold leaf of incredible thinness. There is however one disadvantage from the standpoint of utility. Pure gold, known in the trade as fine gold, is far too soft to be serviceable and is therefore alloyed with other metals which add the needed strength and hardness. Fine gold is termed 24 carat (ct). Gold alloyed with other metals is know by the curious name of carat gold and is designated as so many carats according to the number of parts by weight of fine gold in 24 parts of the alloy. For example, 12 ct gold has a fine gold content of 12/24 or one-half by weight. Thus, while the carat was originally a unit of weight (and still is for precious stones and pearls) it is solely an indication of proportion in relation to gold; it could be replaced by the words 'parts by weight out of 24'. As one would expect, this curious system goes back several centuries. An act of Queen Elizabeth dated 1575 refers to 'golde less in fyness than that of xxii carrottes'. In the USA the correct spelling is 'karat', abbreviated to K or Kt.

Traditionally gold wares are manufactured in certain specified qualities: these are 22, 18, 14 and 9 ct. The higher qualities are more resistant to corrosion and more valuable but may be too soft for a particular purpose. For example, 9 ct gold was considered the most suitable for hand-made spectacle frames.

In the UK, most gold must be 'hall marked' (Hallmarking Act 1973) but the Act does not necessarily apply to spectacle frames because they are classed as Medical Devices under the Medical Devices Regulations of 1994 and are therefore exempt.

The colour of carat gold is largely dependent on the relative proportions of the other metals in the alloy – usually silver and copper. A pink effect is obtained by increasing the proportion of copper. 'White gold' is produced by partly replacing silver with nickel and copper with zinc. A white finish can also be obtained by electroplating yellow gold and rolled gold material with the precious metal rhodium.

## Rolled gold

Rolled gold (RG), is a material designed to provide most of the advantages of gold at a cheaper cost. In the 1970s the escalating price of gold and the demise of the NHS frame (which used rolled gold in all its adult metal frames) reduced the market considerably. The specialised tools and procedures required to produce rolled gold frames reduced their availability further. However, it must be said that rolled gold frames still represent the top end of the 'gold' frame market.

The first stage in the production of rolled gold is to bond a bar of base metal (sometimes using a gold solder) to a close-fitting tube of the gold alloy. This produces a cylinder of about 7 cm diameter and 45 cm long, which is 'rolled', i.e. squashed between rollers until the final diameter and shape is reached. This compression changes the crystalline structure of the gold and the base metal so that they are both harder and springier. The material is then drawn or formed into wire, strip, or tubing having an even covering of carat gold.

Various alloys including bronze have been used for the base metal. For spectacle frames, nickel silver is often preferred because it is more resistant to corrosion should the gold skin become broken or worn.

The gold content of the material is clearly dependent on two factors: the quality of the gold cladding and the proportion of gold covering to base metal. The usual way of specifying these particulars is shown by the example '1/10th 10 ct' which means that the skin is made of 10 ct gold and accounts for 1/10th of the weight of the whole. A less informative description is the number of parts by weight of fine gold in 1000 parts of the material. For example, 1/10th 12 ct gold filled should contain 50/1000 fine gold. This may be verified as follows: only 1/10th of the material or 100 parts in 1000 are carat gold, and 12 ct gold contains 12/24 of fine gold. Hence the total fine gold content is 12/24 of 100 parts in 1000 which is 50/1000. A number enclosed in a circle is a recognised way of marking a rolled gold frame to show the fine gold content per 1000 parts. Another way is to give the more complete specification in the form, for example, of 1/20–10 which means 1/20th of 10 ct gold.

It will be appreciated that the gold skin cannot be very thick. Even in the higher qualities it rarely exceeds one-thousandth of an inch; however, it is claimed to be three to six times thicker than that in other types of plating – a reasonable claim as it would be difficult to obtain a thinner uniform layer by mechanical means. A further advantage of rolled gold is that the base metal, solder (if used) and the gold layer diffuse into each other, preventing the gold from peeling off should the surface of the frame become damaged.

Because of its thickness, it is often possible to solder rolled gold frames using ordinary gas torches without damaging the plating. As the rolled gold is plated before frame production, ornamentation such as open-filigree work cannot be done. In the past, the deep surface impressions created in filigree work caused surface faults, but the shallow impressions used today are not a significant problem. Great care is therefore needed to avoid damage to this very thin covering during the various processes of frame manufacture. This is usually followed by a gold plating process to improve the appearance and restore some of the inevitable losses during manufacture.

## Gold plated

Gold plating has been used for centuries to make both metals and even non-metals look like, and take on the appearance of gold. However, until 1840 the process was mercury based and therefore dangerous and unstable to control.

Even today, whilst mercury is not used the process generates cyanide gas so it is best left to the specialists.

Gold plating is an electrolytic process whereby a layer of gold is deposited on to the surface of a base metal frame. So the bulk of a 'gold' frame is actually the base metal on which the coating is deposited.

The higher the gold content of the alloy coating the softer the 'gold', hence it does not necessarily follow that the higher gold content alloys are better. Equally, low gold content is of little use either. Something in the region of 12–18 ct is often considered optimum.

The question of 'does the quality of the gold coating matter?' is also rather a difficult one to answer. As discussed so far, the answer is an unreserved 'yes'. A thick, even plating with a fairly high gold content and free from faults (say 18 ct) is best. Standards stipulate that the plating should be a minimum of 1 mm thick and a 'fineness' of not less than 18 ct.

As a very high proportion of modern 'gold' spectacle frames actually only used gold to give a nice colour, the term 'gold washed' or 'gold flashed' would not be inappropriate. Therefore, when the frame is new the thickness of the gold alloy layer is almost irrelevant; the layer which protects the frame is not metal at all but some sort of organic 'lacquer'. This is not to say that some of these frames are not better than others in the old 'thickest gold is best' sense. In the case of these frames, it is difficult to decide whether this is a good thing or not. Considered simplistically, any plated frame is like a battery. Gold will act as cathode and the base metal as the anode, with the body fluids as the electrolyte. Instead of protecting the base metal, gold plating actively encourages corrosion when there are any holes in that plating. The lacquer, being an insulator, at worst takes no part in this and also hopefully fills any pores in the gold layer at least when the frame is new. This layer also protects the gold from damage. What makes it difficult to say whether this is better or worse is that we have no idea how good the lacquer is at doing this or how thick it is.

Yellow-lacquered, yellow-alloyed and even gold painted are the most suspect of all 'gold' frames. Yellow lacquering uses a highly polished, silver-coloured metal and covers it with a transparent yellow lacquer. There are many gold look-alikes. Some polished copper alloys can pass as gold. The best known is Pinchbeck (83% copper, 17% zinc). Coat a frame made of this material with a clear lacquer and it will look very much like a gold frame.

Modern lacquers can be utilised so that gold paint takes on the appearance of matt gold plating layer. Unless something exotic such as titanium is being used, then it is likely that this base metal for a gold-plated frame will be one of three basic types:

*Bronze* is an alloy containing principally copper (about 90%) and tin. Minor constituents, often principally phosphorous, are used to improve its mechanical properties. It is springy and therefore often used for sides.

*Monel metal* is an alloy of nickel (about 65–70%) and copper (25–30%) again with traces of other elements. It is relatively hard and inflexible and therefore more suitable for fronts.

*Nickel silver* is a mixture of copper and nickel (and zinc). Ideally this should be about 25% nickel but in practice this is seldom the case. BS 6625 specifies a minimum of 14% by mass of nickel, although 12% is sufficient to disguise the copper colour. Nickel silver is used for all parts of spectacle frames.

The base metal is often chosen for its mechanical as much as its chemical properties, hence the integrity of the surface coating is paramount. However, it is of the utmost importance that the surface of this metal is properly prepared if the frame is to be plated after production. It is also vital that it is compatible with the plating which is to be used. This relates to both the adhesion between the metals and to their mechanical properties. It is little use having a hard, brittle coating on a soft substrate – it would soon crack. Equally two very different thermal expansion coefficients could cause havoc.

In conclusion, it is apparent that we should be very wary of what we mean when we call a frame 'gold'. Somehow though, 'a thin layer of gold–copper–silver alloy on a base metal of copper–nickel–zinc alloy with a protective layer of organic polymer' doesn't roll off the tongue quite as easily.

## Nickel silver

The metal known as nickel silver (formerly as German silver) contains little nickel and no silver. This is, of course, a criticism of the name, not of the material. Nickel silver is an excellent material for many purposes, being fairly resistant to corrosion. It is cheaper than rolled gold but no less serviceable as a material for metal spectacle frames. Although the principal constituent of the alloy is copper, the nickel and zinc with which it is combined have such a bleaching effect that the alloy generally has a white appearance.

Nickel silver frames are generally electroplated with pure nickel after manufacture. They can also be rhodium-plated but this is naturally a more expensive process. Nickel silver frames possess the capability of being adjusted and manipulated very easily. Indeed, parts made from nickel silver fitted to other frames also possess this characteristic.

Due to recent increases in metal sensitivity in the public in general, there has been concern expressed that the nickel content in various products, including spectacle frames, be controlled and identified.

## Stainless steel

Although steel has justly been called the basis of modern civilisation in the material sense, it has the great disadvantage of being highly susceptible to corrosion. Constant protection by painting, electroplating or otherwise is needed to keep rust at bay.

Following its discovery in 1913 by H. Brearley in Sheffield, many types of stainless steel have been developed. One of them, containing about 18% chromium and 8% nickel has the curious property of being non-magnetic despite its large content of iron. It has been used by a number of different firms, in particular for rimless mounts of a design for which other metals would have been unsuitable. Also because of its 'springy' effect, it is very useful for the temple areas of frames.

## Aluminium

Aluminium is widely distributed in the Earth's crust; in fact common garden clay contains a high proportion of it. Unfortunately the cost of extraction from this source is prohibitive.

Aluminium has a number of attractive properties. For example, it is very light, cheap and highly resistant to corrosion. It also lends itself to a beautiful decorative finish by a process known as anodising. This differs from electroplating in which a thin layer of one metal is deposited on an article made of another. In the course of anodising aluminium the surface layer is converted into aluminium oxide which is a much harder substance and therefore acts as a protective coat. It is also capable of being dyed in a number of pleasing shades. Other decorative effects can be obtained at the same time.

Being a good conductor of heat, aluminium is noticeably cold to the touch and this can be a disadvantage. Usually, however, aluminium spectacle sides have plastic end covers so that the bare metal does not make contact with the skin.

## Titanium

Titanium has an almost unique combination of mechanical and corrosion resistant properties that makes it ideal for frame manufacture.

There are three 'types' of titanium frames available: those made from pure titanium, those that are 'clad' in titanium and those that are 'partial' titanium. The 'clad' type are very similar to the gold filled materials already described. The core metal is made of pure titanium and the outside layer from nickel. The 'partial' type of frame has some parts made of pure titanium or 'clad' titanium and other parts are made from other metallic materials. For example, temples and end pieces could be pure titanium and eyerims and bridges nickel copper alloy.

Pure titanium frames can be up to 48% lighter than conventional metal frames. On the other hand, the clad type are 25–37% lighter than more conventional metal frames. Titanium is very resistant to the elements and will not be affected by sea water, perspiration, etc.

Titanium has a melting point of some 1673°C. This can cause problems during manufacturing where frames made partially from titanium and partially from conventional materials have to be soldered, because the softening temperatures of the basic components are vastly different.

Care must also be exercised in maintaining cohesiveness between base metals and the cladding of the titanium clad frames.

To conclude the section on metal frames, mention should be made of the trend towards very bright and colourful 'enamelling' available on these; it can be transfer applied, sprayed or indeed enamelled, to give very interesting results.

## Memory metal

A special blend of titanium and nickel alloy produces a memory metal that permits frames to hold their adjustments after accidental twisting or bending.

Memory metal is generally only used in areas most subject to stress – bridges, top bars and temples. End-pieces, eyewires and pad arms are normally made from conventional rigid metal.

## Plastic and plastics

The word plastic, derived from the Greek *plastikos*, was originally an adjective meaning readily capable of being moulded or shaped. For example, modelling clay is plastic. Other materials such as glass are not plastic under ordinary conditions but become so if raised to a sufficiently high temperature. Later the word was used as a noun to denote a certain type of synthetic material and also as an adjective to characterise an article made of such material. For example, bakelite was termed 'a plastic' and a cup made from this material would be called 'a plastic cup'. Since a bakelite cup is certainly not plastic in the original sense of the word, it was thought that some confusion could arise from this terminology.

Eventually it was decided to allow the word plastic to retain its original meaning and to use the plural form of *plastics* both as noun and adjective for the new meaning. Thus, odd though it sounds at first, we should speak of 'a plastics frame' if we wish to denote a frame made, for example of cellulose acetate. This usage has not met with universal acclaim.

### Natural plastics

Before man-made materials were available it was common to use natural materials, not only for frame making but for other uses as well. In times past, frames have been fashioned from bone, animal horn, ivory and wood. Although the use of horn for spectacle frames is a thing of the past, the familiar term 'horn-rimmed spectacles' – though applied to frames with celluloid rims – testifies to the former popularity of this natural plastics material.

Another natural material, mentioned here for historical reasons, is tortoiseshell. It used to be obtained from the hawksbill turtle. The smallest of marine turtles, it is found in the warmer parts of many oceans. Its mottled shell is made up of a number of plates of varying thickness and colour, the latter ranging from a very dark mottle to a pale amber. The lighter the colour, the more expensive the material became.

Tortoiseshell possessed the remarkable property of bonding to itself under heat and pressure. By this means two or more thin plates could be built-up into a thicker slab of material. The same technique, known as *splicing*, was used to repair a break. A steam kettle for use in this operation was once an indispensable piece of equipment in the spectacle frame workshop.

Thanks to its attractive colours and mottling, its durability, its plastic properties and its ability to take a brilliant polish, tortoiseshell had been a highly prized material for many centuries. Although occasional repolishing was necessary, a 'real shell' frame would outlive several made of imitation material. The hawksbill turtle is an endangered species and is now protected against those who would kill it to obtain its shell.

## Synthetic plastics

The enormous development of the plastics industry has been one of the most striking features of the modern mass-production era. Even though the original spur to invention was the need to find cheaper substitutes for scarce natural materials such as ivory and tortoiseshell, it would no longer be correct to regard all synthetic plastics as inferior substitutes. Some in fact are better in certain respects than the traditional materials which they have displaced.

Nearly all manufactured plastics have certain properties in common. In the first place, they are all made from organic materials associated in some way with animal or vegetable life, e.g. milk, coal and cotton. This feature excludes metals and glass from the accepted definition of plastics, although these materials are certainly plastic in the sense that they can be moulded.

Secondly, the molecules or basic chemical units of which plastics are composed are immensely large. They frequently take the form of long chains built up by a process termed *polymerisation*. Thirdly, in order to improve the working properties of the material, a certain amount of plasticiser is usually added. Numerous different plasticisers are in use, the majority being liquids with a high boiling point. Not all manufacturers of a given material necessarily use the same kind and proportion of plasticiser. This is one of the reasons why different makes of nominally the same material may vary in hardness, brittleness and other physical properties.

In general, synthetic plastics may be divided into two main groups: (1) thermoplastic (or thermosoftening) and (2) thermosetting (or thermohardening). The materials in the first group soften and can be shaped when heated without undergoing any fundamental change. That is to say, the process of heating and cooling can be continued indefinitely without detriment to the plastic properties of the material. On the other hand, the materials of the second group undergo an irreversible chemical change when polymerisation takes place. Additional chemical links in the molecular structure are then forged as a result of which the material loses its plastic properties. Re-heating would lead to the break-up of the material.

Plastics lend themselves to several different methods of fabrication, e.g. machining, compression moulding, injection moulding, vacuum forming, casting, etc. The raw material is usually obtainable in the form of sheets, rods, tubes and extruded section. Granules are normally used for injection moulding, while liquid material is required for casting. Although the majority of spectacle frames are still made from sheet material, injection moulding and casting processes are becoming increasingly used.

Sheet material for spectacle frames is supplied in an enormous range of colours and can be between 4 and 10 m thick. It can also be in different forms. Solid sheet, as its name implies, is all of one piece, whereas laminated sheet consists of two or more layers, usually of different colours, bonded together. Decorative effects are sometimes obtained by metallic or other inclusions in the sheet material.

## Cellulose nitrate

The overview of plastics materials begins with one that is no longer available but because of its importance in the history and development of frame materials, it would be unfair not to include it. Equally important, there are some of these frames still around and some could find their way into the laboratory for reglazing.

Cellulose nitrate, the earliest of the cellulosic plastics, was first produced by Alexander Parkes, a native of Birmingham, in 1855. He named the material Parkesine but failed in his attempts to produce it on a commercial scale. This was successfully achieved by the Hyatt brothers in the USA who manufactured and marketed the material under the trade name Celluloid. Lest Parkes be remembered only for his failures, it should be added that one of his earlier patents was for a method of waterproofing fabrics with a solution of India rubber in carbon bisulphide. Sold to Macintosh & Co., this invention made their name world-famous.

Cellulose, the main constituent of the cell walls of plants, has been estimated to account for about one-third of all the vegetable matter in the world. No other raw material would appear to be so plentiful. As with many other raw materials, however, one is faced with the problem of extracting it in a sufficiently pure or usable form. In practice, cotton has been found to be one of the few satisfactory sources of raw cellulose.

In the manufacture of cellulose nitrate, cotton was used in the form of linters – the short fibres which were left on the cotton seed when the longer fibres suitable for spinning into thread had been removed. After cleaning, purification, bleaching and drying, the linters were heated in a mixture of nitric and sulphuric acids. During this process, which was called nitration, the molecular structure of the cellulose was modified by reaction with the nitric acid, and nitrocellulose was formed. The sulphuric acid took no active part in the reaction beyond assisting it to take place and absorbing the water given off by it. A number of ingenious processes were then employed to remove all traces of sulphuric acid and water from the nitrocellulose.

The next stage of manufacture was to mix the nitrocellulose with a suitable plasticiser at the same time adding the necessary pigments or dyes. It is a very interesting fact that no one ever found a better plasticiser for cellulose nitrate than camphor – the substance used by Alexander Parkes in his poineer efforts over 100 years ago. After thorough mixing and kneading, the 'dough' was filtered and rolled into sheets which were then heated and pressed together to make a large rectangular block. This would then be sliced into sheets of the desired thickness by a machine resembling in principle the carpenter's plane. The production of mottles and other effects required many additional processes too lengthy and complex to be described here.

Cellulose nitrate has many of the properties desired in a material for spectacle frames. It is tough yet easily worked and formed, takes a brilliant polish and retains its shape and stability even in tropical and humid conditions. Its big disadvantage is that it flares up when ignited and burns very rapidly. As a result, its use as a spectacle frame material has been banned in many countries.

In appearance the material is similar to cellulose acetate but it is important that one can distinguish between the two. One method, although not very scientific, was to rub the frame briskly on the arm of your lab coat and then smell it. The camphor content of a nitrate frame would smell bitter, a little like sulphur.

The flash point of nitrate is about 90°C, just a little above its softening point. Care had therefore to be exercised. A flame is a very efficient way of applying heat to the frame but this needed care and some experience. The safest way was to use a hot air blower when handling nitrate material.

## Cellulose acetate

In broad outline the manufacture of cellulose acetate sheet follows the same lines as cellulose nitrate, the essential difference being that nitration is replaced by acetylation with a mixture of glacial acetic acid and acetic anhydride. The other main difference is in the choice of plasticiser. No plasticiser has been found for cellulose acetate having the same undisputed supremacy as camphor for cellulose nitrate. Phthalate compounds are often used with acetone as a solvent.

The commercial production of cellulose acetate began in 1914 pioneered by the Dreyfus brothers in Switzerland. In the UK its use for spectacle frames had largely superseded casein by the early 1930s. This later material, made from milk, had the defect of being rather brittle especially at low temperatures. A sudden spell of cold weather was sure to produce a heavy crop of breakages. Its use for spectacle frames did not last very long after cellulose acetate had established itself for this purpose.

It must be admitted that in some respects cellulose acetate is slightly inferior to nitrate. It absorbs moisture more readily and softens at a lower temperature. For these reasons it is a less suitable material in tropical and sub-tropical climates. On the other hand, it is much less flammable; it does not flare up and burns at a much lower speed than cellulose nitrate.

Through all these waves of innovation cellulose acetate has been no. 1 in the Western world's league table of frame materials. Its ascendancy is waning today, as is the number of manufacturers who supply it. Those who remain active bring out an ever more imaginative and daring selection of colour combinations to tempt frame makers, working more closely with the frame industry and responding faster to market trends. Currently, for example, material ranges are full of variations on natural look themes: wood, horn, natural textiles, leather and shell. Like frames today, material ranges have shorter production life cycles – as a new design may be built round a specific material, this can cause problems for the frame manufacturer who launches a lasting best-seller, especially in more conservative markets like Britain . . . and, in turn, for his customers the dispensers.

### Types of sheet stock cellulose acetate

*Block material.* This is the oldest method of production of optical sheets. Cellulose acetate flake is mixed with solvents, plasticers and pigments and after stirring and kneading it assumes the consistency of rubber and is known as 'dough'. After a number of filtering processes the dough is rolled into sheets known as 'hides' and stacked on to metal base plates. They are then pressed into blocks which undergo long heated curing periods before being sliced into sheets. Depending upon the pigment dispersion within the block and the angle at which the block is sliced, different colour effects can be obtained. The most realistic tortoiseshell effects are created from block material.

More recently, block techniques are being used to obtain very complex veneers which are then laminated on to extruded base material. In this case the sliced sheets of several blocks with different colours and patterns are relayered to form a new block which is reprocessed and resliced. This cycle may be repeated several times before the final laminate is created. The final block will be sliced into thin sheets of approximately 1 mm thick to form the laminate. Quite clearly this is a time-consuming and expensive procedure and other methods of obtaining sophisticated laminated material are developing.

*Extruded material.* As extrusion technology developed this became a much more economic method of producing cellulose acetate sheets and with a much shorter delivery time to the frame producer. Initially these materials were simple. But soon, the ability to extrude two or three colour layers on to a crystal underlayer provided a product that gave the frame manufacturer entirely new scope for creative sculpting of the layers to obtain frame designs with fashion appeal. The problem is that in fine tuning the extruder head at the beginning of each colour production run, a great deal of scrap is produced.

Extrusion remains the production method used for manufacture of the crystal and transparent base materials upon which the more recent complex laminates are bonded. It is also still used to produce a wide range of mottle effects, some in two-tone (e.g. smoke and crystal) made for the more conservative British market.

*Laminated material.* Lamination has a long history in the production of optical cellulose acetate sheet, but since 1990 it has achieved a new vogue with the introduction of some very appealing and complex designs using not only block technology laminates, but also the laminating of screen printed layers between a base extrusion and a top crystal layer. Screen printed multicolour patterns have opened up further new design possibilities. The addition of pearl layers, metallic flecks and various other combinations have given the frame maker the ability to produce stunning colour effects without having to laboriously layer mill the material to obtain them. It has been the Italian manufacturers who have developed these processes in an attempt to maintain a technological and fashion lead on newer producers in the Far East.

*Pressure cast material.* Several Italian manufacturers have been promoting material made by a completely new method. Its advantage is that relatively small quantities of each colour or pattern can be made economically to meet the needs of the current market. In the main the effects most resemble block patterns, either mock tortoiseshell effects or colours that are bright and bold, often designed to appeal to the younger European market. The technology is still developing but appears to offer a genuine alternative for the future. Flakes of various colours are evenly dispersed into a mould of liquid transparent base cellulose acetate. This is compressed under heat and cooled to give a slab of finished material. The material has been marketed under the names Ceblox, Stylebloc and Starbloc.

Cellulose acetate is also available to the frame manufacturers in granule form so that it may be injection moulded rather than cut from sheet. Frame manufacture from acetate sheet is wasteful; after routing and milling, 85% of the material ends as non-recyclable swarf. Though manufacturing methods have been substantially updated, it is hard to eliminate traditional reliance on operative skills and hand finishing; making one frame may involve over 30 separate operations, with inevitable effect on unit costs. (In contrast, frame moulding tooling costs per design are far higher, making short production runs only marginally viable but material wastage, finishing and labour costs per frame are greatly reduced.)

There are still stunningly original effects that a designer can only produce with classical sheet acetate material.

Cellulose acetate softens at about 50°C and although it is not flammable the frame can be damaged by excessive heat, and the surface will bubble, blister or wrinkle. Darker coloured frames require less heat for adjustment than lighter coloured versions.

### Advantages

The specific advantages offered by cellulose acetate as a frame material can be summarised as follows:

*Transparency:* light transmission levels of up to 90% are achieved by some grades giving excellent crystal clarity, a very desirable feature for a product to be worn on the face.

*Natural feel:* cellulose acetate feels comfortably warm to the touch. It is also very tolerant of perspiration and is non-allergenic.

*Stress resistance*: because stresses dissipate rapidly cellulose acetate resists cracking when metal cores are 'shot' into it, metal hinge and joint components are insert moulded or metal joints are ultrasonically welded into it.

*Good impact resistance*: although cellulose acetate has good impact strength it also has the added advantage that if it does break under high impact it will not splinter or shatter, thus reducing any risk of injury to the wearer.

*Self-shining*: whilst cellulose acetate has a relatively soft surface it also has a self-polishing property which helps surface scratches to disappear and the natural sheen to be maintained in use. However, this traditionally useful property is less important now that most frames are finished with a hard, high gloss polyurethane or acrylic lacquer to improve scratch resistance and appearance.

*Colour*: cellulose acetate is very easy to colour using water based dyes to give virtually any colour shade in transparent or opaque form. It is also receptive to decoration by the application of paints, varnishes, enamels and inks. Many special techniques are employed to create attractive colour patterns and effects.

*Resistance to static build-up.*

*Ease of processing*: cellulose acetate can readily be sawn, milled, drilled, formed, blanked, bonded and polished, which is a major reason for its universal use in producing traditional milled frames.

*Ease of adjustment*: cellulose acetate frames can quickly and easily be adjusted by the dispensing optician. The material will become sufficiently pliable for glazing at a temperature of 50°C. This ease of adjustment is, however, also one of the material's major disadvantages. Whether made from sheet or injection moulded, cellulose acetate frames have no elastic 'memory' and are dimensionally unstable. In particular unglazed frames may tend to relax or warp in storage, particularly if originally made from laminated materials.

## Acrylic resins

The acrylic resins are a family of plastics characterised by remarkable transparency (unless deliberately dyed), great stability and a relatively high softening point. In the UK the best known is Perspex, a polymethyl methacrylate manufactured by Imperial Chemical Industries Ltd. This material is available in a number of clear and semi-opaque colours but not in mottled effects. It is, however, possible to produce multitone effects by a process of lamination. Acrylic materials are not so easy to work as the cellulosic plastics and are more brittle. They are resistant to most aqueous solutions and some solvents but have low impact resistance. The material requires about the same amount of heat as cellulose nitrate and although not flammable is easily distorted by excessive heat. Also it generally takes longer to soften than cellulose materials.

## Cellulose materials

Cellulose propionate, made from cellulose flake treated with propionic acid, arrived on the frame market around 1980. It is made into frames by injection moulding. Tooling quality and close control of the moulding cycle is vital for quality of product, as with all moulded ophthalmic frames.

Cellulose propionate frames can be excitingly sculpted as with other moulded frames; colour effects are achieved by dyeing over a pale base shade of the original granules or transfer printing. Finishing technology, glazing and handling properties show only relatively minor differences from those of conventionally made acetate frames. Material is lighter in weight (about 5–6%) than cellulose acetate.

For frame makers, cellulose propionate's future is shadowed by raw material supply problems. For glazing, the material needs a little more heat than, say, acetate but more gently applied. It is considered by some to be slightly brittle. Clean frames using lukewarm water. Never use anything containing alcohol or spirit.

## Optyl

Optyl represents the first serious challenge to acetate's domination of the frame market. It is an epoxy resin. Frames are made from this material in liquid form by a process of casting and subsequent curing. Fronts and sides are made in separate moulds, the joints being inserted at the casting stage. After finishing operations and assembly, the frames are dyed in essentially the same way as CR39 lenses. Polishing is by immersion in a bath of polyurethane.

The material itself – the first ever developed specifically for ophthalmic frame making – and the technology are owed to Austria's Wilhelm Anger Group. The finished product looks different – it can be elaborately sculpted and shaped. At the Optyl launch in Vienna a technician brought the house down by tying a frame in knots under heat, then letting it relax back unharmed into its initial shape on cooling.

Like all moulded frames, styles in Optyl were designed for production to a built-in 'base curve'; they did not require to be bumped and bowed to shape like frames cut from flat slab material and they had no betraying flat shape 'memory' to return to. The material, combined with the manufacturing technology, enabled things to be done in frame design that had never before been possible.

The softening temperature of Optyl is around 80°C but this is not critical and there is no danger of overheating under normal circumstances, since it can be heated to 200°C and still return to its normal condition. (The manufacturers say that it can even be heated to 350°C for a short time without permanent damage.) Optyl should be cooled in water.

The material is useful as it can be considered hypo-allergenic.

When edging lenses, it helps if they are slightly oversize to ensure best fit. Adjustment can take longer and is best achieved using a hot air blower with a narrow opening. Heat and adjust one part at a time. Sides can even be lengthened by heating until soft and gently stretching. Caution, however, in very warm weather as the material may resume the original moulded shape and lose individual adjustments!

## Nylon

Nylon has so far found only a limited use for spectacle frames, chiefly for sunglasses, sports and safety wear. It is lightweight, hypo-allergenic and relatively unbreakable. The material is really far more suitable for injection moulding than for the traditional method of manufacturing spectacle frames from sheet material.

To provide a wide range of colours might also be a problem. It is only produced in opaque colours, so frames are often spray coloured, coated and baked to provide a variety of colouration. Nevertheless, nylon does undoubtedly offer many advantages for certain types of spectacle frames. Because of its high degree of 'plastic memory' it cannot be adjusted after manufacture except when a metal wire is inserted into the ends of the sides for this purpose.

Nylon can be difficult to glaze because of the high heat required. It is best to cut lenses as close as possible to final size and shape. Nylon tends to dry out so patients should be advised to 'soak' their spectacles in water on a monthly basis.

# SPX

Up to the 1980s, the polyamides (nylon materials to the layman) were found wanting. Then, in 1982, Silhouette launched their own heavily researched superpolyamide, SPX. It has the advantages that had always attracted materials scientists: it is ultralight, strong, mouldable, colourable, comfortable and safe to wear, flexible for adjustment and virtually unbreakable. With SPX, Silhouette seemed to have overcome the problem of atmospheric water absorption that had affected the performance of previous polyamides.

It has established itself as a real contribution to the modern library of frame materials but has also influenced the whole trend of frame design through its suitability for light, fine-rimmed styles. Other new generation enhanced polyamides have now followed SPX out of the mass market sunglass sector into quality frame making.

## Carbon fibre

The material used to make frames is a blend of carbon fibres and other ingredients such as nylon or copolyamide.

Carbon fibre graphite is extremely durable; it is essentially the same material that has been used in golf clubs, tennis rackets and skis. It has proved to be stronger than steel and lighter than aluminium, which makes it an ideal substitute for metal components.

When applied to eyewear, carbon is used to mould an extremely thin frame that won't bend or stretch out of alignment as can metal. Since carbon fibre graphite has a very high melting point, carbon frames are heat resistant; they do not lose their shape at high temperatures as plastics frames sometimes do.

At the same time, carbon makes for a remarkable lightweight frame and because carbon can be fashioned into such a thin frame, carbon designs tend to be lighter than plastics ones.

For best results when glazing a frame without closing joints, check the size of lenses before inserting them. It is important that they be cut accurately with regard to both size and shape. Most glazers would advise glazing 'cold', i.e. no heat applied prior to insertion of lens in frame.

# Chapter 4

# Spectacle frame nomenclature

## An important glossary

Much of this chapter is based on British Standard (BS) 3521 Part 2 (1991) – Spectacle Frames – Glossary of Terms and the author would strongly recommend that the reader obtains a copy of this together with the accompanying ISO 13666 (1998) – Spectacle Lenses – Vocabulary.

## Main classifications

### Classification by type

Most of the devices used to hold spectacle lenses in their correct position before the eyes can be classified as either frames or mounts. The distinction is that in a frame the lenses are secured by rims which completely surround them, whereas in a mount the rims (if any) do not completely surround the lenses and the lenses are therefore held in by some other means.

Another important distinction is between spectacles and eyeglasses. These terms strictly relate to the complete appliance including the lenses, the difference being that spectacles have not only a front but sides which fit over or round the ears or at least extend towards them. Eyeglasses, on the other hand, have no sides and usually depend on gripping the nose as a means of support. Today eyeglasses, which once enjoyed considerable popularity, are now uncommon, so much so that BS 3521 no longer even mentions eyeglasses as a separate item.

There are a few miscellaneous devices which cannot be classified as either spectacles or eyeglasses. For example, there are various attachments to spectacles permitting additional lenses or prisms to be worn for occasional or experimental use. The most common of these is known as a 'clipover' and is attached by means of hooks, sometimes supplemented by spring action. Although clipover is a commonly used terminology it has been replaced in British Standards by 'clip-on'. There are also *monocles* (a single lens, with or without a rim, designed to be held between the brow and cheek) and *lorgnettes* (described as eyeglasses for occasional use, held between the eyes by a handle into which the lenses may fold when not required). An even rarer item would be a *lorgon* (more commonly known as a *quizzer*) which is similar to a lorgnette but has only one lens. It could be said that it is similar to a monocle but with a handle.

### Classification by material

According to the material from which their main parts are made, spectacle frames and mounts are described as 'metal', 'plastics' or 'combination'. The latter term applies to frames which cannot be said to be predominantly of either material. For example, a combination frame may have metal rims connected by a metal bridge, but hoods (concealing the upper part of the rims) and sides of a plastics material.

### Subsidiary classifications

A few other broad classifications relating to various parts should be mentioned at this stage. If the bridge or rims are fitted with pads designed to rest on the sides of the nose, the frame is said to be of the 'pad bridge' type (*Figure 4.1*).

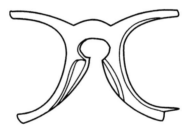

**Figure 4.1** A pad bridge.

The height of the joints connecting the front and the sides determines whether the frame is classed as a 'central joint', 'high joint' or 'low joint' pattern (*Figure 4.2*). For a central joint, the joint must be positioned on or near the centre line. For a high joint it should be positioned substantially above the centre line and for a low joint it should be positioned substantially below the centre line.

Spectacle sides are classified into three main types to which self-explanatory names have been given: 'curl sides', 'drop-end sides' and 'straight sides' (*Figure 4.3*).

## Metal frame nomenclature

There are two principal ways of adding a decorative effect to what would otherwise be 'plain' gold filled or nickel silver frames. One is to cover the rims with removable plastic surrounds. The sides also may be partly covered with plastics material to match. The other method is to manufacture the main parts of the frame from wire or strip having a

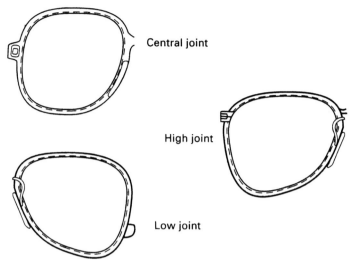

Central joint

High joint

Low joint

**Figure 4.2** Joint positions.

decorative pattern. A frame so made is described as *engraved* even though the pattern has usually been impressed on the material by a stamping process. The main parts of metal frames are listed below.

## The bridge

In the metal pad bridge frame, the rims are connected by a bar which is not intended to rest on the nose. Instead, the weight of the frame is borne on two small pads which are usually made of a plastics material but have a metallic insert for attachment to the pad arm. The latter usually

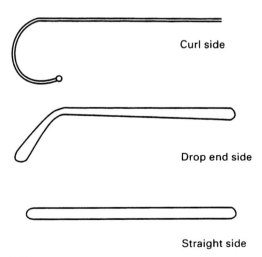

Curl side

Drop end side

Straight side

**Figure 4.3** Types of side.

incorporates a loop or is otherwise designed to permit adjustment of the pad position by pliering. The pads themselves are usually attached by some means which allow them to pivot and so adjust themselves to the slope of the nose. Pads of this type are known as 'rocking pads' to distinguish them from 'rigid pads' which are sufficiently described by their name. One can even have a 'twinned pad' fitted, more commonly referred to as a *flexibridge*. It is like two pads but joined at the top to help distribute the weight of the frame more evenly (*Figure 4.4*). The flexibridge is normally made from silicone. Most rocking or rigid pads are made in acetate with the silicone variety being available as an extra.

**Figure 4.4** A flexibridge.

The pad arm is often an extension of the bridge bar, in which case only two soldering points (one on each rim) are necessary to attach the entire bridge assembly. Sometimes, however, the pad arms are quite separate, in which case there are four soldering points.

To give extra strength and rigidity when special circumstances require, an additional bar is sometimes soldered to the rims above the main bridge assembly. This is known as a brace bar (*Figure 4.5*).

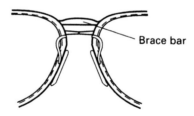

**Figure 4.5** The Brace bar.

## The rims

The rims of a metal spectacle frame are made from eyewire which is obtainable in various sections, two of which are shown in *Figure 4.6*. The band rims type lends itself to engraving when in vogue.

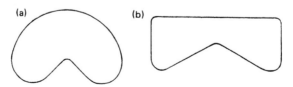

**Figure 4.6** Eyewire sections in common use: (a) round section; (b) flat section (band rim).

## The joints

The joints of the metal frame often serve a double purpose – to provide a pivot for the side and a means of closing the rim on the lens to hold it securely in position. Sometimes the joint will perform both of these functions using one securing device, the closing block screw, more commonly referred to as the joint screw (*Figure 4.7*).

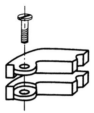

**Figure 4.7** Joint suitable for closing of rim and allowing pivoting of side, all by one screw.

Sometimes, the fixing for securing the rims together and allowing the sides to open and close are achieved separately. A closing block screw is still used in conjunction with a dowel screw, sometimes referred to as a pivot screw (*Figure 4.8*).

The dowel screw on some frames is replaced with a dowel pin sometimes referred to as a pivot pin. This is secured in the joint by riveting.

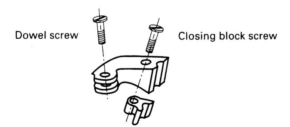

**Figure 4.8** Joint where closing of rim and pivoting of side is achieved by separate screws.

## The sides

The principal parts of a metal spectacle side are shown in *Figure 4.9*.

One other type of side meeting a fortunately limited need remains to be mentioned. This is the loop-end side, used on spectacle frames for babies and very young children. It has a short straight butt ending in a loop to which tape or ribbon is attached, enabling the spectacles to be tied on so that the child cannot remove them.

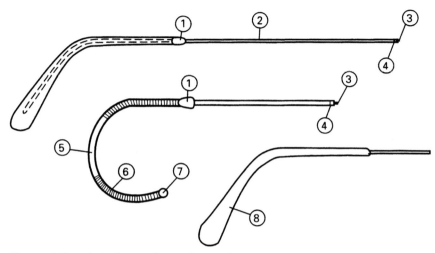

**Figure 4.9** The principal parts of a metal spectacle side: (1) collet; (2) butt; (3) knuckle; (4) half joint; (5) core; (6) spinning; (7) ball tip; (8) end cover.

## Plastics frame nomenclature

### Thickness of material

The majority of frames made from sheet material will come from rectangular slabs of between 6 and 8 mm thick. The more fashionable non-budget type frame tends to be made from the 8 mm thickness as this allows sculpturing and engraving to be performed, giving the frame much more cosmetic appeal. Plastics frames of substantially heavier weight and appearance are known by the generic term *library*.

### The bridge

As with metal frames, plastics frames are made with two essentially different types of bridge, the pad bridge and the regular bridge. A regular bridge is defined as a bridge without pads designed to rest on the nose over a continuous area. The regular bridge and two of its variants are shown diagrammatically in *Figure 4.10*. Normally the bridge is curved outwards (by a process known as *bumping*) to form a projection, which is measured from the back of the rim as indicated by the arrows in *Figure 4.10a*. In certain cases, however, such as when the brows are unusually prominent or the bridge of the nose poorly developed, an inset bridge is needed to throw the rims forward. This construction is illustrated in *Figure 4.10b*. As will be seen, the projection is a minus quantity and is, in fact, indicated by prefixing a minus sign to the dimension shown by the arrow. Additional material has to be cemented to the back of the slab from which the front is made in order to produce such a bridge. The saddle bridge is illustrated in *Figure 4.10c*. This has a positive (forward) projection but like the inset bridge requires additional material at the back to enable it to extend further round the nose, thereby increasing the

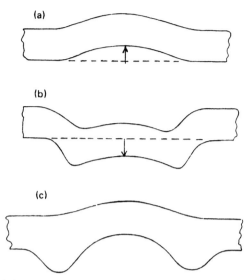

**Figure 4.10** Types of plastics spectacle bridges (diagrammatic view from above): (a) regular bridge; (b) inset bridge; (c) saddle bridge.

area of the bearing surface. A flush bridge has zero projection, the bumping process being simply omitted. It should be noted that the term 'saddle bridge' encompasses regular, flush and inset bridges.

Alternatively, a pad bridge is defined as having two specific and limited bearing areas. The greater majority of pad bridge plastics frames have rigid pads of the same material cemented to or integral with the rims. It is, however, possible to fit rocking pads mounted on adjustable pad arms pinned or otherwise attached to the front.

A varient of the ordinary pad bridge which is sometimes useful is termed the keyhole pad bridge and is illustrated in *Figure 4.11*. Its purpose is to reduce the distance between the rims in relation to the distance between the edges of the lenses.

Some metal frames have a bridge similar to a pad bridge found on plastic frames but adopted to either clip or be firmly cemented to the two rims (*Figure 4.12*).

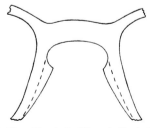

**Figure 4.11** The keyhole pad bridge. The dotted lines indicate the position of the rims in the normal pad bridge.

**Figure 4.12** Bridge suitable for fitting to metal frame.

## The joints

The sole purpose of a joint on a plastics frame is to provide a means of attachment for the sides on which the latter can pivot. When the dowel screw is removed, the joint falls into two halves, one of which is attached to the front and the other to the side. The main parts of each half-joint are the 'plates' (which are drilled with two or more holes for the fixing rivets) and the charnier(s) through which the pivot screw passes. The minimum number of charniers is three (two on one half-joint and one on the other) but joints are also made with five (*Figure 4.13*).

The joint is attached to the front of an extension termed a lug. These are of various forms such as mitred, radiused and swept-back (*Figure 4.14*). For this latter style a special type of joint is required.

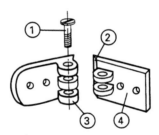

**Figure 4.13** The joint on a plastics frame. (1) dowel screw; (2) mitre; (3) charniers; (4) front plate.

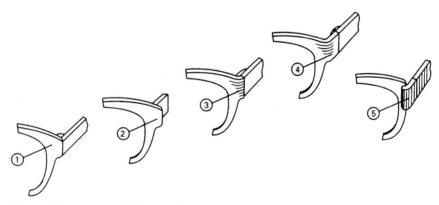

**Figure 4.14** Types of lug: (1) mitred; (2) overhang; (3) radiused; (4) swept-back; (5) wrap-round.

## The sides

Since the introduction of cellulose acetate spectacle frames, the great majority of sides have incorporated a reinforcing wire. This serves the double purpose of strengthening the side and making it easier to adjust. Decorative effects are sometimes added by engraving or electroplating the wire (*Figure 4.15*).

The drop-end type of side is by far the most popular (*Figure 4.15*). Curl sides fitted to plastics frames are usually made by soldering a super-comfort curl to the reinforcing wire in the butt, the end of which may be fitted into a collet to improve the appearance.

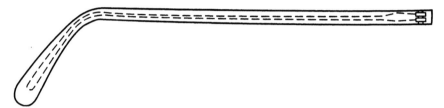

**Figure 4.15** Side complete with reinforced wire.

## Rimless and supra spectacles

Rimless styles can be subdivided into either those that are truly rimless where the lenses are held in position by screws or slotting to a bridge piece, joints and sides, or a semi-rimless where there is a rim around part of the lens, normally a brow bar and the lenses are again held in position by screws or slotting. The number of holes drilled in each lens to accommodate the bridge and joints can be between two and four. It is not unknown to combine rimless spectacles (or mounts as they are sometimes called) with facetted lenses to give an interesting appearance.

Another form of semi-rimless has its own distinct category, *supra*. The rims do not totally surround the lenses, the lenses being held in position, not by screws or slots but by a thin nylon cord attached to the rims that rests in a groove on the lens edge.

## Vocational frames and mounts

To conclude this chapter it may be of interest to the reader to consider the more 'unusual', or should we say 'specialist', type of eyewear available for specific vocational/medical needs (*Figure 4.16*).

### Half eyes

Normally worn when only a reading correction is required. Patient looks over the top of the spectacles for distance vision. There are many types, straight-top, crescent-top, fully rimmed, nylon-supra or a full-rim with a

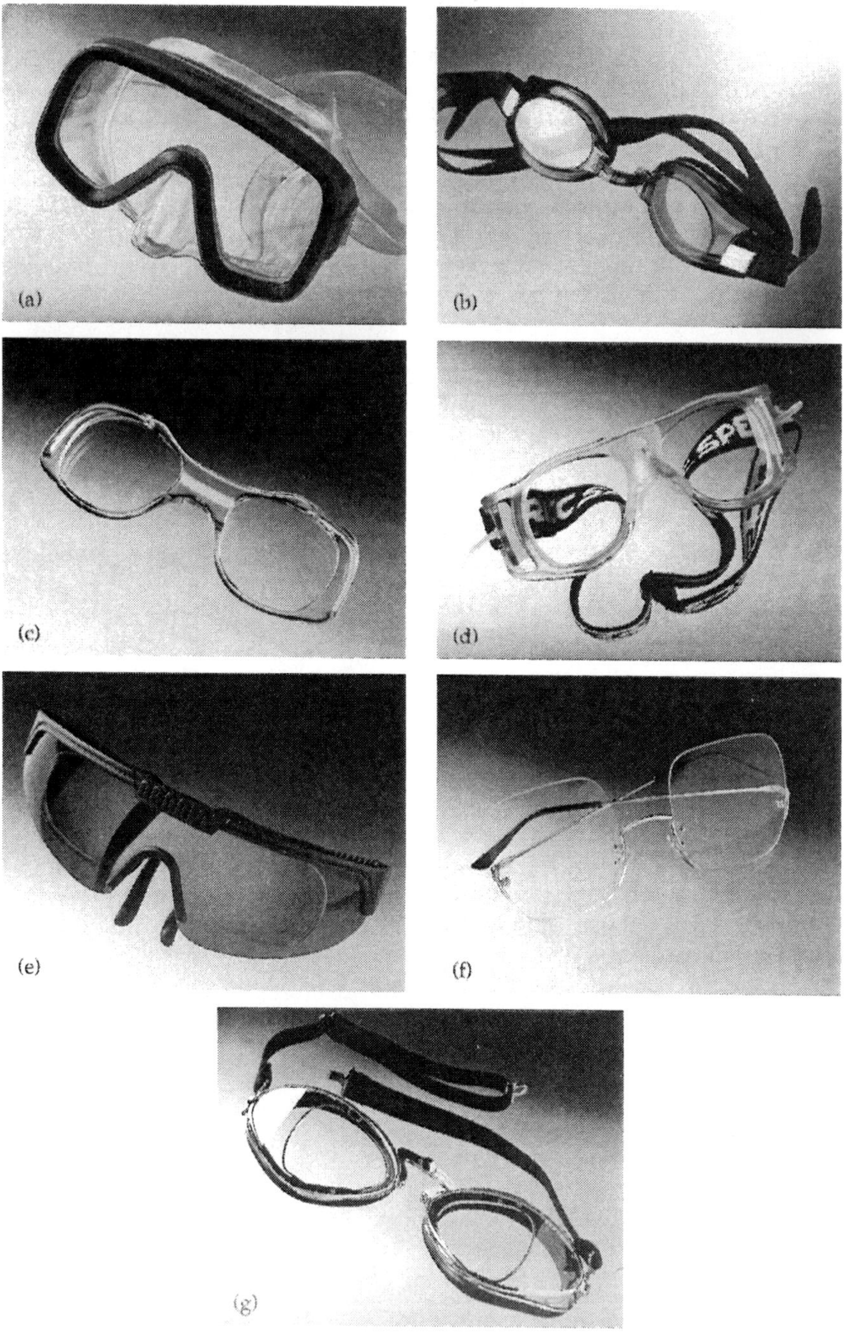

**Figure 4.16** Examples of different vocational frames and mounts. (a) Diving mask.
(b) Swimming goggles. (c) Special Rx insert for diving mask. (d) Sports goggles typically
used for squash. (e) Wraparound with Rx insert for various uses. (f) Snooker spectacles.
(g) Motorcycle goggles – can also be used as 'classic car' or aviator goggles. Rx insert
included. (Pictures courtesy of Norville Optical.)

lens in the lower half only. Very occasionally a request for a 'reversed half eye' is received with lenses only being glazed in the top portion.

## Lorgnette

Eyeglasses for occasional use, held before the eyes by a handle into which the lenses may fold when not required. Care must be taken to ensure lens curvatures allows folding or closing where applicable.

## Quizzer

One lens mounted on a handle (like a lorgnette but only one lens instead of two).

## Dress-clips

Similar to lorgnettes, but to be worn on a dress when not being used to assist vision. The handle is often jewelled to form a brooch. Usually folds to grip on the dress.

## Monocle

Single lens, with or without a rim, designed to be held between the brow and cheek.

## Folding spectacles

As well as the joints connecting the front to the sides, there are three further joints, one on the bridge and one halfway along each side enabling the spectacles to be folded away for easy storage. Care must be taken to ensure lens curvature allows folding to take place.

## Hinged-front spectacles

Spectacles may be made with a second front hinged at the tops of the rims. The outer front holds a pair of supplementary lenses which can be swung away when not needed.

## Make-up spectacles

A frontal bar is made up to which each eyerim is independently fixed by a hinge. One rim can then be raised or lowered to enable the wearer to apply eye cosmetics while viewing through the other. Some designs consist of one eyerim (normally glazed with spherical lens) that can be positioned in front of each eye in turn.

## Snooker spectacles

Can be made with swivel joints so that the angle can be varied to give the visual axis normal to the lens surfaces. Also they can be made with fixed low-set joints giving a retroscopic joint angle. As the line of vision is through the top half of the lens, the optical centres should be raised to take this into account. Rimless or supra style mounts are often used as with no restriction regarding rims, lenses can be made deeper making them ideal for this purpose.

### Recumbent spectacles

Designed where a patient is bed-ridden and wishes to read while lying down. A pair of reflecting prisms are included so that the patient can look upwards and rest the book on their chest.

### Telescopic spectacles

Patients with low visual acuity may have their prescription incorporated into telescopic spectacles to increase the magnification enabling them to make the best use of the limited vision they have available. The telescope is of Galilean design and is either screwed to a back-plate or bonded to a carrier lens.

### Ptosis spectacles

Ptosis is a condition where the upper eyelid droops due to the inability of its muscles to keep it open. The ptosis spectacle supports the lid by means of an extension or gallery fixed to the upper half of the rim.

### Safety spectacles

Frames used to give protection to the eyes must be very robust and must not disintegrate when being worn in an environment where danger of impact exists. To give additional protection side-shields are fitted.

### Hearing-aid spectacles

For patients requiring hearing aid as well as vision aid, the two requirements are combined into a spectacle frame normally with the hearing aid(s) fitted unobtrusively behind the ear(s).

### Diving mask

Where a patient wishes to have a prescription added to enable them to see while wearing a diving mask, a pair of lenses are made up with one side plano and all the power on the other side. These are then bonded to the inside of the faceplate of the mask. Some masks even permit the glazing of a limited prescription range into the mask itself. Instead of a faceplate they have two separate eyeshapes. The plano lenses are removed and replaced by prescription. These replacement lenses will normally require special edging to ensure watertight fit and the prescription lenses will need to be toughened.

Before attempting to deal with any diving mask, always inspect closely to ensure it is suitable for either the bonding or glazing of prescription lenses. Be careful, many are not! An alternative to bonding lenses to a faceplate is to use a spectacle front insert that is glazed in the normal manner and then fitted inside the mask.

## Swimming goggles

It is possible to fit a pair of prescription lenses to a swimming goggle, the first priority naturally is to keep the goggle waterproof and it is best to examine the goggle before commencing work to ensure that this is possible.

## Squash goggles

Because of the danger of eye injury from the ball, eyesize must be smaller than the diameter of the ball. Lenses would normally be made of polycarbonate to give maximum impact resistance and goggle held securely in position by a tight headband.

## Gun sights

A lens to prescription can be glazed into a gun sight so that a marksman need not wear spectacles. Lens is usually in flat form and may be tinted to act as a contrast filter to help facilitate viewing.

## Shooting spectacles

Front consists of a browbar from which suspends a rim holding the patient's correction for the eye used for sighting. Usually fitted with curl-sides to hold frame securely in place.

## Ski goggles

Prescription lenses can be glazed to a supplementary front which clips inside the ski goggle. Lenses may have to be made with steeper curves to match that of the wrap-around goggle.

## Over specs

Protection can be given by wearing over-specs which fit in front of the prescription lenses in a standard frame.

## Motorcycle goggles

Prescription lenses can be bonded to the inside surface of the front faceplates of motorcycle goggles. Lenses have plano contact surfaces with all the power surfaced on the other side. Care must be taken with centration as goggles are very wide. Some goggles have an insert facility, so only this has to be glazed, removing the need for bonding.

## Welding goggles

To give protection from very bright light experienced in this process, and also the welding splatter. Some goggles allow prescription lenses to be glazed. Whilst lens material can be toughened glass, they do tend to retain the welding splatters which in time prevent clear vision. Better to use resin or polycarbonate material which allows the splatter to 'bounce' off the lens surface thereby giving the goggles a longer working life.

## Cycling spectacles

Where a cyclist wishes to wear eye protectors and also needs a correction, prescription lenses can be fitted to the spectacles, normally using inserts.

## Ultra-violet sunspecs

Where a patient is extremely susceptible to ultra-violet light, special wrap-around sunspecs are available to screen sunlight from front and sides.

## Reversible spectacles

Can be used when a patient uses one eye only, and requires a different prescription for distance and for reading. The distance Rx is fitted to one eye and the reading Rx to the other. The bridge of the frame is of swivelling or fixed pad design and the sides with revolving butts. The round or oval eyed frame can then be turned over to give desired lens in front of the sighted eye.

## Respiration spectacles

Designed to be worn under a gas mask, this round-eyed metal frame has flat butted curl-sides and is wholly functional.

# Chapter 5

# Spectacle frame dimensions

## Standards

The agreed system of spectacle measurement in the UK is based on the British Standard BS 3199 (1992) (ISO 8624). Readers would be advised to obtain a copy along with BS EN ISO 12870 (1998) which details general requirements and test methods for the marking of spectacle frames. BS 3521 Part 2 (1991) – *Glossary of Terms Relating to Spectacle Frames* – would also be useful.

The original measuring system used in Britain until 1992 was the *Datum system* with many of the measurements being taken on or around a position referred to as the datum line or from the datum centre. The UK has now moved to use the more popular international method referred to as the *Box system*.

Many years of work were devoted to standardisation of spectacle frame measuring, particularly concerning the system by which we design, define and identify frames centred on the rationalisation of these two similar but conflicting systems of measurement. They use much the same terminology but are capable of generating two distinctly different locations for such fundamental points as the 'reference' centre of the lens shape, or indeed its size.

Taking the latter (its size) to a diagrammatic illustration, it is necessary to define the position of the 'old' datum line. It was a line midway between and parallel to the horizontal tangents to the lens shape at its highest and lowest points (*Figure 5.1*). Its length was equal to the datum length. The Box system uses the widest parameters of the shape to determine its size. So, as can be seen from *Figure 5.1*, a frame could have two eyesizes yet be one size!

As referred to earlier, there was also the problem that the reference centre could be in two different positions depending upon the system used (*Figure 5.2*). This could have confusing results as it is this point that is used as a starting point for lens positioning.

For many years, the UK in particular, had in circulation frames from both the Datum and the Box systems, causing inevitable confusion.

1992 marked an important occasion when the Box system was recognised as the only one for defining the dimensions of a spectacle frame front.

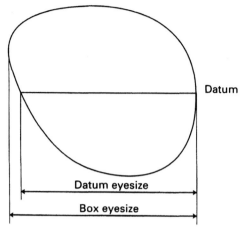

**Figure 5.1** Difference between box and datum eyesizes.

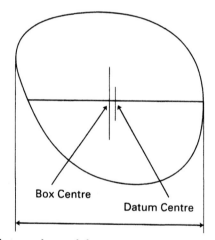

**Figure 5.2** Difference between box and datum centres.

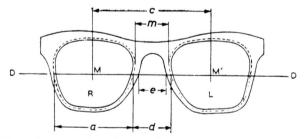

**Figure 5.3** Datum references. Dimensions applying to fronts. The dotted curves represent peak of bevel or bottom of groove. DD = Datum line of frame; M = Datum centre of right lens; M' = Datum centre of left lens; $a$ = Datum length of lens; $c$ = Datum centre distance; $d$ = Distance between lenses; $e$ = Distance between rims (dat); $m$ = Minimum between lenses.

Old habits die hard so it will be some years yet before all of the 'old' Datum terminology is cleansed from the system. Old brains may still refer to *datum* when they should be referring to *horizontal centre line*.

Finally, for historical reference purposes only, some of the old datum references are shown in *Figure 5.3*.

## Basic frame dimension

There follows a description of the primary frame dimensions that the reader should be familiar with.

*Horizontal centre line (Figure 5.4)*. A line drawn through the geometrical centres of the rectangular boxes that just encompass/enclose the two lenses.

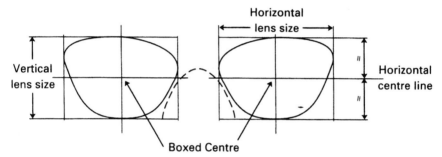

**Figure 5.4** Position of horizontal centre line, boxed centres, vertical and horizontal lens sizes.

*Distance between centres*. The distance between the boxed centres *(Figures 5.4)*.

*Boxed centre*. Intersection of the horizontal and vertical centre lines *(Figure 5.4)*.

*Horizontal lens size*. Distance between the vertical sides of the rectangle which circumscribes the lens *(Figure 5.4)*.

*Boxed lens size (Figure 5.5)*. The horizontal and vertical dimensions formed by the box that circumscribes the lens.

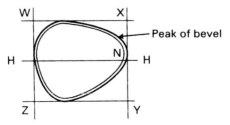

**Figure 5.5** Boxed lens size. ZY × WZ = Lens size; HH = Centre line; WXYZ = Limiting rectangle defining the boxed lens. *Note*: the letter N denotes the nasal side of the lens shape.

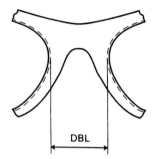

**Figure 5.6** Distance between lenses (DBL).

*Vertical lens size.* Distance between the horizontal sides of the rectangle which circumscribe the lens (*Figure 5.4*).

*Distance between lenses (DBL) (Figure 5.6).* The minimum distance between the two lenses.

*Distance between rims (DBR) (Figure 5.7).* The distance between the rims measured at a stated level (*x*) below the midpoint of the bridge.

For example, DBR 19 at 10 mm below crest. In this instance $x = 10$ mm. For pad bridges the DBR would be expressed as a horizontal measurement taken either along the horizontal centre line or above or below it, instead of in relation to the midpoint of the lower edge of the bridge.

*Bridge width (Figure 5.8).* The minimum distance between the pad surfaces measured along the bridge width line which is positioned 5 mm below the horizontal centre line.

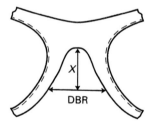

**Figure 5.7** Distance between rims (DBR). *x* = level below midpoint of bridge.

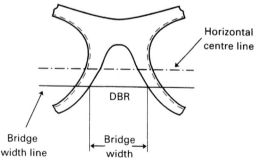

**Figure 5.8** Bridge width.

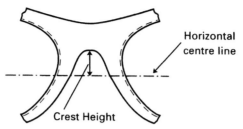

**Figure 5.9** Crest height.

*Crest height (Figure 5.9).* The vertical distance from the horizontal centre line of the frame to the midpoint of the lower edge of the bridge.

*Length to bend (TB) (Figure 5.10).* The distance between the dowel point and the ear point.

On a curl side frame there is a *length to tangent* instead of length to bend (*Figure 5.11*).

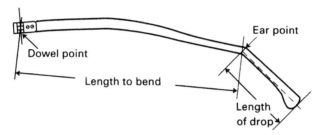

**Figure 5.10** Drop-end side – dowel point, length to bend, ear point and length of drop.

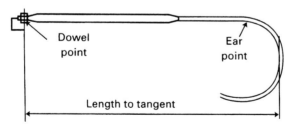

**Figure 5.11** Curl side – dowel point, ear point and length to tangent.

Drop-end, curl sides and straight sides can also be measured as a total length (*Figure 5.12*). This is measured again from the dowel point but now to the very end of the side. For curl sides the curl would have to be straightened to measure this.

*Angle of side (Figure 5.13).* The angle between a normal to the back plane of the front and the line of the side when open. Unless otherwise stated this is normally an angle downwards.

The remaining measurements are depicted in *Figure 5.14*.

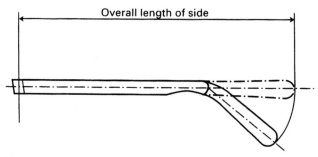

**Figure 5.12** Drop-end sides – total length.

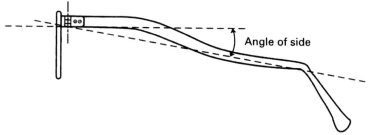

**Figure 5.13** Angle of side.

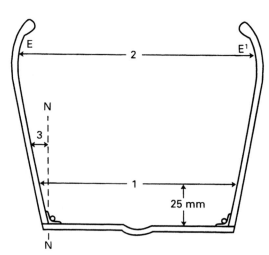

**Figure 5.14** Remaining measurements. (1) Temple width – measured 25 mm behind the back plane of the front. (2) Head width – measured between the ear points. (3) Angle of let back – horizontal angle between the inner surface of the fully opened side, adjacent to the joint and a normal to the back plane of the front.

## Marking of frames

BS 6625 Part 2 (ISO 9456) requires manufacturers to make certain minimum information available concerning measurements and sizing (*Figure 5.15*).

It is also important to note that the stated dimensions should be marked on the relevant component (i.e. front size on the front, side length on a side). The side length marked shall be the overall length as a minimum. If the manufacturer wishes to mark length to bend, it must be in addition to overall length.

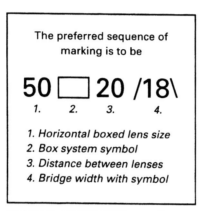

**Figure 5.15** Extract from BS 6625 Part 2 (ISO 9456) regarding measurements and sizing.

Other obligatory markings that must be present for compliance are manufacturer's identification, model, colour and some identification of the materials used. It is acceptable for this to be in some kind of code but the manufacturer will be obliged to make a key to that code available. The standard also sets out certain other information that the manufacturer should make available either with the frame or separately, on request.

1 Range available, i.e. size/colour combinations.
2 Components available separately.
3 Lens area in square millimetres.
4 Mass of frame for an identified frame size.
5 Bridge height.
6 Effective lens diameter uncut size necessary to glaze the frame.

# Chapter 6

# Lens shapes and sizes

## Uncut lenses

An uncut is a finished lens that has not been cut or edged to the eyeshape of a spectacle frame. All mass produced stock single vision lenses are uncuts. A lens that has been specially surfaced is also referred to as being in uncut form until it is glazed.

The modern prescription house will normally have two different types of customer. Those who order uncuts because they have their own cut, edge and fit workshop and those who require 'glazed orders', when the prescription house performs all the various tasks and sends a finished pair of spectacles to the optician. In Europe the trend is towards all prescription house work being of the uncut variety, the opticians fitting the lenses via their own workshops.

Over the years the dimensions of uncut lenses have gradually increased to match the trend toward larger frames. In the 1920s, 47 mm diameter was the average uncut size. Today it is nearer 70 mm, with blanks as large as 85 mm being available if required.

A further development, thanks to computer technology, is the facility for a practice to digitally trace the eyeshapes of a chosen frame. This along with prescription details can then be transmitted to the Rx house who will not only supply or make the lenses, but edge them to the correct size and shape. Upon receipt at the practice they have only to be inserted into the chosen frame. Valuable time is no longer lost 'in the post', as the need to send the frame to the Rx house has been eliminated.

## Glazing

The process of fitting a lens to a spectacle frame is known as glazing. It normally includes the prior operation of reducing the uncut lens to the desired shape and size while imparting the required form to its edge. Spectacle frames with a completely surrounding rim for each lens require the lens to have a bevelled edge to fit into a retaining groove. For other types of spectacles the lenses may need to be flat edged, grooved, or given different edge forms in different parts of the periphery.

An important aspect of glazing is concerned with achieving excellent optical accuracy; the optical centre of the edged lens should be located at the correct position and the axis of the cylinder, if any, in the specified orientation. Segments on multifocal lenses, fitting crosses on progressives, must all be correctly positioned to match the prescriber's specifications.

## Lens shapes

The term lens shape may be defined as the outline of the lens periphery, with the nasal side and the horizontal indicated. The reason for defining it in this way is seen from *Figure 6.1* in which HH is a horizontal line relative to the spectacle frame or mount and N denotes the nasal side of the lens. Shape (b) is obtained by lifting up and turning over shape (a), while shape (c) is shape (b) turned through 15°. Nevertheless, they are regarded as different.

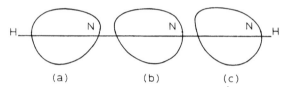

Figure 6.1 Lens shape with nasal and horizontal centre line indicated.

## Finished lens dimensions

For many centuries, lens shapes were restricted to the simplest geometrical forms, principally round and oval (elliptical). Both of these have an obvious geometrical centre at which the optical centre of the lens would normally be placed or used as a 'starting point' for any decentration to be obtained.

Most lens shapes are now asymmetrical and require an agreed system of measurement for specifying not only the dimensions of the lens but also the standard optical centre position. An additional requirement of the measuring system is a horizontal reference line for certain vertical dimensions of the finished spectacles.

In the UK, a solution was provided by the Datum system put forward in 1935 by J. Cole and A. Blackburn. With some loose ends tied up, this became the basis of the British Standard for spectacle measurement, that is until 1992 when the Box system was officially adopted.

The *datum line*, mentioned in Chapter 5, was defined as the line midway between and parallel to the horizontal tangents to the lens shape at its highest and lowest points. In *Figure 6.2*, these tangents are represented by HH and JJ, the datum line being DD. In passing, it should be noted that for the purpose of this and other definitions, the periphery of the lens is taken to be the peak of the bevel, if any.

The datum lens size was specified by two dimensions in millimetres. The first was the datum length, represented by AB in *Figure 6.2*. It was

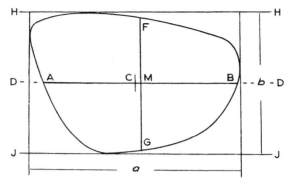

**Figure 6.2** Relationship between box and datum eyesizes and standard optical centre position.

defined as that portion of the datum line bounded by the lens periphery. The midpoint of AB, denoted by M, was of particular importance and was therefore given a name – the *datum centre*. The vertical line FG through the datum centre and bounded by the periphery of the lens specified its vertical dimension, termed the mid-datum depth.

This has now been superseded by an alternative method known as the Box system. According to this the boxed lens size is expressed by the length *a* and the height *b* of the rectangle with horizontal and vertical sides all tangential to the lens periphery. In the Box system the geometrical centre of the box, denoted by C in *Figure 6.2*, is the standard optical centre position, whereas in the Datum system it is the datum centre M.

It should be noted that the datum line and the equivalent in the Box system, *horizontal centre line*, are in exactly the same position but from there the similarity ends.

## Shape difference

The difference in millimetres between the horizontal and vertical dimensions of a lens is known as the shape difference (termed 'lens difference' in the American Standard). There is one point about the shape difference that is worthy of notice. In any true-to-scale enlargement or reduction, the dimensions of a figure are changed but not its proportions. Thus, two rectangles of dimensions 40 × 32 and 50 × 40 both have the same ratio of length to height but not the same shape difference.

## Lens size of unglazed frames

The rims of metal frames cannot be stretched and plastics frames can be stretched only within narrow limits. Generally speaking, a rimmed frame is therefore intended to be fitted with lenses of a predetermined size and shape. The stated lens size of an unglazed frame indicates the dimensions of this shape.

Measuring the lens size of an empty frame presents a point of difficulty because the peak of the bevel corresponds to the bottom of the groove in the rim which is not accessible to measurement by any simple means. The best one can do is to measure the clear aperture of the rim and make an allowance for the depth of the groove at each extremity. To a close approximation, the lens size can generally be taken as the clear aperture plus 1 mm.

## Effective lens diameter

As described in Chapter 5, it is recommended that frame manufacturers state the effective lens diameter to glaze a particular frame, sometimes referred to as the ELD or simply ED (effective diameter). If this figure is not available it is easy enough to ascertain (*Figure 6.3*). Once one has located the box centre, measure the distance to the farthest point and double it. This will give the ELD before any decentration is taken into account. It is normal to add on a glazing allowance, say 2 mm, to the ELD.

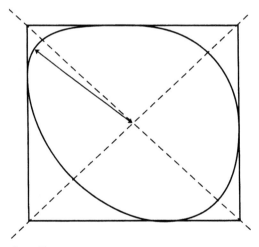

**Figure 6.3** Effective lens diameter.

A good 'rule of thumb' method for single vision is to take the decentration required for one lens, double it and add this figure to the ELD already calculated, to arrive at the minimum size uncut. By way of an example, let us suppose the distance from the box centre to the farthest point on the lens periphery is 32 mm. Double this to arrive at an ELD of 64 mm. Add 2 mm glazing allowance which now gives a figure of 66 mm. Let us suppose there is a requirement to decentre the lens 3 mm in. Double this (6 mm) and add to the 66 mm already obtained. This gives an ELD of 72 mm.

One cannot apply such a simplistic approach with multifocals or progressives due to the consideration of segment top/fitting cross position when glazed and the position of the segment/fitting cross, both vertically and horizontally within the semi-finished blank.

## Classification of lens shape

The bewildering variety of modern lens shapes, complicated by the use of different trade names for substantially the same shape, makes any systematic classification very difficult. One can, however, single out various shapes and families of shapes which can either be clearly defined or have been given generally accepted descriptive names.

### Geometrical shapes

*Round* (*Figure 6.4*)

This is one of the most ancient of lens shapes, possibly because a circle is the obvious shape for a centred spherical lens, making the edge thickness the same all round. Round lenses fitted in 'horn-rimmed' spectacles enjoyed a tremendous vogue shortly after World War I when, not unnaturally, they were considered an improvement on the small oval shapes which had prevailed for many decades previously. Like most fashion trends the round eyeshape comes and goes with the fickle nature and demands of the spectacle-wearing public.

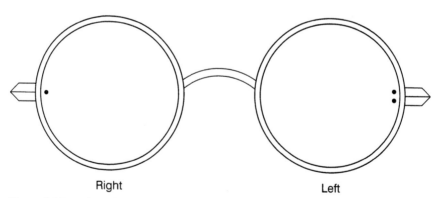

Right                                Left

**Figure 6.4** Round eyeshape.

Because of its round shape the nasal edge of the lens is not easily determined, so care must be exercised when the lens is fitted into the frame that the centration is in the correct direction. To avoid possible problems, BS 2738 Part 1 (1998) suggests that the setting position of round lenses (except those of thermally toughened glass) should be identified by means of permanent marks placed next to the joint on the back lens surface. They should consist of one mark on the joint line for the right eye, and two marks placed symmetrically, one either side of the joint line, for the left (as indicated on *Figure 6.4*).

### Oval (*Figure 6.5*)

The word 'oval' has several meanings including egg-shaped. Applied to a lens shape however, it means elliptical – the shape produced by cutting through a circular rod in any plane oblique to its axis. This shape, too, is very ancient and may be seen in some of the earlier artistic representations of spectacles.

Since an ellipse can be made with any shape difference, the term oval does not so much define a shape as a family of lens shapes.

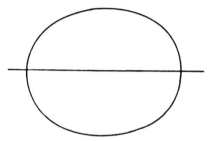

**Figure 6.5** Oval eyeshape.

### PRO (*Figure 6.6*)

Written in full, the term denoted by this abbreviation is *pantoscopic round oval*. It denotes a family of lens shapes formed by the lower half of a circle and the upper half of an ellipse with the same horizontal diameter. In practice, the outline thus obtained may be subtly modified in order to produce a more pleasing effect. PRO shapes can be made with any shape difference, depending on the proportions of the ellipse used.

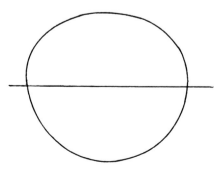

**Figure 6.6** PRO eyeshape.

The PRO has played an important part in the evolution of modern lens shapes because it was the first step towards the recognition of both functional and aesthetic factors. As a lens shape it is undoubtedly more pleasing than the round. At the same time the advantage of the large field of view of the round shape is retained, the portion sacrificed being in an area where vision is, in any case, limited by the brows.

Although the terminology PRO no longer appears in British Standards it has an accepted place in the optical world.

### Perimetric shapes (*Figures 6.7 and 6.8*)

It will be noted on closing one eye that the field of view is not symmetrical in shape, the nasal side being much more restricted than the opposite (temporal) side.

The 1930s saw the introduction of the first lens shapes modelled on the eye's own field of view. A shape of this type which he termed 'perimetric' had been suggested as far back as 1897 by the American ophthalmologist, J. Thorington. The name given is an allusion to the instrument (the perimeter) with which the boundary of the eye's field of view can be traced. In the UK the term *contour* was once used and accepted as a generic name for this family of shapes.

There is no simple geometrical formula whereby such shapes can be defined and in the course of time numerous variations on the original theme have appeared. Originally, the shape was quite rounded as in *Figure 6.7* like the PRO from which it developed.

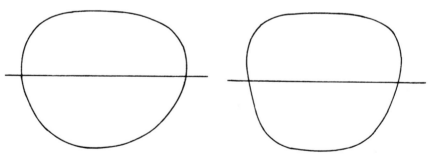

**Figure 6.7** A rounded contour eyeshape.    **Figure 6.8** A squarer contour eyeshape identified as a Quadra.

Later, a squarer vision as in *Figure 6.8* gave rise to numerous slightly different shapes. This squarer version has a generic term of *quadra* which can be defined as a family of lens shapes characterised by four recognisable sides of shallow curvature joined by arcs of shorter radius. There is no fixed shape difference. The general trend has been towards more elongated shapes but the vagaries of fashion are not predictable.

## Pilot shapes (*Figure 6.9*)

This shape used to be referred to as 'aviator' shape but should now be termed *pilot*. It's a family of lens shapes essentially triangular, characterised by a nasal cut-away and a pronounced fullness in the lower temporal quadrant.

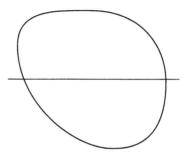

**Figure 6.9** A pilot eyeshape.

## Upswept shapes

The term upswept has come into general use to describe any shape with a top sloping upwards towards the temple, as in *Figure 6.10*. The gradient may vary from the slight to the very pronounced.

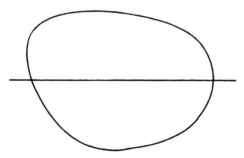

**Figure 6.10** An upswept eyeshape.

## Rimless

As described in Chapter 4, rimless styles can be either truly rimless, semi-rimless or supra. As there are no shape limiting rims the possibilities are endless. *Figure 6.11* illustrates a traditional rimless shape used on the more conservative styles.

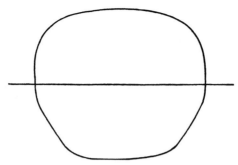

**Figure 6.11** A typical rimless eyeshape.

## Half-eye shapes

The object of these shapes (*Figures 6.12* and *6.13*) is to enable the wearer to use a correction for near vision only and to enjoy a useful field of distance vision over the top. They can also be employed, upside down, to provide corrected distance vision and unaided near vision. *Figure 6.13* illustrates what is often termed crescent shaped.

Rarely seen today are half eyes that have a straight top and 'sharp' corners, as depicted in *Figure 6.14*. Lenses of this shape often had to be 'hand edged' to obtain the final fit, hence 'rounded' corner (*Figure 6.12*) gained popularity. The trend has changed further with many half eyes not only having 'rounded' corners, but tops as well (*Figure 6.15*), as this allows edging machines to be used without the need for further hand edging by skilled technicians.

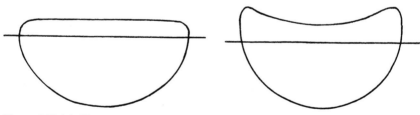

**Figure 6.12** A half eye.

**Figure 6.13** Crescent shaped half eye.

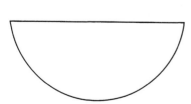

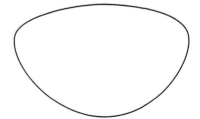

**Figure 6.14** A half eye with a straight top and sharp corners.

**Figure 6.15** A half eye with rounded corners and tops.

# Chapter 7

# The prescription order form

This is the document that provides sufficient information for suitable uncut or mounted spectacle lenses to be manufactured or supplied which comply with the prescription requirements of a particular patient. Considering its importance it is one of the most abused pieces of paper in the profession and industry!

Designs will vary from company to company, some allowing the details to be completed by hand, whilst others are generated via computer or word processor. It is essential that it is completed in the correct manner to ensure requirements are clearly understood and not open to mis-interpretation. Although as stated earlier, designs vary, one can detect a general theme running through them. BS 2738 Part 3 (1991) gives guidance on the subject of the prescription order form.

Unless written in full the letters R and L are used to identify the patient's lens data for the right and left eyes respectively. The term 'BE' (both eyes) can also be used to identify data applicable to lenses that are identical to both eyes of the patient. When writing a prescription order it is conventional for the details of the right lens to precede the details for the left.

For all data relating to focal power two digits should be included after the decimal point, and if the power is less than 1.00, a zero should be placed before the decimal point. Some examples follow.

| Correct method | Incorrect method |
|---|---|
| 0.25 | .25 |
| 1.00 | 1 |
| 10.00 | 10 |
| 1.50 | 1.5 |
| 10.00 | 10.0 |

If a lens has a plano sphere it can be written as either 'plano' or '0.00'. Sometimes the initials DS after the sphere value may be seen, e.g. +2.00 DS, indicating 'dioptre sphere'. You may also see the initials DC after the cylinder value, e.g. +1.00 DC, indicating 'dioptre cylinder'. All dioptric powers with the exception of plano should have either a + or − sign preceding the value.

If a cylinder is incorporated into a prescription then an axis value should be stated to enable correct orientation of the lens before the eye. On no account should a degree sign (°) be used.

A system referred to as Standard Axis Notation (*Figure 7.1*) is used. It is taken from an observer's point of view so the right eye is on the observer's left, and the left eye on the right. It works on a 0–180 notation in an anti-clockwise direction.

For vertical or horizontal prisms we use the Greek capital delta sign (Δ) followed by the base direction, i.e. $2^\Delta$ base-up or $1^\Delta$ base-in. Alternatively, prism directions can be stated solely by axis. For example, $2^\Delta$ base-up could be given as $2^\Delta$ base 90. $2^\Delta$ base-down would therefore be $2^\Delta$ base 270 (working this time on a 360 notation, unlike cylinder axis which works on a 180 notation).

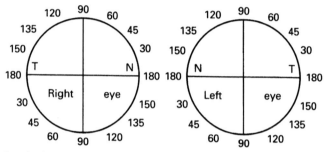

**Figure 7.1** Standard Axis Notation.

If prism in two directions is required it could be specified as $R3^\Delta$ base-down and $4^\Delta$ base-in or $R5^\Delta$ base 323, which is the resultant prism and axis of the two separate prism values. (Chapter 13 gives detailed information on prisms.)

For multifocal and progressive lenses the prism will be assumed effective across the whole lens unless otherwise stated.

Other information required on the prescription order includes the materials in which it is to be fabricated and, where relevant, the manufacturer's name and in the case of multifocals, the segment size and/ or shape. All multifocals and progressives will have an addition, commonly called the *add*. It represents the magnitude of the power which, when added to the distance portion, gives the power of the near or an intermediate portion. For example, a patient may require a distance correction of +2.25 DS –1.00 DC × 90 and a reading correction of +5.00 DS –1.00 DC × 90. The patient is therefore deemed to require a +2.75 near addition (the additional power required to take the +2.25 DS element up to +5.00 DS).

The centration distance (the distance between the patient's pupil centres) needs to be stated. This can be in the form of a total centration distance between the two eyes or as a monocular measurement if patient's eyes are asymmetrically placed.

For example, the distance between the patient's eyes may be 66 mm. That could be expressed in monocular terms as R33 mm, L33 mm but as they are both equal it is more likely to be expressed as 66 mm. However, the patient could have R32 mm and L34 mm. In this instance the eyes are still a total of 66 mm apart but not equally, the right being 2 mm closer to the centre of the bridge of the frame than the left.

By way of an example to try and clarify the above, assume that the patient chooses a frame that has a distance between its centres of 72 mm. The patient has monocular distances of R32 mm L33 mm, that is to say from the centre of the frame bridge to the centre of the right eye is 32 mm and the left 33 mm. To position the lenses correctly in the frame so that the optical centres are in front of the patient's pupils and not central to the eyeshape, a small calculation has to be made. This is shown diagrammatically in *Figure 7.2*.

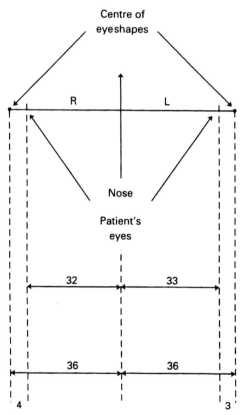

**Figure 7.2** Relationship between box centres, distance between centres, monocular centres and decentration.

The right lens would have to be decentred 4 mm in and the left 3 mm in to position the optical centres of the lens in front of the patient's pupil.

If the lens is a multifocal then the position of the segment top in relation to the horizontal centre line will also need to be stated. This measurement can be above or below so it is necessary to state which, although it is generally assumed to be below unless indicated otherwise.

As progressives do not have segments it is normal to talk in terms of their 'fitting cross' being above or below the horizontal centre line. Segments and fitting crosses are also stated as positions from the bottom rim, or more precisely from the lens periphery at its lowest point including any bevel. However, this system is open to misinterpretation. Many incorrectly measure to the point directly below the segment, which may not be the lowest point. *Figure 7.3* illustrates the correct and incorrect method if stating segment position by height rather than in relation to horizontal centre line.

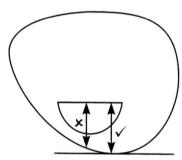

**Figure 7.3** Correct and incorrect method if stating segment position by height rather than in relation to horizontal centre line.

If using this method it is also difficult to make an allowance on a bevelled lens due to the depth of the groove. For this reason BS 2738 Part 3 (1991) states 'the previous use of the measured height from the lower rim of the lens is now deprecated'.

There is no misunderstanding as to the position of the horizontal centre line and therefore no error if measurements are based around this rather than something less tangible.

Multifocals have visible segments and therefore it is important that not only are they fitted correctly in the vertical meridian by means of the segment top position, but horizontally by means of what we term geometrical inset, which is defined as a distance between vertical lines through the distance centration point and the midpoint of the segment diameter (*Figure 7.4*).

As with most other measurements in optics there are other ways of specifying the same information. For example, a patient may have a distance of 66 mm between their eyes when viewing distance objects. When his or her eyes converge for reading this could reduce to 62 mm. The difference between these two figures is 4 mm so the eyes effectively move a total of 4 mm in when reading and as both eyes appear to be symmetrically placed, this means that each eye moves in by 2 mm, i.e. 2 mm geometrical inset.

The same applies even if the patient has asymmetrical centres. For example, for distance viewing the patient may have monocular

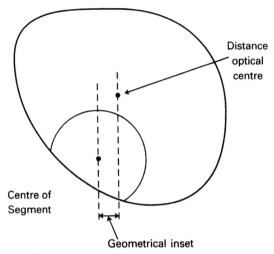

**Figure 7.4** Geometrical inset.

measurements of R32 mm L34 mm. When viewing near objects this measurement becomes R30 mm and L31 mm. Taking each eye separately, the right eye has moved 2 mm in and therefore the lens is said to have a geometrical inset of 2 mm. The left lens has moved 3 mm in and therefore is said to have a geometrical inset of 3 mm. Even though the figures were originally given in a different way, it is possible to convert them into geometrical insets.

It should be noted that for the purpose of geometrical inset it is assumed that the optical centre of the segment is in the middle of the segment. This is not the case in most instances! However, as it is frequently impossible to control the optical centre within the segment, it is convenient to 'assume' it is central. It should be stated that in many instances the optical centre of the segment may not even be on the lens!

Occasionally the term 'optical inset' is used and this is truly the horizontal distance between the distance optical centre and the near optical centre but for the reasons stated above, it is often not a practical or even possible measurement to work to.

Other information required on the prescription order form would involve details of any tints, coatings, anti-reflection requirements, etc., along with frame details. It is generally accepted that an uncut prescription order normally contains less information than a glazed prescription order.

Traditionally, because uncuts have been ordered by stating the diameter required, details such as distance centres, segment top position and frame details have been omitted from the prescription order. However, with newer technology now available to the industry it is possible on uncut orders (where no frame is included) to scan a drawing of the eyeshape to which the lenses will eventually be fitted so that, as with glazed work, a lens can be designed, not just to a diameter, but to the individual frame. For this as much detail as possible is needed. The result is that lenses produced by this method will be of the minimum substance.

In conclusion, there is what could be termed 'distance edging' (see Chapter 6) which is neither a glazed nor an uncut order, but due to computer technology allows the Rx house to edge a lens accurately to the correct settings for a frame being held at another location.

# Chapter 8

# Spherical lenses

## Definitions

Simple errors of refraction unaccompanied by astigmatism are corrected by spherical lenses. This term does not refer to the shape of the lens but to the form of its surfaces. A spherical lens is one in which each surface forms part of the surface of a sphere. One surface may be flat or plane, in which case it may be considered as part of a spherical surface of infinite radius.

Spherical surfaces are either convex, concave or plane. A convex surface is one that bulges: a straight edge placed across it will touch at only one point and will therefore rock. On the other hand, a concave surface is hollow: a straight edge placed across it will touch at each extremity (*Figure 8.1*).

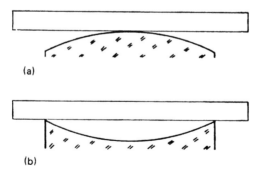

(a)

(b)

**Figure 8.1** (a) A convex surface; (b) a concave surface.

The radius of curvature of a spherical surface is the radius (that is, half the diameter) of the sphere of which it forms part. The centre of curvature is the centre of that sphere. The imaginary line joining the two centres of curvature of a lens' surface is termed the optical axis. If one surface is plane, the optical axis is the straight line perpendicular to that surface which passes through the centre of curvature of the other surface. These terms are all illustrated in *Figure 8.2*.

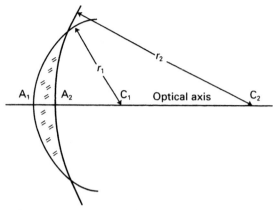

**Figure 8.2** Section through a spherical lens. $C_1$ and $C_2$ are the centres of curvature; $r_1$ and $r_2$ are the radii of curvature; $A_1$ and $A_2$ are the front and back vertices.

A spectacle lens is always mounted so that its less convex or more concave surface is next to the eye. The lenses shown in *Figure 8.3* are all drawn correctly positioned with respect to an eye to the right of them. The surface that is placed nearer the eye is termed the back surface, the other being the front surface. The two points at which the optical axis intersects the surfaces, denoted by $A_1$ and $A_2$ in *Figure 8.2* are termed the front vertex and back vertex respectively.

There is a theoretical point on the optical axis of any spherical lens having the property that if any ray passes through it, the direction of the ray on emerging from the lens is parallel to its direction before reaching the lens. This point is termed the optical centre. It is usually very close to one surface and in ophthalmic practice is taken as coincident with either vertex $A_1$ or $A_2$.

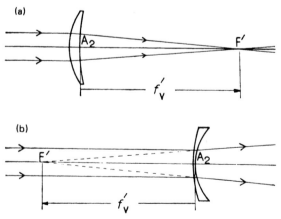

**Figure 8.3** Second principal focus (F') and back vertex focal length ($f'_v$) of a spherical lens: (a) plus; (b) minus.

# Plus and minus lenses

Spherical lenses may be divided into plus (or converging) and minus (or diverging). This classification is a fundamental one because it is based on the most important optical properties of lenses.

Objects are seen by virtue of the light which they emit (if they are self-luminous) or reflect into our eyes. Rays of light are imagined to spread out from every point of a visible object in straight lines. A narrow cone of rays is termed a pencil and its apex the focus. If the object is sufficiently distant, the rays of any given pencil proceeding from it may be regarded as parallel to one another. It is the effect of a lens on a parallel pencil of rays that not only determines whether it is plus or minus but also provides a means of specifying its power.

If a parallel pencil is directed along the optical axis of a plus lens (*Figure 8.3*), the latter causes it to converge to a point F' on the axis termed the *second principal focus*. On the other hand, when an axial parallel pencil passes through a minus lens it is made to spread out or diverge and then appears to be proceeding from a point F' on the axis in front of the lens. This point is also termed the second principal focus.

If an object is placed in front of a minus lens, the image is always erect (the right way up), diminished in size and nearer to the lens than is the object itself. To illustrate this general law, *Figure 8.4* shows a minus lens, an object PQ, its image P'Q', and the path of the rays from P and Q which enter the eye, appearing to come from the image points P' and Q'. Although the image is nearer than the object, it may nevertheless appear to be further away simply because it is smaller. This same effect is seen very strikingly when one looks through a telescope or field glass the wrong way round.

The image formed by a minus lens is termed virtual because the rays by which it is formed do not actually pass through it. This point is brought out in *Figure 8.4*.

Unlike the minus lens, a plus lens forms images of two entirely different types according to the distance of the object. If the latter is far enough away, a plus lens forms an inverted image which is termed real in order to distinguish it from a virtual image. The characteristic feature

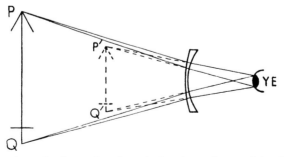

**Figure 8.4** Image formation by a minus lens. A virtual erect image of the object PQ is formed at P'Q'.

of a real image is that the rays of light by which it is formed actually pass through it, which means that the image can be received on a screen. This type of image formation has already been demonstrated in Chapter 1.

The other type of image formation by a plus lens is shown in *Figure 8.5*. When the object PQ is brought close enough to the lens, the divergence of the rays becomes too great for the lens to overcome. However, although the pencils cannot be made to converge to form a real image behind the lens, they are rendered less divergent than before. As a result, the image P'Q' is formed at a greater distance in front of the lens than the object itself. On the other hand, the image is larger than the object which hence appears to be magnified. This is, in fact, the principle of the simple magnifier.

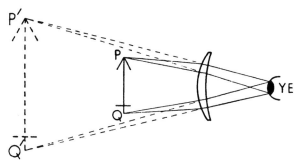

**Figure 8.5** Formation of a virtual image by a plus lens. An erect image of the object PQ is formed at P'Q'.

## Lens power

The distance from the back vertex of a lens to its second principal focus (*Figure 8.3*) is termed the back vertex focal length ($f'_v$). In the case of a minus lens, this distance is seen to include the centre thickness.

Lenses were at one time specified in terms of their focal lengths but this method had several disadvantages, the main one being that focal lengths are not additive. A much more convenient notation is now in general use throughout the world. According to this system the basis of numbering is the power of the lens: more strictly, its back vertex power ($F'_v$). This is found by dividing the back vertex focal length expressed in millimeters into one thousand. Expressed mathematically

$$F'_v = \frac{1000}{f'_v} \text{ (mm)}$$

The unit of focal power is the *dioptre*, denoted by the symbol D, a lens of power 1 D having a focal length of exactly 1 m. A plus or minus sign must always be prefixed to the power to show whether the lens is plus (converging) or minus (diverging). Focal lengths should also be prefixed with a plus or minus sign to indicate whether they refer to plus or minus powered lenses.

A few examples may be useful. If a plus lens has a back focal length of +125 mm, its back vertex power is 1000/125 or +8.00 DS. A minus lens with a focal length of −400 mm has a power of 1000/−400 or −2.50 DS.

If the focal length is given in centimetres rather than millimetres then one should divide into 100 instead of a 1000, to arrive at dioptric power. If the focal length is given in metres, then divide into 1 to arrive at dioptric power.

Although rare, if focal length is expressed in inches then divide into 39.37 to arrive at dioptric power. An example of when this could occur would be when a non-ophthalmic request is made. A company may have the need to replace a lens in a machine that has been broken. The machine is no longer made but the specifications state that a lens with a focal length of $x$ inches is used.

It is also worthwhile knowing that the calculation work in reverse. Earlier it was seen that a lens of +125 mm focal length was equivalent to +8.00 DS (1000/125). Alternatively, one can determine the focal length of a specific powered lens by dividing the power into 1000 to obtain the answer in millimetres, i.e. 1000/8 = +125 mm. If the answer is required in centimetres divide the dioptric power into 100. For an answer in metres divide the dioptric into 1, for an answer in inches divide the dioptric power into 39.37.

It is normal to express powers in steps of 1/4 dioptre. Powers must always be written in decimal notation. To prevent confusion it is important to form the habit of always writing two figures after the decimal point, even if they are both noughts and, if necessary, a nought in front of it. Otherwise it is very easy for mistakes to occur. For example, +1.0 might be mistaken for +10 if the decimal point were not clear, −.5 misread as −5, and so on. By writing +1.00, −0.50, etc., such errors would be prevented (see also Chapter 7). On rare occasions lenses are prescribed 1/8 dioptre intervals. In such cases the figure 5 in the third decimal place is dropped and the prescriber merely writes 0.12, 0.37, 0.62, and so on.

The power of a lens of given centre thickness and surface radii of curvature varies with an optical property of the material known as refractive index. This is determined by the velocity with which light passes through it and varies with the wavelength of the light. At the shorter (blue) end of the visible spectrum, the refractive index may be (for example) 1.529, decreasing to 1.520 at the longer (red) end of the spectrum. It is therefore necessary to specify the wavelength used to determine the mean refractive index to which the nominal power of a lens is related. Traditionally a wavelength in the middle (yellow) region of the spectrum has always been used for this purpose in the UK: 587.6 nm (Helium d-line). However, the Americans prefer 589.3 nm (Sodium D-line), whilst the rest of Europe prefers 546.1 nm (Mercury e-line). (The abbreviation 'nm' denotes the nanometre, one-millionth part of a millimetre.) The controversial subject of which wavelength should be used to harmonise the different systems has been and still is the source of much heated discussion.

## Surface power

Each of the surfaces of a lens has its own surface power which contributes to the power of the lens as a whole. The surface power ($F$) is determined by two factors: the radius of curvature ($r$) and the mean refractive index ($n$) of the lens material. In the workshop radii of curvature are generally measured in millimetres, in which case the expression for surface power becomes

$$F = \frac{1000(n-1)}{r}$$

As one would expect this expression shows that the shorter the radius or the steeper the curve, the greater the surface power. It can also be put in the form

$$r\ (mm) = \frac{1000(n-1)}{F}$$

giving the radius of curvature needed for the desired surface power. The mean refractive index (for wavelength 587.6 nm) of the hard crown glass used for spectacle lenses is 1.523, but 1.525 if the wavelength 546.1 nm is adopted. For most optical resins it is within the range 1.49–1.50, although polycarbonate has the higher value of about 1.586 and high index resins can have up to 1.7. No doubt with improved technology even higher indices will become available in resin.

One must not forget that glass is also available in 1.6, 1.7, 1.8 and even 1.9 indices.

The power of a convex surface in air is always positive, that of a concave surface always negative. When the two surface powers of a lens are added together algebraically, the result is usually a close approximation to the back vertex power of the lens as a whole. For example, a lens with surface powers of +6.00 D and −8.00 D has an approximate back vertex power of −2.00 DS. It is only the thickness of the lens that introduces a complicating factor and makes the simple addition of surface powers inexact.

## Standard lens forms

Since the two surface powers of a lens add up to approximately the power of the lens as a whole, it follows that a lens of given power can be made in an unlimited number of different surface power combinations or lens forms. In simple terms, it is just a matter of how the total effect desired is distributed between the two surfaces. For convenience in manufacture, however, spherical lenses are normally produced in a limited number of standard forms.

The standard forms of plus lenses are shown in profile in *Figure 8.6* and are as follows.

### Equi-convex (*Figure 8.6a*)

This is a symmetrical form, both surfaces having the same curvature and power. Although in common use for several centuries, today it is now virtually obsolete.

### Plano-convex (*Figure 8.6b*)

The back surface is plane, all the power being provided by the front surface. This form is not mass produced but it is often employed for specially worked lenses of high power.

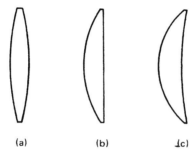

(a)              (b)              (c)

**Figure 8.6** Standard forms of plus spherical lenses: (a) equi-convex; (b) plano-convex; (c) plus meniscus.

### Plus meniscus (*Figure 8.6c*)

The essential feature of all meniscus lenses is that whereas the front surface is invariably convex, the back surface is invariably concave. This is the form in which mass-produced lenses are now made. To rationalise production, the entire range of powers is divided into several groups and all the lenses in each group have one surface power in common. For example, all the lenses in the range of powers from +2.00 DS to +3.00 DS may have a common front surface power of +6.00 D.

The standard forms used for minus lenses are shown in profile in *Figure 8.7* and are as follows:

### Equi-concave (*Figure 8.7a*)

This symmetrical form, like the equi-convex, is virtually obsolete.

### Plano-concave (*Figure 8.7b*)

The front surface is plane and the power of the lens is that of the back surface. This form is frequently used for specially worked lenses of high power.

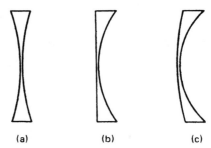

(a)                    (b)                    (c)

**Figure 8.7** Standard forms of minus spherical lenses: (a) equi-concave; (b) plano-concave; (c) minus meniscus.

### Minus meniscus (*Figure 8.7c*)

This is now the only mass-produced form. Lenses of meniscus form with the front surface appreciably convex and the back surface appreciably concave are popularly known as curved to distinguish them from the earlier standard forms which are termed flat.

### Periscopic

Mention should perhaps be made of another form that is still used occasionally though no longer mass-produced. This is a very shallow meniscus form termed periscopic. All the plus lenses have a back surface curve of −1.25 D and all minus lenses have a front surface curve of +1.25 D.

## Nominal/actual base curves

A little confusion in terminology begins to creep in here. The prescription house would normally refer to the front curve as the *base* that the lens is being supplied on. Other optical textbooks would suggest that the base is the surface that has the lowest numerical curve. For example, if the lens was made up on surface powers of

$$\frac{+6.00}{-4.00}$$

the minus 4.00 D curve would be referred to as the base. This subject will be developed further in Chapter 10.

In view of possible confusion perhaps it would be better, in our example, to refer to the lens as being made on a '+6.00 D sphere curve' or a '−4.00 D sphere curve'.

Despite the above it is generally accepted terminology in the prescription industry that the term base be used to describe the curve that the semi-finished manufacturer uses to describe his product and for the purpose of this book we shall also assume this.

As pointed out earlier, the back vertex power of a lens is affected by its centre thickness and is not the exact sum of the two surface powers. In order to compensate for the effect of thickness, it is usual to make some adjustment – termed a vertex power allowance – to the front surface power of a curved lens.

Plus base curves quoted by manufacturers are generally nominal base curves; that is to say, the surface powers that would be employed if no vertex power allowance were made. For example, a meniscus lens of power +4.00 DS on base +9.00 D would have surface powers of +9.00 D and −5.00 D if the effect of thickness could be ignored. In practice, such a lens would probably have a front surface power in the neighbourhood of +8.75 D. It could nevertheless be described as being a nominal +9.00 D base. The +8.75 D surface power would be referred to as the 'actual curve'.

A useful table of vertex power allowances, together with a simple method of calculation, can be found in Appendix 1.

## The spherometer formula

The technique of measuring the radius of curvature of a spherical surface is termed spherometry and a spherometer is an instrument designed for this purpose.

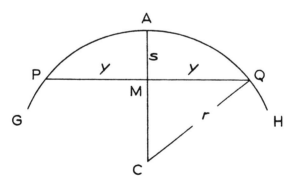

**Figure 8.8** Derivation of the spherometer formula.

Spherometers are based on the elementary geometry of the circle. In *Figure 8.8* GAH is the arc of a circle with its centre of curvature at C and PQ is a chord of length $2y$. The quantity $y$ is usually termed the *semi-aperture*. A line from C drawn perpendicular to the chord PQ intersects it at its midpoint M and meets the surface at A. The distance AM is the sagitta (for brevity, the sag) of the curve over the aperture $2y$. It is denoted by the symbol $s$.

It is evident that, given the value of $2y$, the sag varies only with the radius of curvature $r$. To find the exact relationship consider the right-angled triangle CMQ. Pythagoras' theorem gives

$$CQ^2 = CM^2 + MQ^2$$

or

$$r^2 = (r - s)^2 + y^2$$

so that

$$2rs = y^2 + s^2$$

giving

$$r = \frac{y^2 + s^2}{2s} = \frac{y^2}{2s} + \frac{s}{2}$$

If the radius of curvature is large in relation to the sag, a simple but possibly acceptable approximation can be obtained by neglecting the last terms $s/2$ in above equation which then becomes

$$r = y^2/2s \text{ (approx)}$$

To put this relationship in terms of surface power the following formula should be used

$$F = \frac{2000(n - 1)s}{y^2} \text{ (approx)}$$

It now becomes apparent that for given values of $y$ and $n$, the surface power is approximately proportional to the sag.

## The lens measure

The power of a lens surface may be found to a fair degree of accuracy with an instrument known as a lens measure. This is a simple form of three-legged spherometer, the legs being of circular cross-section with the ends tapering off to virtual points. Only the middle leg is movable, the outer pair marking off, in effect, a chord of predetermined length $2y$ (*Figure 8.9*). The middle leg is spring-loaded so that a three-point contact can be maintained on the steepest concave surface within the scope of the instrument. As shown in the diagram, what the instrument does is to measure the sag $s$ corresponding to a fixed semi-aperture $y$, the dial being calibrated so as to record the result directly in terms of surface power. This can refer only to one selected refractive index, normally 1.523.

A lens measure should be held perpendicularly to the lens surface in order to prevent avoidable errors. Care should also be taken not to damage the surface by abrupt or sliding contact with the points of the legs. A recommended technique is to hold the instrument between forefinger and thumb, extending the second finger until it makes contact with the lens surface to act as a steady. By this means, the points can be

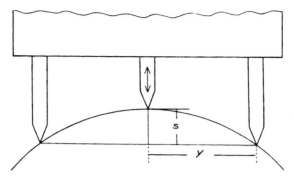

**Figure 8.9** Principle of the lens measure.

brought into gentle and controlled contact with the surface to be measured.

From time to time it is advisable to check the zero reading on a plane surface, such as a piece of plate glass. Most lens measures incorporate some means of adjustment to correct zero errors.

## High-precision spherometers (sag gauges)

The lens measure is a comparatively simple instrument and should not be expected to record surface powers to an accuracy better than about 0.06 D. Even this may be optimistic. More accurate measurements can be achieved by using a suitably mounted engineer's dial gauge (*Figure 8.10*). This normally records the sag of the surface at 0.01 mm intervals. Conversion to surface power for the appropriate refractive index can then be made from tables or by computer. Gauges giving a digital readout of

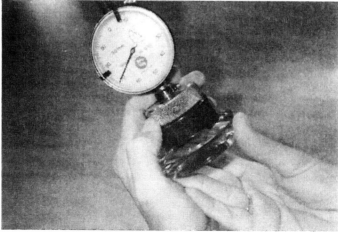

**Figure 8.10** A sag gauge fitted with a 'bell' housing.

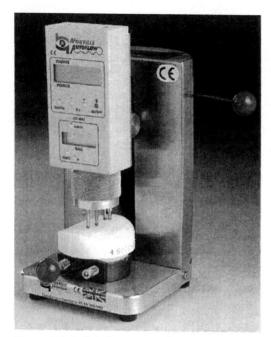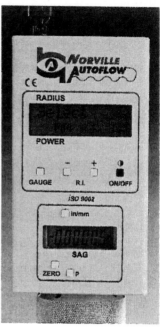

**Figure 8.11** A digital sag gauge showing sag, radius and power surface.

surface power are now also available (*Figure 8.11*). Even high-precision spherometers do not purport to be entirely free from errors, especially if used over a wide range of surface curves. A set of master curves of known power, enabling the instrument to be used as a comparator, is one method of maximising accuracy.

It should also be realised that gauges are available in different sizes, that is to say, the distance between the two fixed outer legs. The 'standard' sag gauge is normally referred to as a 40 mm gauge (40 mm between the two fixed legs). Gauges of 34 and 20 mm are also available for checking smaller areas, for example, the distance portion of a solid bifocal or perhaps a lenticular aperture.

Some gauges are designed for quick and easy checking of spherical surfaces and are often fitted with what many term a 'bell' housing rather than the more conventional 'legs'. However, one is limited to checking spherical surfaces only. There is often a cut-out incorporated enabling the gauge to clear any protruding segment which would invalidate the reading obtained should any part of the gauge come into contact with the segment area. Some gauges also come in different versions for checking plus or minus curves. A gauge designed for checking minus curves would normally have a longer centre leg to reach down into the concave surface, whereas a gauge designed for plus curves would have a shorter middle leg to allow it to rise up on the convex surface.

It should also be realised that the sag value for, say, a −6.00 D curve would be exactly the same as that for a +6.00 D curve as they have the same radius of curvature and are simply opposites.

## The sag formula and its uses

It may be of help at this stage to develop a little further the concept of the sag of a lens. In practice, sags are used for two apparently different purposes. Firstly, to check the accuracy of a curve and secondly to assist in the calculation of either centre or edge substance.

So, how can it be of assistance in checking the accuracy of a curve? As seen in *Figure 8.9* any curve will produce a certain movement of the middle leg in comparison to the two fixed outer ones. If the curvature is steeper it will produce more movement and if it is shallower it will produce less movement. If it is known how much movement there will be for a specific curve, then if that curve is wrong (too steep or too shallow) it will cause the leg to register a different value on the gauge.

In practice, as mentioned earlier, charts or computers are used to calculate the values and/or convert the value on the dial to dioptric surface power equivalents. Assume that charts and computers are not available! Suppose a check is required that a curve of $-5.75$ D on a crown glass lens is correct. Assume a 40 mm sag gauge is used. The sag value for a 5.75 D curve therefore needs to be calculated. Using the sag formula

$$s = r - \sqrt{r^2 - y^2}$$

where

$s$ = sag
$r$ = radius of curve to be checked
$y$ = radius of the checking instrument (in our example it is a 40 mm gauge and therefore $y = 20$ mm)

$r$ can be calculated from

$$r = \frac{1000(n - 1)}{F}$$

where

$n$ = refractive index
$F$ = surface power

The radius of a 5.75 D curve is therefore

$$r = \frac{1000(n - 1)}{F}$$

$$r = \frac{1000(1.523 - 1)}{5.75}$$

$$r = \frac{523}{5.75}$$

$$r = 90.96$$

Now, substitute this into the sag formula

$$s = r - \sqrt{r^2 - y^2}$$
$$s = 90.96 - \sqrt{90.96^2 - 20^2}$$
$$s = 90.96 - \sqrt{8273.72 - 400}$$
$$s = 90.96 - \sqrt{7873.72}$$
$$s = 90.96 - 88.73$$
$$s = 2.23$$

The sag gauge should read 2.23. To put it another way, the centre leg will move 2.23 mm when placed on a curve of 5.75 D.

Suppose the sag guage instead of reading 2.23, actually reads 2.28. Using the following formula one can convert this back to a radius value and then a dioptric value in order to determine the amount of error. In practice charts or computers would be used.

$$r = \frac{y^2 + s^2}{2s}$$

$$r = \frac{20^2 + 2.28^2}{2 \times 2.28}$$

$$r = \frac{400 + 5.20}{4.56}$$

$$r = \frac{405.2}{4.56}$$

$$r = 88.86 \, mm$$

If this figure is then substituted into the following formula, we arrive at the dioptric power of the surface

$$F = \frac{1000(n - 1)}{r}$$

$$F = \frac{1000(1.523 - 1)}{88.86}$$

$$F = \frac{523}{88.86}$$

$$F = 5.89 \, D$$

Therefore, compared with the curvature required (5.75 D) we have an error of 0.14 D (see also Appendix 2 for sag charts and accompanying

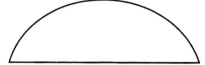

**Figure 8.12** Theoretical flat plus powered lens.

data). Checking the accuracy of curvatures is one use of the sag formula.

What about its use in calculating substance? Take any flat plus lens with minimum edge substance (often referred to as knife edge). It could look something similar to *Figure 8.12*.

If a sag gauge were large enough it could be positioned so that the two fixed outer legs just touched the edges of the lens (*Figure 8.13*). The plus curve would cause the middle leg to move. So, the thickness of the lens would be equal to the sag of the curve. Put into another way

  *t* (thickness) = *s* (sag)

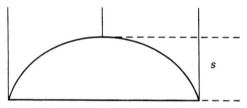

**Figure 8.13** Theoretical flat plus powered lens imagined to have a sag gauge applied to the convex surface.

The same principle would apply to a flat minus lens. As it was assumed the plus lens had no edge substance, assume the minus lens has no centre substance (*Figure 8.14*). If a sag gauge were large enough it could be positioned so that the two fixed outer legs just touched the edges of the lens (*Figure 8.15*). The minus curve would cause the middle leg to move. Therefore, the edge thickness of the lens would be equal to the sag of the curve. Put another way

  *e* (edge) = *s* (sag)

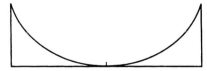

**Figure 8.14** Theoretical flat minus powered lens.

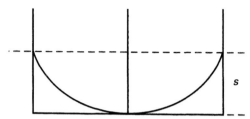

**Figure 8.15** Theoretical flat minus powered lens imagined to have a sag gauge applied to the concave surface.

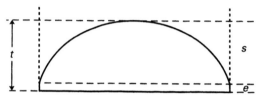

**Figure 8.16** Flat plus powered lens with allowance for edge substance and thereby demonstrating the centre thickness $t$ is equal to the sag of the curvature plus the edge thickness.

In practice of course, plus lenses have edge substance and minus lenses have a centre substance. If an allowance is made for this, the plus lens now looks like *Figure 8.16*.

So, the expression

$$t = s$$

changes to

$$t = s + e$$

or

$$e = t - s$$

Similarly the minus lens would now look like *Figure 8.17*. Subsequently, the expression

$$e = s$$

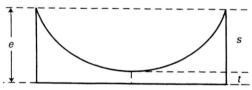

**Figure 8.17** Flat minus powered lens with allowance for centre substance thereby demonstrating that edge thickness $e$ is equivalent to the sag of the curvature plus the centre substance.

changes to

$$e = s + t$$

or

$$t = e - s$$

Here are two examples. For the purpose of this exercise the contribution that the substance factor makes to the power of the lens will be ignored.

*Example 1*: A +8.00 DS flat lens, 54 mm diameter, 1 mm edge and made in crown glass. What will the centre substance be?

$$t = s + e$$

is to be used but first $s$ has to be determined. Therefore

$$s = r - \sqrt{r^2 - y^2}$$

Before this can be used, the value of $r$ must be ascertained

$$r = \frac{1000(n - 1)}{F}$$

$$r = \frac{1000(1.523 - 1)}{8}$$

$$r = \frac{523}{8}$$

$$r = 65.38 \, \text{mm}$$

Therefore

$$s = 65.38 - \sqrt{65.38^2 - 27^2}$$
$$s = 65.38 - \sqrt{4274.5 - 729}$$
$$s = 65.38 - \sqrt{3545.5}$$
$$s = 65.38 - 59.54$$
$$s = 5.84$$

So

$$t = 5.84 + 1$$
$$t = 6.84 \, \text{mm}$$

*Example 2*: A –14.00 DS flat lens, 50 mm diameter, 2 mm centre substance and made in CR39. What will the edge substance be?

$$e = s + t$$

is to be used but first $s$ has to be determined. Therefore

$$s = r - \sqrt{r^2 - y^2}$$

Before this can be used, the value of $r$ must be ascertained.

$$r = \frac{1000(n - 1)}{F}$$

$$r = \frac{1000(1.498 - 1)}{14}$$

$$r = \frac{498}{14}$$

$$r = 35.57\,\text{mm}$$

Therefore:

$$s = 35.57 - \sqrt{35.57^2 - 25^2}$$
$$s = 35.57 - \sqrt{1265.22 - 625}$$
$$s = 35.57 - \sqrt{640.22}$$
$$s = 35.57 - 25.30$$
$$s = 10.27$$

So

$$e = 10.27 + 2$$
$$e = 12.27\,\text{mm}$$

Up to now it has been assumed lenses are flat form. What then happens in the case of meniscus (curved) lenses which of course is the form that the majority of lenses are made in?

A meniscus lens has two curved surfaces, unlike a flat that only has one. The front sag is referred to as $s1$ and the back as $s2$, so the expression for plus powers $t = s + e$ (flat form) now becomes $t = s1 - s2$ (curved form). This can be confirmed from *Figure 8.18* which represents a meniscus lens with no edge substance (knife edge).

Because, in practice, lenses have an edge substance, $e$ has to be included in the formula, so it now becomes $t = s1 - s2 + e$.

A similar principle has to be applied to minus powered meniscus. They also have two curved surfaces. As with plus powered meniscus, the front

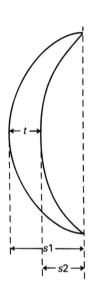

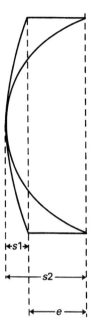

**Figure 8.18** Theoretical meniscus plus powered lens showing relationship between s1, s2 and t.

**Figure 8.19** Theoretical meniscus minus powered lens showing relationship between s1, s2 and e.

is termed $s1$ and the back $s2$, so the expression for minus powers $e = s + t$ (flat form) now becomes $e = s2 - s1$ (curved form). This can be confirmed from *Figure 8.19* which represents a meniscus lens with no centre substance. Because in practice lenses have a centre thickness, $t$ has to be included in the formula, so $e = s2 - s1 + t$.

Here are two examples. For the purpose of this exercise the contribution that the substance factor makes to the power of the lens will be ignored.

*Example 1*: +8.00 DS meniscus lens, 60 mm diameter, 1 mm edge, made in crown glass on a −3.00 D curve. What will the centre substance be?

First establish what nominal curve will be needed on the front surface, so if −3.00 D is on the back, +11.00 D is needed on the front to produce a total of +8.00 DS.

$t = s1 - s2 + e$ is to be used but firstly $s1$ and $s2$ must be determined.

Therefore

$$s1 = r - \sqrt{r^2 - y^2}$$

from

$$r = \frac{1000(n - 1)}{F}$$

the radius can be found

$$r = \frac{1000(1.523 - 1)}{11.00}$$

$$r = \frac{523}{11}$$

$$r = 47.55\,\text{mm}$$

Therefore

$$s1 = 47.55 - \sqrt{47.55^2 - 30^2}$$
$$s1 = 47.55 - \sqrt{2261 - 900}$$
$$s1 = 47.55 - \sqrt{1361}$$
$$s1 = 47.55 - 36.89$$
$$s1 = 10.66$$

$$s2 = r - \sqrt{r^2 - y^2}$$

From

$$r = \frac{1000(n - 1)}{F}$$

the radius can be found

$$r = \frac{1000(1.523 - 1)}{3}$$

$$r = \frac{523}{3}$$

$$r = 174.33\,\text{mm}$$

Therefore

$$s2 = 174.33 - \sqrt{174.33^2 - 30^2}$$
$$s2 = 174.33 - \sqrt{30390.95 - 900}$$
$$s2 = 174.33 - \sqrt{29490.95}$$
$$s2 = 174.33 - 171.73$$
$$s2 = 2.64$$

Therefore

$$t = s1 - s2 + e$$
$$t = 10.66 - 2.64 + 1$$
$$t = 9.02 \, mm$$

*Example 2*: A –10.00 DS meniscus lens, 66 mm diameter, 1 mm centre substance made in crown glass on a +2.00 D curve. What will the edge substance be?

First establish what nominal curve will be required on the back surface. If a +2.00 D is on the front, a –12.00 D is needed on the back to produce a total of –10.00 DS.

$$e = s2 - s1 + t$$

is used but firstly s1 and s2 must be determined. So

$$s1 = r - \sqrt{r^2 - y^2}$$

From

$$r = \frac{1000(n - 1)}{F}$$

the radius can be found

$$r = \frac{1000(1.523 - 1)}{2}$$
$$r = \frac{523}{2}$$
$$r = 261.5 \, mm$$

Therefore

$$s1 = 261.5 - \sqrt{261.5^2 - 33^2}$$
$$s1 = 261.5 - \sqrt{68382.25 - 1089}$$
$$s1 = 261.5 - \sqrt{67293.25}$$
$$s1 = 261.5 - 259.41$$
$$s1 = 2.09$$
$$s2 = r - \sqrt{r^2 - y^2}$$

From

$$r = \frac{1000(n - 1)}{F}$$

the radius can be found

$$r = \frac{1000(1.523 - 1)}{12.00}$$

$$r = \frac{523}{12}$$

$$r = 43.58\,\text{mm}$$

Therefore

$$s2 = 43.58 - \sqrt{43.58^2 - 33^2}$$
$$s2 = 43.58 - \sqrt{1899.2 - 1089}$$
$$s2 = 43.58 - \sqrt{810.2}$$
$$s2 = 43.58 - 28.46$$
$$s2 = 15.12$$

Therefore

$$e = s2 - s1 + t$$
$$e = 15.12 - 2.09 + 1$$
$$e = 14.03\,\text{mm}$$

## In conclusion

There are two further factors that need to be considered before this chapter on spherical lenses can be concluded.

The first factor is: how is it known what semi-finished base curve should be used for a particular power? There are general rules for this but certainly not hard and fast ones. The semi-finished manufacturer would normally provide charts or a computer program to help on base selection.

A typical chart is shown below.

| Nominal base | To work powers | | |
|---|---|---|---|
| +2.00 | −9.25 | to | −12.00 |
| +3.00 | −6.25 | to | −9.00 |
| +4.00 | −2.25 | to | −6.00 |
| +6.00 | −2.00 | to | +1.00 |
| +7.00 | +1.25 | to | +3.00 |
| +8.00 | +3.25 | to | +4.00 |
| +9.00 | +4.25 | to | +5.00 |
| +10.00 | +5.25 | to | +6.00 |

The second factor for consideration is the problem that, as stated earlier, the power of a lens is not simply the sum of its surface powers; the substance has an influence on the matter. Manufacturers of semi-finished lenses normally compensate by labelling the lens one curve (nominal) but put a different compensated (actual) curve on it.

There follows a brief explanation of how this complex problem can be tackled. Emphasis is placed upon plus powers as of course minus powers have very little centre substance to effect the power. There is always somewhat of a 'catch 22' situation concerning plus powered lenses. Calculations cannot be made for the surface curvatures without the centre substance but this cannot be calculated without knowing the surface curvatures!

The following is a good general guide that should assist the reader with the problems and go some way to resolving them. However, it should be stated that it is only an overview and cannot be considered as the definitive answer to all optical problems.

Firstly, what are the consequences of not compensating one of the lens surfaces to allow for the substance factor? If a lens of power +6.00 DS was required in crown glass, the nominal curves could be +10.00/−4.00. Assume the substance is calculated to be 6 mm (substance calculation will be developed later). A lens of this substance and curvature as stated would actually result in a power of +6.41 DS. This is +0.41 D stronger than required.

The formula used to derive this is

$$F'_v = \frac{1000}{\dfrac{1000}{F1} - \dfrac{t}{n}} + F2$$

where

$F'_v$ = back vertex power
$F1$ = nominal front surface
$F2$ = nominal back surface
$t$  = thickness in millimetres
$n$  = refractive index

If figures are substituted from the example, the results are

$$F'_v = \frac{1000}{\dfrac{1000}{10.00} - \dfrac{6}{1.523}} + (-4.00)$$

$$F'_v = \frac{1000}{100 - 3.94} + (-4.00)$$

$$F'_v = \frac{1000}{96.06} + (-4.00)$$

$$F_v' = 10.41 + (-4.00)$$

$$F_v' = 6.41 \text{ DS}$$

In terms of front surface compensation it becomes evident that it must be somewhat less than +10.00 D to give correct power. Alternatively, if a +6.00 DS is to be obtained with a front surface of +10.00 D, the back surface must be somewhat more than −4.00 D.

For the front surface compensation (termed vertex power allowance) the following formula should be used

$$F1 = \frac{1000FN}{1000 + \dfrac{t}{n}FN}$$

where

    $F1$  = compensated front curve
    $FN$ = nominal front curve
    $t$    = thickness in millimetres
    $n$   = refractive index

Substituting figures from the above example gives

$$F1 = \frac{1000 \times 10}{1000 + \dfrac{6}{1.523} \times 10}$$

$$F1 = \frac{1000}{1039.4}$$

$$F1 = 9.62$$

This is the compensated front curve which should be used. Put another way, a vertex power allowance (VPA) of 0.38 D has been made (10.00–9.62).

With reference to lenses finished on the front, where the prescription house will be processing the back, a different formula has to be used.

$$\text{VPA} = \frac{t\,F1^2}{1000n - t\,F1}$$

where

    $t$   = thickness in millimetres
    $F1$ = actual front curve
    $n$   = refractive index

*Example*: It is required to produce a +1.25 lens in crown glass using +7.00 D nominal, +6.87 D actual base with a centre thickness of 3 mm.

$$\text{VPA} = \frac{3 \times 6.87^2}{1000 \times 1.523 - 3 \times 6.87}$$

$$\text{VPA} = \frac{141.6}{1502.4}$$

$$\text{VPA} = 0.09$$

This is the allowance that must be added to the nominal inside curve.

If the front actual curve is +6.87 D then the back nominal curve to achieve +1.25 DS must be −5.62 D, to which a VPA of 0.09 must be added. Therefore −5.71 D is arrived at which in practice would be rounded to −5.75 D. This is the curve that would have to be worked on the lens to arrive at the correct power of +1.25 D.

Hopefully, the link between the manufacturer's nominal and actual bases can now be seen. It was a nominal base of +7.00 D. If one continues to work in nominal curves, what curve would have to be worked on the inside to give a power of +1.25 DS?

Answer: −5.75 D. This is the same answer which was arrived at using the formula. In this instance it is clear that the manufacturer's allowance was sufficient. This will not always be the case. By designating the lens a +7.00 D base (but knowing that it is really +6.87 D) simple subtracting can be performed to arrive at the inside curve. Before the days of the computer this was the accepted method of calculating the inside curve, based on a simple calculation from the nominal front curve. The industry has now advanced beyond this, with computers making far more accurate calculations. 'Why not continue to calculate from the manufacturer's nominal curve?', one may ask. The compensation made by the manufacturers cannot possibly be accurate for every combination of power and thickness. For example, a +6.00 D base semi-finished lens could be used to produce any power from −0.50 DS through to possibly even +3.50 DS. There is a significant difference in centre substance between these two powers. How can the compensation made by the manufacturer be accurate for all powers? Hence the need for calculation to obtain the correct power first time, every time.

One can calculate for what exact substance the manufacturer has made a compensation. Additionally one can also calculate what range of substances would be permissible up to a pre-determined power tolerance.

For example, imagine a semi-finished resin lens ($n = 1.498$) in a packet marked +10.00 base (nominal) which has an actual curve of +9.62 (i.e. 0.38 difference between nominal and actual curves).

To find what exact substance this compensation has been calculated for, we use the following formula.

$$t = \left( \frac{1000}{F1 \text{ Act}} - \frac{1000}{F1 \text{ Nom}} \right) \times n$$

where

F1 Act    = actual front curve
F1 Nom = nominal front curve
$n$          = refractive index.

Substituting values into the formula gives

$$t = \left(\frac{1000}{9.62} - \frac{1000}{10}\right) \times 1.498$$

$$t = (103.95 - 100) \times 1.498$$

$$t = 3.95 \times 1.498 = 5.92\,\text{mm}$$

Therefore, providing the final lens substance is required to be 5.92 mm, the 0.38 compensation made by the semi-finished manufacturer is exactly correct.

In practice it is highly unlikely that every powered lens produced on this base will be required to be 5.92 mm thick! So, by using the same formula we can calculate how much the substance can vary within preset limits.

Suppose we are prepared to have a power error of ±0.12 D on any lens made on this base (this is quite reasonable as powers made on this base would fall into power category '+6.00 to +9.00' and according to BS EN ISO 8980 Part 1 (1997) a tolerance of ±0.12 D is permissible).

Using the same formula as above but adding and subtracting the 0.12 D tolerance it is possible to find the range of substances that would give a maximum error ±0.12 D.

$$t = \left(\frac{1000}{9.62} - \frac{1000}{10.12^*}\right) \times 1.498 \quad (\text{*nominal base plus } 0.12)$$

$$t = (103.95 - 98.81) \times 1.498$$

$$t = 5.14 \times 1.498 = 7.7\,\text{mm}$$

So the thickest the lens can be without affecting the power by more than 0.12 D is 7.7 mm.

$$t = \left(\frac{1000}{9.62} - \frac{1000}{9.88^{**}}\right) \times 1.498 \quad (\text{**nominal base minus } 0.12)$$

$$t = (103.95 - 101.21) \times 1.498$$

$$t = 2.74 \times 1.498 = 4.1\,\text{mm}$$

So the thinnest the lens can be without affecting the power by more than 0.12 D is 4.1 mm.

This means that one can use the nominal front curve to arrive at the inside curves by simple subtraction with a maximum error of ±0.12 D providing the substance of finished lens is between 4.1 and 7.7 mm.

Another area of difficulty is that the different semi-finished manu-facturers cannot agree on what compensation should be made on each different base. Subsequently, for example, a prescription house may have a selection of +6.00 D nominal base semi-finished lenses in stock. They may not necessarily be bought from the same supplier. Perhaps three different suppliers are used. In this instance all the blanks will be labelled as '+6.00 base' (nominal) but because different manufacturers make different VPAs, the situation could arise whereby some lenses have actual curves of +5.93 D, +5.87 D and +5.81 D. All this would have to be taken into account when calculating inside curves. (See also Appendix 1 for VPA chart and accompanying data.)

It needs to be re-emphasised that the correct centre thickness of a plus lens cannot be calculated easily without knowing the exact curves, but that the correct curves cannot be calculated without knowing the substance. A good 'rule of thumb' method is to find the sag of the power that is required and to this add a 1 mm allowance for glazing. This will give a reasonable estimation of centre thickness.

For example, if a +8.00 DS crown glass lens in a 60 mm blank is required, the sag of 8.00 over 60 mm can be calculated from

$$s = r - \sqrt{r^2 - y^2}$$

The radius must first be determined from

$$r = \frac{1000(n - 1)}{F}$$

$$r = \frac{1000(1.523 - 1)}{8}$$

$$r = \frac{523}{8}$$

$$r = 65.38 \text{ mm}$$

Therefore

$$s = 65.38 - \sqrt{65.38^2 - 30^2}$$
$$s = 65.38 - \sqrt{4274.5 - 900}$$
$$s = 65.38 - \sqrt{3374.5}$$
$$s = 65.38 - 58.09$$
$$s = 7.29$$

*Add* 1 mm = 8.29 mm

One could now proceed to calculate curvatures based on this centre substance.

# Chapter 9

# Astigmatic lenses

Straightforward cases of hypermetropia (long-sighted) and myopia (short-sighted) can be corrected by spherical lenses as described in Chapter 8. Most spectacle wearers, however, also suffer from what is termed astigmatism. They require a correcting lens whose powers vary in different meridians. The lens effectively gives a minimum power in one direction, gradually changing to a maximum power in the other, at right angles to the first. These meridians of minimum and maximum power are referred to as the principal meridians of the lens. In simplistic terms, a lens that includes a cylindrical element in the prescription requirements is astigmatic.

A spherical surface is equally curved in all principal meridians and so a spherical lens, being made up of spherical surfaces, is symmetrical about its optical axis. For example, a camera lens could be rotated in its housing without apparent effect. It is because of this axial symmetry that a spherical lens is capable of bringing a pencil of rays to a focal point. On the other hand, an astigmatic lens does not possess this degree of symmetry. In the first place, pencils refracted by such lenses assume a more complicated form. Secondly, astigmatic lenses are optically affected by rotation and hence have to be correctly set with respect to the eye. This is the principal reason why a notation for specifying different meridians is required.

The simplest form of astigmatic lens has one spherical and one cylindrical surface. Although this form is now largely obsolete, a great part of accepted lens terminology is based on it. It is therefore logical to begin with a brief study of the cylindrical surface, illustrated in *Figure 9.1*.

## The cylindrical surface

Only a relatively small portion of the surface would be used, such as that enclosed by the dotted outline. The imaginary line YY, about which the cylinder would rotate without wobbling, is its axis of revolution. Any line AA on the surface that is parallel to YY is an axis meridian. The direction PP at right angles to AA is a power meridian. If a lens measure were applied to a cylindrical surface and rotated about its middle leg so as to examine the curvature in different meridians, the reading on the dial would be found to

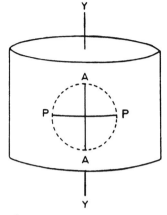

**Figure 9.1** The cylindrical surface.

vary continuously from zero in the axis meridian to a maximum in the power meridian. A section through the cylinder in this latter meridian would, of course, be circular. It is the radius of this circle which, together with the refractive index of the material, determines the power of the surface in accordance with the formula already given for a spherical surface. Hence, the highest reading given by an accurate lens measure on a cylindrical surface can be taken as the power of that surface.

Cylindrical power is expressed in dioptres in exactly the same way as spherical power. As with spherical surfaces, a plus sign denotes a convex surface and a minus sign a concave surface. The symbol DC (dioptres of cylindrical power) is used to prevent confusion with spherical power (DS).

## The sphero-cylindrical lens

A lens with one spherical and one cylindrical surface used to be termed a flat sphero-cylinder, or *spherocyl* for brevity. It had two principal meridians which intersected at the optical centre of the lens. The first was the axis meridian – one of the lines along which the cylindrical surface has zero curvature. The second principal meridian was at right angles to the first.

Spherocyls were used to correct eyes which, apart from any defect of long or short-sightedness were also astigmatic. To neutralise the eye's astigmatism, the lens had to be correctly set: any rotation from the correct setting impaired its efficiency. The method used to specify the setting was to state the desired position of the axis meridian in standard notation. A prescription for a spherocyl lens hence had three components: the spherical power, the cylindrical power and the axis direction. For example:

+3.25 DS +1.75 DC × 30

## Principal powers

All astigmatic lenses including sphero-cylinders have two principal powers, each associated with a different principal meridian. Along the axis meridian, a cylindrical surface is flat; consequently, the power of the lens in this meridian is that of the spherical surface alone. In the other principal meridian, the cylinder does contribute to the total power of the lens. If the spherical power can be denoted by S and the cylindrical power by C, the principal powers of any sphero-cylinder may thus be tabulated as follows:

| Meridian | Power |
| --- | --- |
| Axis meridian | S |
| Meridian at right angles to axis | (S + C) |

In adding S and C together, regard must be paid to their signs: that is to say they must be added algebraically. For example, consider the prescription +1.50 DS +1.00 DC × 90. An optical cross representation would be as depicted in *Figure 9.2*. The principal powers are +1.50 D and +2.50 D. Along its axis a cylinder has no power, so any power must be due to the sphere only. In the example the axis is at 90 and therefore at 90, only the sphere (+1.50 D) is effective.

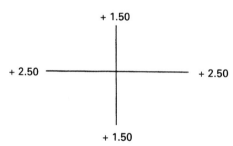

**Figure 9.2** An optical cross representation of a +1.50 DS +1.00 DC × 90 powered lens.

At right angles to the axis the spherical element still has influence but now the cylinder also contributes. So at 180 there is a total of both the sphere (+1.50 D) and the cylinder (+1.00 D), making a total of +2.50 D.

The authors have always found the rule *the cylinder has no power along its axis* a concept that tends to confuse some students of optics. It would be better to turn the expression around to a simple statement: the last number (axis) informs where the first number (sphere) is effective. Therefore, of course, at right angles to the axis the power is equivalent to the sphere and the cylinder combined, remembering to obey the signs of each element.

It was seen in connection with spherical lenses that their power is related to the back vertex focal length. Exactly the same is applicable for sphero-cylinders, except that they have two principal powers and have two separate foci. An attempt to depict the type of image formation characteristic of the astigmatic lens is made in *Figure 9.3*. This shows in relief a parallel pencil of axial rays before and after refraction by the lens +4.00 DS −1.50 DC set with its axis vertical. The dotted line XX represents the optical axis, $A_2$ the back vertex of the lens, AA the extremities of the incident pencil in the axis meridian and PP its extremities in the other principal meridian.

In the axis meridian the principal power is that of the sphere alone, namely, +4.00 D, corresponding to a focal length of 1000/4 or 250 mm. The rays in this meridian are therefore converged to a focal point $F'_A$ on the optical axis at a distance 250 mm from $A_2$. If the rays were traced in other sections of the lens parallel to AA, it would be found that they were brought to a focus at the same distance from the lens as $F'_A$ but on either side of it, thus building up the focal line JJ at right angles to AA.

In the other principal meridian PP, the power of the lens is that of the sphere and cylinder combined, that is to say, +2.50 D. This corresponds to a focal length of 1000/2.5 or 400 mm; the rays in meridian PP are brought to a focus $F'_P$ on the optical axis, 400 mm from $A_2$. With this focus is associated a second focal line KK, at right angles to the first.

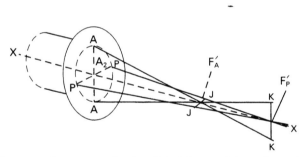

**Figure 9.3** Diagrammatic representation in relief of the pencil formed on refraction by an astigmatic lens.

Although *Figure 9.3* does not convey a complete picture of the rather complicated geometry of an astigmatic pencil, it does bring out the fact that the pencil nowhere gives rise to a single focal point. On the contrary, it forms two mutually perpendicular line foci. The term *astigmatic*, meaning *without a point*, is hence well chosen. If the lens were rotated about its optical axis, the two focal lines would clearly rotate with it.

It therefore becomes very evident that the positioning of an astigmatic lens before the eye is critical, and as the cylindrical power increases so does the requirement to set the lens 'on axis' become more important.

Present standards allow a cylinder of power up to 0.50 DC to have a tolerance of + or − 7 degrees, but a cylinder, say 2.00 DC, has only

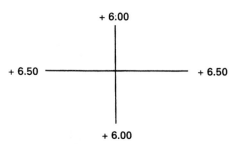

**Figure 9.4** An optical cross representation of a +6.00 DS +0.50 DC × 90 powered lens, showing only 0.50 dioptres between the principal meridians.

a tolerance of 2 degrees. Why should there be such difference between the tolerances? It can again be explained by the use of an optical cross. If the prescription +6.00 DS +0.50 DC × 90 is used, the optical cross representation would be like that in *Figure 9.4*.

Whilst obviously it would be desirable for the lens to be set 100% correctly before the eye, realistically this is not always achievable, which is why standards are available to give guidance. The difference between the two meridians is only 0.50 D and therefore if the lens was set up to 7 degrees off axis it would cause very little power error as there is only 0.50 D between the two meridians. If, on the other hand, the lens – 7.00 DS + 2.00 DC × 180 (*Figure 9.5*) was set 7 degrees off axis, serious problems would occur. By way of illustration, a 7 degree error on the lens depicted in *Figure 9.4* would cause a power error of only 0.04 of a dioptre. On the lens depicted in *Figure 9.5*, an error of 0.16 dioptres would be introduced.

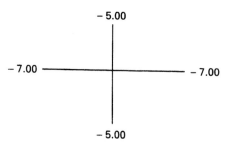

**Figure 9.5** An optical cross representation of a –7.00 DS +2.00 DC × 180 powered lens, showing a 2.00 dioptre difference between the principal meridians.

If the principal meridians of the lens are not aligned correctly with the main meridians of the eye, the patient will not be receiving the correct power. The lens in *Figure 9.5* has 2.00 D difference between the meridians. Any axis error will therefore have a more detrimental effect than on the previous example, hence present standards only allow a 2 degree error.

# Transposition

It can now be shown that an astigmatic lens of specified principal powers can always be made up in two different spherocyl forms. Suppose that the principal powers required are as follows:

in the 30 degree meridian +2.00 D
in the 120 degree meridian +5.00 D.

First, a spherical surface of power +2.00 D could be used, combining it with a +3.00 D cylindrical surface with its axis at 30 degrees so as to build up the power of +5.00 D in the 120 degree meridian, as required.

Alternatively, a +5.00 D spherical surface could be used combined with a −3.00 D cylinder with its axis at 120 degrees, so as to reduce the power to +2.00 D in the 30 degree meridian as required.

Expressed in the conventional manner, the first lens would be

+2.00 DS +3.00 DC × 30

whereas the second would be

+5.00 DS −3.00 DC × 120

These two prescriptions, which are optically equivalent, are termed *alternative transpositions*. The word transposition is also applied to the process of converting a prescription from one possible formulation to another. Thus, when a prescription written out in the plus cylinder form is changed to the equivalent minus cylinder form, or vice versa, it is said to be transposed.

The choice of transposition in which a prescription is written is immaterial. What the prescription really does is to specify the two principal powers required. However, it must be said that as the majority of lenses today are made in minus cylinder form it would seem logical to express the prescription in minus cylinder form as well.

# Rules of transposition

It is sometimes necessary to change a written prescription from one transposition to another. The reasons why will be explained later.

Transposition can be rapidly carried out by means of the following rules.

1 Add the sphere and cylinder together taking into account their signs.
2 Change the sign of the cylinder.
3 Alter the axis by 90 degrees – that is to say, if the original axis is 90 degrees or less, add 90 degrees to it. If the original axis is over 90 degrees, subtract 90 degrees from it.

The following examples may be of use

+3.50 DS +0.75 DC × 30

*Rule 1*   Add the sphere and cylinder together taking into account their signs (+3.50) + (+0.75) = +4.25 ⌐
*Rule 2*   Change the sign of the cylinder. At the moment it is a + therefore it becomes a − ⌐
*Rule 3*   Alter the axis by 90 degrees. Therefore 30 + 90 = 120 ⌐

The lens is now transposed from   +3.50 DS +0.75 DC × 30
to +4.25 DS −0.75 DC × 120

*Another example*:

−5.50 DS +1.25 DC × 110

*Rule 1*   Add the sphere and cylinder together taking into account their signs (−5.50) + (+1.25) = −4.25 ⌐
*Rule 2*   Change the sign of the cylinder. At the moment it is a + therefore it becomes a − ⌐
*Rule 3*   Alter the axis by 90 degrees. Because it is over 90, 90 is subtracted. 110 − 90 = 20 ⌐

The lens is now transposed from   −5.50 DS +1.25 DC × 110
to −4.25 DS −1.25 DC × 20

It could be useful to prove that one transposition is equal to another, for after all most of the numbers seem to change so how can they be the same? By the use of optical crosses (*Figures 9.6–9.9*) and a rule mentioned earlier: 'the last number informs where the first number is effective', it becomes very easy to demonstrate.

Using the prescription +6.00 DS +4.00 DC × 90 as an example, utilisation can be made of the rules of transposition to arrive at its alternative form of +10.00 DS −4.00 DC × 180.

Now to prove that they are indeed equal. Commencing with +6.00 DS +4.00 DC × 90 and applying the rule 'the last number informs where the first number is effective', the first part of an optical cross can be constructed (*Figure 9.6*). If at 90 the power is +6.00 D then at right angles to this (180) the power must be the sphere and the cylinder combined, +10.00 D (*Figure 9.7*).

Now take +10.00 DS −4.00 DC × 180. Applying the rule 'the last number informs where the first number is effective', the first part of an optical cross can be constructed (*Figure 9.8*). If at 180 the power is +10.00 then at right angles to this (90) the power must be the sphere and the cylinder combined, i.e. +6.00 (*Figure 9.9*).

As can be seen both optical crosses are identical, therefore +6.00 DS +4.00 DC × 90 must equal +10.00 DS –4.00 DC × 180 (*Figure 9.7* equals *Figure 9.9*).

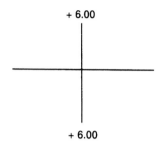

**Figure 9.6** Optical cross with one power meridian shown.

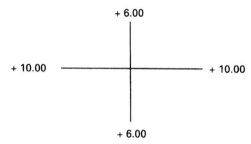

**Figure 9.7** Optical cross with both power meridians shown.

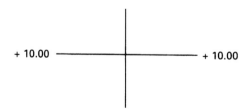

**Figure 9.8** Optical cross with one power meridian shown.

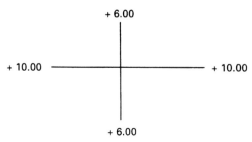

**Figure 9.9** Optical cross with both power meridians shown.

By way of summary the four reasons for the transposition process are outlined. The first is that traditionally stock single vision lenses have been boxed/stored with the prescription written in plus cylinder form. Therefore, if it is required to find the location of a stock lens, and the prescription is written in minus cylinder transposition, it is necessary to transpose to plus cylinder form in order to locate the correct lens box/packet. A visit to most prescription houses will prove this point. Stock lens manufacturers have started to print both forms of transposition on their lens packets but for stock/location purposes the plus cylinder transposition is still mostly used.

The second reason is that for determining the correct price of a particular lens. The prescription house will either price a prescription in its + or − cyl form, or indeed some will price in either, depending upon whether the prescription is plus or minus. Although in practice it is normal for a computer to ensure correct pricing, the ability to transpose is still required. For example, a prescription house may receive a telephone enquiry regarding how much a particular lens will cost. If not given in the correct transposition, it will be necessary to transpose to give the caller the information they require.

The third reason for transposition is to convert the lens into the same form as it is going to be worked. For example, if a prescription in plus cylinder form is received and it is going to be manufactured in minus cylinder form (as will be the case in most instances) it must be transposed in order that the curve calculations can be made.

The fourth and final reason for transposition is to allow the 'range' of a lens to be determined. Manufacturers express the available power ranges of their lenses in different ways. The ability to be able to transpose allows determination of range regardless of the format used.

Earlier in this chapter reference was made to the fact that it really does not matter in which transposition the prescription house receives an order because in the production they will apply the rules of transposition to suit their requirements.

# Chapter 10

# Toric lenses

## The toroidal surface

Just as flat spherical lenses have been superseded by those of curved meniscus form, so have flat plano and sphero-cylinders, by curved forms known as toric. This term derives from the Latin word torus (a protuberance) used in architecture to denote a rounded portion at the base of a column.

Like meniscus lenses, torics have one convex and one concave surface but only one of these is spherical. The other, which incorporates the required astigmatic effect, is of a type known as toroidal.

A toroidal surface is generated by rotating the arc of a circle VAV about an axis of revolution RR which lies in the same plane as the arc but does not pass through its centre of curvature G (*Figures 10.1* and *10.2*).

If the axis of revolution RR lies on the side of G remote from the vertex A of the generating arc, the toroidal surface so produced is of tyre formation (*Figure 10.1*). On the other hand, if RR lies between A and G, the resulting surface is of a barrel formation (*Figure 10.2*).

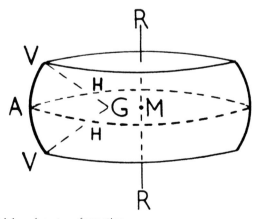

**Figure 10.1** Toroidal surface: tyre formation.

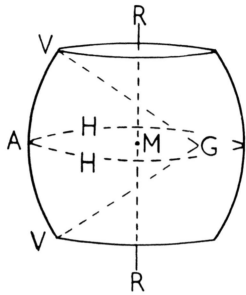

**Figure 10.2** Toroidal surface: barrel formation.

## Toric lenses

A toric lens has one convex and one concave surface, either of which is toroidal. As with meniscus lenses there is no standardisation of base curves.

It is necessary to develop an understanding of the term toric. In principle, whatever is added to one surface has to be added to the other. Take the prescription +3.00 DS –1.00 DC × 90. If made in flat form then it could have the following surface powers (assuming at this stage we are working on nominal not actual curves):

$$\frac{+3.00}{\text{Plano} \times 180\ –1.00 \times 90}$$

If we add 4.00 dioptres to each surface, that is to say +4.00 to the front and –4.00 to the back, we obtain:

$$\frac{+7.00}{–4.00 \times 180\ –5.00 \times 90}$$

The lens still has the same power but in toric rather than flat form. In established optical terms the base curve is the lowest numerical curve on the toroidal surface (–4.00 D). However, in prescription house practice the base curve would be the +7.00 D surface when working minus cylinder form.

British Standards 3521 Part 1 (1991) tries to clarify the situation. The base curve on a spherical lens is defined as the power of *either* surface selected to determine the form of the lens, or in the case of a range of lenses of different powers, a surface power common to all the lenses in the range. BS 3521 makes the distinction between *base curve* and *nominal base curve*, the latter being the base curve stated by the manufacturer for identification purposes. In reference to toric lenses, it is classed as the lowest numerical curve on the toroidal surface.

Those working in lens surfacing departments will certainly refer to the –4.00 D curve in our example as the base curve with the –5.00 D being termed the cross curve. The difference between the base and the cross curve is equal to the cylinder power. In the example the difference between –4.00 D and –5.00 D is –1.00 D, hence a 1.00 D cylindrical power is obtained. This assumes that the calculations and the smoothing/ polishing tools have been made for the same index as the lens material itself. That is to say, a prescription house may have a range of tools calibrated for 1.498 material. In many instances they would be able to also use these tools for surfacing, for example, 1.60 material, but because of this change of refractive index a re-calculation of curvatures is required. As a result of this, the difference between the base curve and the cross curve will no longer equal the cyl power even though the end result as read by a focimeter will be correct.

For example, assume calculations have been performed and we are required to produce inside curves of –6.00 –7.00 on 1.60 index material, but using tools calibrated for 1.498. The tool used would be –5.00 –5.75 (the exact curves required are –4.98 –5.81 but the nearest tool would be selected). Because of the use of higher index material it is possible to reduce the inside curves, yet still obtain the required powers. Also note the difference between the base curve and the cross curve is only 0.75, but because material is of higher index, this 0.75 difference will produce a 1.00 cyl.

To determine the curvature change when using material of one index and tools calibrated for another is relatively simple.

If lens curve calculations are performed in the same index as the material, as in our example, the inside curves required are –6.00 –7.00.

Using

$$r = \frac{1000\,(n-1)}{F}$$

determine the radius of both the –6.00 and –7.00 curvatures

$$r = \frac{1000\,(n-1)}{F} = \frac{1000\,(1.60-1)}{6.00}$$

$$= \frac{600}{6.0} = \underline{100\,\text{mm}}$$

$$r = \frac{1000\,(n-1)}{F} = \frac{1000\,(1.60-1)}{7.00}$$

$$= \frac{600}{7.0} = \underline{85.71\,\text{mm}}$$

If the two radii (100 and 85.71 mm) are now substituted into the following formula for 1.498 tooling, it is easy to arrive at the tool required.

$$F = \frac{1000\,(n-1)}{r}$$

$$F = \frac{1000\,(n-1)}{r} = \frac{1000\,(1.498-1)}{100}$$

$$= \frac{498}{100} = 4.98 \text{ (rounded to } \underline{5.00})$$

$$F = \frac{1000\,(n-1)}{r} = \frac{1000\,(1.498-1)}{85.71}$$

$$F = \frac{498}{85.71} = \underline{5.81} \text{ (rounded to } \underline{5.75})$$

Returning to our example at the start of this section on toric lenses (+3.00 DS –1.00 DC × 90) and assuming tooling is calibrated for the index of the lens, although now rare, the cylindrical surface can also be incorporated on the front.

This would be the case, for example, with solid bifocals. A lens of nominal curves

$$\frac{+\,8.00 \times 90 + 9.00 \times 180}{-\,6.00}$$

will still give a power of +3.00 DS –1.00 DC × 90 (transposed +2.00 DS +1.00 DC × 180).

Now this will be developed a little further to try to appreciate why the curves stated in either minus cylinder toric form or plus cylinder toric form produce the correct power.

Commencement was made with a lens of power +3.00 DS –1.00 DC × 90. The principal powers of this lens are depicted in *Figure 10.3* (see Chapter 9 for confirmation).

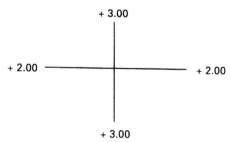

**Figure 10.3** Optical cross.

Firstly look at the minus cylinder toric form:

$$\frac{+7.00}{-4.00 \times 180 \ -5.00 \times 90}$$

The front surface is common to both principal powers but the back surface changes from a minimum curvature in one direction to a maximum at right angles to this.

Considering the +7.00 D front curve in relation to the –4.00 D curve, this equals the principal power of +3.00 D ((+7.00 D) + (–4.00 D) = +3.00 D). Considering the +7.00 D front curve in relation to the –5.00 D curve, this equals the principal power of +2.00 D ((+7.00 D) + (–5.00 D) = +2.00 D). It can immediately be seen how the two different back curves, combined with the common front curve equals the principal powers. Working through the same procedure for the plus cylinder toric, the answers will be the same.

If a lens measure is applied to a toroidal surface and rotated, the reading on the dial will gradually change from a minimum in the base curve meridian to a maximum in the cross curve meridian at right angles to the former. In this respect the toroidal surface possesses a fundamental similarity to the cylindrical surface. In fact, the latter could be imagined as a toroidal surface with a base curve of zero.

## Use of semi-finished blanks

To cope with prescriptions outside the range of mass-produced lenses, semi-finished blanks in both glass and resin materials are extensively used. Having one surface already optically worked, leaves only the other side to be finished by the prescription house. Semi-finished single vision lenses many years ago used to be made in what was termed 'rough torics', that is to say the front surface incorporated a base and cross curve, the prescription house only having to surface a spherical surface on the inside to finish the lens.

These lenses presented a problem because they necessarily incorporated an arbitrary vertex power allowance. In deciding on this allowance, the manufacturer could only base them on an assumed average centre thickness of the finished lenses most likely to be made from each different blank. For example, a plus base toric blank having a nominal base curve of +9.00 D and a cross curve of +10.50 D may have actual curves of +8.77 D and +10.19 D, based on an assumed finished centre thickness of 4.5 mm. If, in a particular case, the finished lens thickness varies appreciably from this accepted value, the power of the lens may be incorrect beyond permitted tolerances. This type of semi-finished has now been replaced by lenses that are spherical on the front surface, the cylinders being worked on the inside by the prescription house surfacing base and cross curves accordingly.

Multifocals and progressives are also produced in a similar way, that is to say, supplied with the front surface finished. The exception to this would be glass solid bifocals that are traditionally supplied with a finished minus spherical curve on the inside with any cylinder having to be incorporated on the front. Even so, the manufacturers of these lenses have recognised that this lens form is going against the trend for back surface torics and have started to make them available with spherical front surfaces.

## Why curved lenses

Remarks in this section apply to spherical as well as to astigmatic lenses, but it is convenient to deal with the subject here.

An ideal lens would reunite all the rays emanating from each point on the object and bring them to a focus at the corresponding point on the image. The image would also be an exact-to-scale reproduction of the object.

In actual fact, a simple lens does not behave in this way but is subject to various aberrations which impair the quality of the image. Although a detailed study of lens aberrations demands advanced mathematics, their effects may be summarised quite simply: they are loss of definition (blurring), distortion (e.g. straight lines appearing curved) and chromatism (colour fringes). Each of these defects may be observed on viewing some fine print through a strong magnifying lens. Towards the edges of the field of view there will generally be a marked deterioration in the quality of the image.

Spectacle lenses are subject to similar aberrations which the wearer may notice, especially when looking through them obliquely. The amount of each aberration depends not only on the power of the lens, but also on the form in which it is made. It is because of their superior performance (i.e. their greater freedom from aberrations) that curved lenses have largely superseded the old flat forms.

A great deal of study and calculation has been devoted to the problem of determining the theoretically most suited base curve for every lens power. Unfortunately, in the field of optical design, it is seldom possible to achieve one's aims entirely. The base curve required to eliminate one aberration may not deal so successfully with others. There are also differences of opinions as to which aberration is the most objectionable and should hence be given prior consideration. Since the beginning of the century a number of lens designers in various countries have formulated different combinations which they consider ideal. A series of lenses produced in accordance with such a scheme are generally termed best-form.

Best-form series may employ as many as a dozen different base curves to cover the mass-produced range of spherical powers, say from –8.00 D to +8.00 D. The base curves may vary from +3.00 D or even shallower to +12.5 D or thereabouts on the strongest plus powers.

The term best-form is rather misleading inasmuch as there is no universally agreed principle of design but a number of different best-forms, each based on a different theoretical approach or satisfying a different ideal. Nevertheless, the term is firmly established in the English literature on the subject. In the USA the term 'corrected curve lenses' is used, but this too is not entirely apt: it is not the curves which are corrected but the aberrations.

There is a conflict here between optical and cosmetic requirements. The thinnest lens one can make is flat form; however, off axis vision suffers. As a general statement, lenses produced on much higher curves give good vision at both centre and edge but have rather a bulbous appearance and are not cosmetically flattering. The approach has therefore been to adopt a 'middle of the road' stance. That is to say, curved meniscus and toric lenses although thicker than flat form, are reasonable from a cosmetic point of view and provide good all round vision.

Aspheric lenses (see Chapter 25) are an interesting development. They are less curved than conventional meniscus or torics, that is to say approaching a flattish appearance but due to the aspheric surface, maintain the vision obtained from much more curved lenses. The end result is that patients obtain flatter, thinner lenses but with good all round vision. When this is combined with high index materials, the appearance of the lens can be improved to an even greater degree.

In Chapter 8 the sag concept was developed to a stage whereby it could be used to calculate the centre and edge substances of various lenses. The sag at the front was referred to as $s1$ and the back, $s2$. The same approach can be applied to calculations for toric lenses.

For minus spherical lenses it has been shown that

$$e = s2 - s1 + t$$

but a toric lens has two curves on one of the surfaces. As the majority of lenses made today are produced with spherical front surfaces and toroidal back surfaces, examples will be shown in this form.

As there are now two curvatures on the back surface, this explains why a toric lens, unlike a meniscus, will have a thick and thin edge. It also means that $s2$ has two values which are termed $s2$ base and $s2$ cross.

As an example the prescription $-5.00$ DS $-2.00$ DC $\times$ 90 made on a $+4.00$ D sphere curve would have surface powers

$$\frac{+4.00}{-9.00 \times 180 \ -11.00 \times 90}$$

The principal powers of this prescription, represented by an optical cross are shown in *Figure 10.4*. The lowest power, $-5.00$ D, is a result of a combination of the $+4.00$ D front curve and the $-9.00$ D base curve. The highest power, $-7.00$ D, is a result of the combination of the $+4.00$ D front curve and the $-11.00$ D cross curve. The expression

$$e = s2 - s1 + t$$

changes to

$$e \text{ thin} = s2 \text{ base} - s1 + t$$
$$e \text{ thick} = s2 \text{ cross} - s1 + t$$

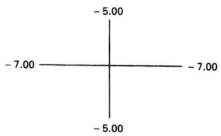

**Figure 10.4** Optical cross.

The meridian of lowest power will have the thinnest edge and the meridian of highest power will have the thickest when referring to minus powered lenses.

Using the sage formula (Chapter 8) calculate the sags of all curvatures in our example (4.00 D, 9.00 D and 11.00 D). Assume glass 1.523 index 60 mm diameter, centre thickness 1.00 mm. Your answers should be:

| Curve | Sag |
|-------|-------|
| 4.00 D | 3.49 |
| 9.00 D | 8.34 |
| 11.00 D | 10.66 |

Putting these into the formulae stated above

$$e \text{ thin } = 8.34 - 3.49 + 1 = 5.85 \text{ mm}$$

$$e \text{ thick } = 10.66 - 3.49 + 1 = 8.17 \text{ mm}$$

In the above example $t$ is given as 1.00 mm because this is the generally accepted minimum substance for high minus powered glass lenses. Ordinary resin (1.498 index) is normally worked to a minimum of 2.00 mm although some higher index resins can be as thin as 1.00 mm. For glass minus powered lenses the following expression is normally used:

$$t = 2 + 0.2F$$

where

$t$ = centre thickness
$F$ = focal power.

As an example take a − 1.50 DS and apply the formula to it

$$t = 2 + (0.2 \times -1.50)$$

$$t = 2 + (-0.3)$$

$$t = 1.7 \text{ mm}$$

If the lens was astigmatic, for example

−7.00 DS +3.00 DC

one would transpose to minus cylinder form (−4.00 DS −3.00 DC) and apply the centre substance formula to the sphere element.

With reference to plus powered lenses, there are again two curvatures on the back surface, $s2$ base and $s2$ cross. From Chapter 8 it was shown that for a meniscus

$t = s1 - s2 + e$

As with the minus powered toric this has to be modified.

Using the prescription +5.00 DS −1.50 DC × 180 made on a +9.00 D sphere curve, the surface powers would be

$$\frac{+9.00}{-4.00 \times 90 \ -5.50 \times 180}$$

The principal powers represented by an optical cross are shown in *Figure 10.5*. The lowest power, +3.50 D, is as a result of the combination of the +9.00 D front curve and the −5.50 D cross curve. The highest power, +5.00

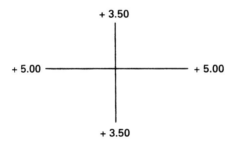

**Figure 10.5** Optical cross.

D, is as a result of the +9.00 D front curve and the −4.00 D base curve. It is the curve that gives us the highest power that is controlling the centre thickness on a plus lens, therefore our expression

$t = s1 - s2 + e$

changes to

$t = s1 - s2 \text{ base} + e$

Using the sag formula (Chapter 8) calculate the sags of 9.00 D and 4.00 D. Assume glass 1.523 index, 60 mm diameter, minimum edge substance 1.00 mm. The answers should be

| Curve | Sag |
|-------|------|
| 9.00 D | 8.34 |
| 4.00 D | 3.49 |

Substituting these into the formula stated

$$t = 8.34 - 3.49 + 1 = 5.85 \, \text{mm}$$

Although the normal requirement for a plus lens is to know the centre thickness, and for minus the edge thickness, occasionally the thick edge substance on a plus powered toric is also needed. On the example above the minimum edge is already deemed to be on average 1 mm but of course this only applies along the meridian of highest power. What will be the edge thickness along the meridian of lowest power?

In Chapter 8, the sag relationship for flat lenses, was shown to be

$$e = t - s$$

When applied to a meniscus this became

$$e = t - (s1 - s2)$$

When applied to torics (assuming minus cylinder form) it becomes

$$e \text{ thick} = t - (s1 - s2 \text{ cross})$$

In the example previously calculated $t$ was found to be 5.85 mm and the sag of s1 8.34. To use the $e$ thick formula, the sag of s2 cross has to be determined. The answer should be

| Curve | Sag |
|-------|------|
| 5.50 D | 4.86 |

Substituting the figures into the formula stated

$$e \text{ thick} = 5.85 - (8.34 - 4.86) = 2.37 \, \text{mm}$$

As with spherical lenses there is still the consideration of which semi-finished base to use for a particular power. Manufacturers' charts are available for this purpose although in most instances the prescription house will hold the information on its computer files.

There is also the problem of considering the effect of lens thickness on the final power of the lens. This was outlined in Chapter 8 and is applicable to torics.

The formula

$$\text{VPA} = \frac{tF1^2}{1000n - tF1}$$

gives the compensation that must be added to the inside curve of a meniscus lens. The same formula is used even for torics as the resulting answer is applicable to both the base curve and the cross curve.

Assuming the inside *nominal* curves have worked out to be

−5.62 −6.62

and the VPA allowance calculated out as 0.09, then this figure is simply added to both curves, giving

−5.71 −6.71

which, in practice, would normally be rounded to

−5.75 −6.75

There is no need to perform the calculation twice. This is another reason why minus cylinder torics are preferred against plus cylinder torics where it is necessary to calculate the base curve and cross curve separately.

In Chapter 8 the 'chicken and egg' situation was mentioned that exists on plus powered lenses. Calculation of plus lens thickness cannot be made without knowing the exact curves but the correct curves cannot be calculated without knowing the exact substance.

The 'rule of thumb' method described is equally as applicable to torics. However, it must be remembered to use the sphere power when the lens is in its minus cyl transposition. For example, to determine the thickness of a +4.00 DS +2.00 DC lens it has to be transposed to +6.00 DS −2.00 DC. Use the sag of +6.00 D over the required diameter plus 1 mm edge to arrive at a centre thickness.

It is, however, possible to refine the substance calculation even further. With today's computer technology it is easy to make many complex calculations in a fraction of a second. Lens design programs have a system often referred to as 'looping' because of the 'chicken and egg' situation regarding substance and curvature calculations, the computer making some initial assumptions and then, through 'looping', goes on to achieve a more accurate calculation.

By way of an example, to determine the substance of a +11.00 DS +1.00 DC lens (1.523) to be made in flat form with minus cyl on the back surface, 54 mm diameter, 0.5 mm minimum edge thickness, first transpose so that sphere power is in its highest form i.e. +12.00 DS −1.00 DC.

Then determine sag of +12.00 over 54 mm diameter (see Appendix 2), which is found to be 9.37, and add to this the minimum edge substance of 0.5 mm, which gives 9.87 mm.

Up to now this would have been considered the correct centre substance of the lens; however, using 'looping' we can achieve a more accurate figure. To arrive at 9.87 mm substance, the calculation was based on the sphere power being +12.00 and the front surface of the lens being +12.00; however, in practice it has been learnt from the proceeding chapters that the front surface would be something less than +12.00 to allow for the substance of the lens (vertex power allowance).

Begin 'looping' by first determining the VPA of +12.00 at 9.87 mm thickness (see Appendix 1). The value is 0.87. The compensated front surface will therefore be (rounded to nearest 0.06) approximately +11.12 (12.00 – 0.87).

Determine sag of +11.12 at 54 mm by either calculation or 'guesstimate' from Appendix 2. The answer is 8.52 mm. Add on the 0.5 mm minimum edge substance to give a figure of 9.02 mm.

This is the centre substance that the lens should be made to and all calculations based around this figure rather than the 9.87 mm first determined. For the readers benefit the curve calculations for the lens will be completed so that the process may be considered in context.

Determine VPA of +12.00 at 9.02 mm substance (see Appendix 1). A value of 0.79 is obtained. Subtract this from the +12.00 to give 11.21.

The curvatures required are therefore

$$\frac{+11.21}{\text{Plano} \times 90 - 1.00 \times 180}$$

at a centre substance of 9.02 mm.

The procedures described in Chapters 8, 9 and 10 are not meant as definitive answers to all optical calculations problems. For example, no consideration has been given to the thickness of shaped (edged) lenses. It is not the purpose of this book to explore all these factors. There are already very good optical textbooks available on such topics.

# Chapter 11

# Chapter revision

Having detailed information on spherical, astigmatic and toric lenses, it may be as well to briefly pause to ensure that the reader has absorbed the complex factors involved in the world of optics.

To commence, transpose the following powers into their alternative sph/cyl form. (All answers end of chapter.)

1 +2.00 DS +1.75 DC × 5
2 −3.00 DS +3.00 DC × 95
3 Plano −2.00 DC × 110
4 +0.25 DS −1.50 DC × 70
5 −4.00 DS −0.25 DC × 180
6 +2.00 DS −1.75 DC × 45

In the prescription +4.00 DS −5.00 DC × 90:

7 What is the power in the horizontal meridian?
8 What is the power in the vertical meridian?

9 What is the medical term for 'longsighted'?
10 What is presbyopia?
11 With the aid of a diagram explain 'standard notation'.
12 Give names to the lens forms shown in *Figure 11.1*.

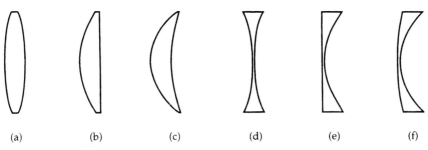

(a)    (b)    (c)    (d)    (e)    (f)

**Figure 11.1** Lens forms.

13 Calculate the sag of a 3.25 D curve on a glass lens (1.523) over a diameter of 67 mm.

14 Draw a simple diagram to illustrate a myopic eye.

15 Draw a simple diagram to illustrate how myopia can be corrected by using a lens.

16 What is the name given to the condition when a cyl has to be incorporated into the prescription?

17 What does '$n$' denote?

18 Name the two methods by which the length of a curl side can be specified.

19 What is the preferred method of specifying the position of a segment top or fitting cross when fitting to a frame?

20 Explain the terms 'nominal' and 'actual' in relation to a semi-finished spherical front surface lens.

21 What is an aphakic eye?

22 How is refractive index determined, i.e. what formula?

23 Draw a diagram to illustrate head width.

24 By what other method could prism base down be expressed.

25 Assuming 1.498 material, what is the radius of a +8.25 D curve?

26 Assuming 1.498 material, what curve would have a radius of 90.55 mm?

27

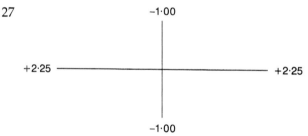

Expressed on an optical cross the principal powers are as shown. Express these powers in conventional sph/cyl/axis form.

28 A 40 mm sag gauge measures 2.34 when placed on a lens of 1.498 material. What is the curve of the lens expressed in dioptres?

## Answers

1 +3.75 DS −1.75 DC × 95

2 Plano −3.00 DC × 5

3 −2.00 DS +2.00 DC × 20

4 −1.25 DS +1.50 DC × 160

5 −4.25 DS +0.25 DC × 90

6 +0.25 DS +1.75 DC × 135

7 −1.00

8 +4.00

9 Hypermetropia

10 Presbyopia: the crystalline lens becomes less flexible with age and therefore the eye finds it difficult to focus at normal reading distance. The condition begins to show itself at around 40–45 years of age. The result is that help with reading, normally in the form of bifocals, trifocals or progressives, is required.

11

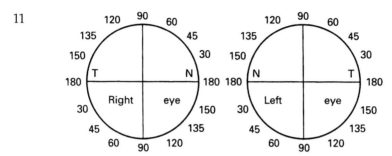

**Figure 11.2** Standard notation.

12 (a) Bi-convex, or if both curves equal, equi-convex.
   (b) Plano-convex.
   (c) Plus meniscus.
   (d) Bi-concave, or if both curves equal, equi-concave.
   (e) Plano-concave.
   (f) Minus meniscus.

13 3.53

14

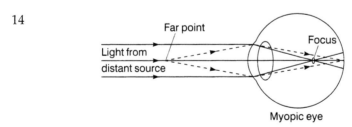

**Figure 11.3** A myopic eye.

15

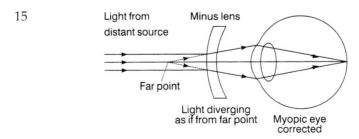

**Figure 11.4** How myopia can be corrected by using a lens.

16  Astigmatism.
17  Refractive index.
18  Total length. Length to tangent.
19  Above or below the horizontal centre line.
20  'Nominal' is the 'rounded' curve by which the lens is known. 'Actual'
    represent the *actual* curve on the lens when vertex power allowance is
    taken into account, which in turn is made to compensate for the
    finished lens substance.
21  One that has had the crystalline lens removed.

22  $n = \dfrac{\text{Speed of light in air}}{\text{Speed of light in medium}}$

23

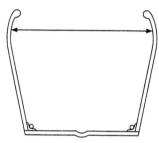

**Figure 11.5** Head width.

24  Base 270
25  60.36 mm
26  5.50
27  −1.00 DS +3.25 DC × 90 or +2.25 DS −3.25 DC × 180
28  5.75 D

# Part Two

# Chapter 12

# Optical centration

## Optical centre of a lens

Elementary optical theory is greatly simplified by assuming lenses to be 'thin', meaning without any thickness. They can be represented in diagrams by straight lines, as in *Figure 12.1*, which shows a plus spherical lens with the centres of curvature of its two surfaces at $C_1$ and $C_2$. By definition, the line XX on which these lie is the optical axis of the lens. The line representing the lens is drawn at right-angles to it.

The point O at which the thin lens intersects the optical axis is regarded as its *optical centre*. Any ray such as JOK or MON that is incident at the optical centre passes through the lens without being deviated. This property is of great importance and is not shared by any other point on the lens.

When the thickness and form of a lens are taken into account the definition of the term 'optical centre' becomes a little more complicated, and its precise position – though always on the optical axis – may even be external to the lens. In ophthalmic lenses, however, the optical centre is regarded as coinciding with the vertex of either surface.

It is very important that the optical centre of each lens should occupy the desired position relative to the pupil of the wearer's eye. This means, in turn, that the optical centre of the edged lens should be correctly positioned relative to the lens shape. Unless other instructions are given, the optical centre of each lens is expected to be placed at the standard optical centre position.

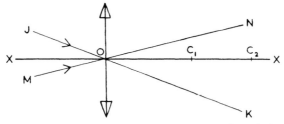

**Figure 12.1** Diagrammatic representation of a 'thin' lens. Rays through the optical centre O are undeviated.

## Decentration

Vertical decentrations are expressed as *up* or *down* according to the direction in which the optical centre is moved from its standard position. For example, the prescriber may require the optical centres to be placed 4 mm above the horizontal centre line. He/she could specify either 'decentre each lens 4 mm up' or 'optical centres 4 mm above horizontal centre line'.

Horizontal decentrations are expressed as *in* or *out; in* means that the optical centre is shifted towards the nose, and *out* means the opposite. Again, there are two different ways of giving the necessary instructions. One method is to state the amount and direction of decentration for each lens, as in the example 'decentre right lens *x* mm in'.

In the other method, the desired decentration follows by implication from certain other dimensions. To consider these, attention must now be turned from the individual lens to the spectacle frame and its wearer.

## Interpupillary distance and centration distance

A factor having a very important bearing on horizontal centration is the distance between the centres of the patient's pupils. This is known as the interpupillary distance or PD. It is normally measured with the eyes looking straight ahead as in distance vision, unless of course single vision lenses are being prescribed for intermediate or reading purposes in which case, as the eyes converge, a narrower distance between them would be expected compared with those for distance vision.

With regard to terminology clarification, whilst a patient will have an interpupillary distance, a pair of spectacles will have a centration distance; these should under normal circumstances be equal to one another.

Since the face is often asymmetrical, it is sometimes necessary, particularly when fitting progressive lenses, to consider each eye separately. In this event, the horizontal distances from the centre of the bridge of the frame to each pupil centre are recorded as right and left monocular centres.

There is a relationship between decentration, interpupillary distance, centration distance and certain frame dimensions which has to be understood.

As an example, a patient has a frame with a distance between its box centres of 72 mm. The distance between the patient's pupils may be 62 mm (interpupillary distance). For a prescription house to position the lenses correctly they have to convert this to a decentration value. It is not possible to simply set the optical centres at 62 mm! We have to have a starting point (box centre). In our example the difference between the box centres is 72 mm whilst the patient's eyes are 62 mm apart. The difference is 10 mm. Put another way, the optical centres of the lens have to be set 10 mm narrower apart than the frame box centres. Thinking in the term of two eyes, this means that each optical centre will need to be set 5 mm narrower than the box centres. This is therefore the decentration required to obtain the correct centration distance. *Figure 12.2* may be of assistance. The distance between the box centres (designated by C) is 72 mm. If each optical centre is moved 5 mm inwards (designated by *) then the distance between them is 62 mm.

As mentioned earlier, not all patients' faces are symmetrical. The distance from the centre of the bridge of the frame to each eye may be different. In this instance monocular centres may be requested.

Remaining with the same frame from our previous example, but now being used on a patient with monocular pupillary distances of R34 L32: the patient's eyes are 66 mm apart in total but not equally positioned. This is not uncommon.

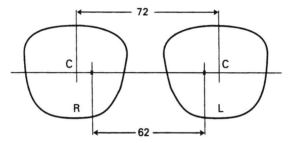

**Figure 12.2** Relationship of distance between boxed centres and patients' interpupillary distance.

To determine the decentration that this represents, firstly halve the distance between the box centres of the frame. In our example this is equal to 36 mm. In other words from the centre of the bridge to each box centre is 36 mm. If the right pupil centre is 34 mm from the centre of the nose, the difference is 2 mm and therefore the optical centre should be decentred 2 mm in to position it correctly. If the left pupil centre is 32 mm from the centre of the nose, the difference is 4 mm and therefore the optical centre should be decentred 4 mm in to position it correctly.

The relationship between all the different factors can now be seen. Effectively the position of the optical centre can be ordered in three different ways:

1 as a bodily decentration
2 as a total interpupillary distance
3 as a monocular distance

the latter two requiring conversion to a decentration value.

## Prismatic effect of a spherical lens

*Figure 12.3* represents a thin plus spherical lens, the line XX being its optical axis and O its optical centre. A fundamental property of spherical lenses is that incident rays parallel to the optical axis are made to pass

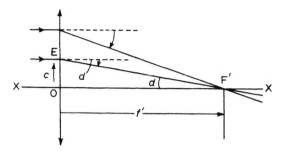

**Figure 12.3** Prismatic effect of a spherical lens, showing it to increase with the distance from the optical centre.

through (or to appear to diverge from) an axial point F', known as the second principal focus. This evidently requires the rays to undergo different amounts of deviation, according to the distance of the point of incidence from the optical centre. Since deviation is the characteristic effect of a prism, the action of a lens in deviating incident rays is termed its prismatic effect.

In the diagram, consider the ray incident at the point E at a distance $c$ (centimeteres) from the optical centre. The deviation $d$ undergone by the ray is equal to the angle EF'O. Hence, the prismatic effect $P$ in prism dioptres is

$$P = 100(c/f')$$

if $f'$ is also in centimetres. Finally, since the power $F$ of a thin lens is equal to $100/f'$ where $f'$ is the focal length in centimetres

$$P = c \times F$$

For example, the prismatic effect of a +6.00 DS lens at a point 3 mm (0.3 cm) from its optical centre is $0.3 \times 6.00$ which is $1.8^\triangle$.

This simple formula is known as Prentice's rule after the American, Charles F. Prentice, one of the foremost experts of his day in the field of ophthalmic lenses and prisms. It was Prentice who introduced the idea of the prism dioptre, though he was not responsible for its unfortunate name.

All lenses could be considered as having a prismatic element, for what are they but 'prisms with curves' (*Figure 12.4*). A plus lens is like two prisms placed base to base whilst a minus is like two prisms placed apex to apex. When viewing through the points at which they meet (optical centres) there is no induced prismatic element, but there will be whilst looking through any other point on the lens.

It now remains to consider the base–apex direction in which prismatic effects of spherical lenses are exerted.

In the case of a spherical lens with its optical centre at O (*Figure 12.5a*), the prismatic effect at any point Q has its base–apex line in the meridian QO. If a section through the lens along this meridian is visualised, the

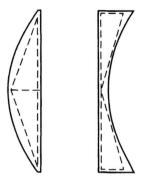

**Figure 12.4** Diagrammatic representation showing prismatic elements in lenses.

position of the base can be readily determined. For example, a plus spherical lens has its thickest point at the optical centre, the thickness decreasing towards the edge. Consequently, the base of the prism is always towards the optical centre. At a point Q immediately above the optical centre, the prismatic effect is base down, as shown in *Figure 12.5a*. At R the base is to the left (in or out according to whether the lens is for the right or left eye). At S the base is up, and at T it is to the right.

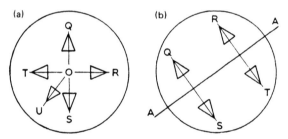

**Figure 12.5** Base direction of prismatic effects: (a) plus spherical lens; (b) plus plano-cylinder.

The same principle would apply to any point U in some oblique meridian: UO would be the base–apex line, the base of the prism being towards O.

On the other hand, a minus spherical lens has its thinnest point at the optical centre, and so the prismatic effect at any point would have its base in the opposite direction to that of a plus lens.

Earlier it was seen that looking through a point 3 mm away from the optical centre of a +6.00 DS lens caused $1.8^{\Delta}$ prism. To put this into context, *Figure 12.6* illustrates what happens if a right lens is not positioned correctly in front of the eye (plan view). In relation to the eye's line of vision the optical centre (or base of prismatic element) is positioned outwards and therefore a base out prism effect has been created.

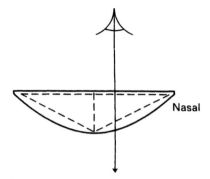

**Figure 12.6** Diagrammatic representation of a base out prismatic effect.

The situation with a minus lens can be seen from *Figure 12.7*. In relation to the eye's line of vision the optical centre (or apex of prism element) is positioned outwards and therefore the base of the prismatic element is towards the nasal, subsequently a base in prism effect has been created.

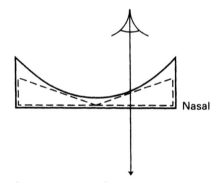

**Figure 12.7** Diagrammatic representation of a base in prismatic effect.

## Prismatic effect of a plano-cylinder

*Figure 12.5b* represents a plus plano-cylinder with its axis meridian along AA. Any section through the lens parallel to AA would have the form of a flat parallel plate, but the thickest of all these sections would be that along AA itself. Consequently, the prismatic effect of such a lens can be determined by visualising the lens as two prisms joined base to base along the axis meridian.

The base–apex line is invariably at right-angles to the cylinder axis. Suppose the latter to be at 30 degrees. At the points Q and R, for example, the prismatic effect of the lens would be base down at 120 degrees, whereas at S and T it would be base up at 120 degrees.

As with spherical lenses, the magnitude of the prismatic effect at any point follows from Prentice's rule but in this case $F$ is the cylinder power and $c$ the perpendicular distance in centimeters from the point in question to the cylinder axis AA.

The same principles apply to minus plano-cylinders. With these lenses, however, the minimum thickness is along the axis meridian and so a minus plano-cylinder can be visualised as two prisms joined apex to apex along the cylinder axis. Consequently, the prismatic effect at any point is at right-angles to the axis meridian, the base of the prism being turned away from it.

## Combining a prism with a lens

*Figure 12.8* shows a base down plano prism and a plus spherical lens as they might be placed before the eye at the end of a sight-test. Only one lens is needed to combine the effect of these two elements. In *Figure 12.9* consider first the plano-convex lens alone. The centre of curvature of its curved surface is at $C_1$. A line drawn through this point so as to meet the plane surface normally (that is, perpendicularly) is the optical axis XX of the lens and its intersection O with the front surface can be taken as its optical centre. If a plano prism is now affixed to the lens as shown, the combination is equivalent to another planoconvex lens with a different back surface. The normal X'X' to this surface passing through $C_1$ becomes the new optical axis and O' the new optical centre.

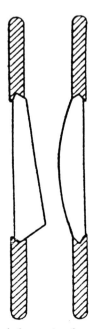

**Figure 12.8** Trial lens combination of plano prism base down and plus spherical lens.

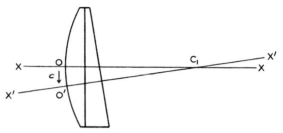

**Figure 12.9** The prism displaces the optical centre of a plus lens towards the base of the prism.

The effect of the added prism has been to shift the position of the optical centre towards the base of the prism. This is true for any plus lens.

With any minus lens, the effect of adding a prism is to shift the optical centre towards the apex of the prism, as shown in *Figure 12.10*. In this case it is the back (second) surface of the lens which is curved and so its centre of curvature has to be denoted by $C_2$.

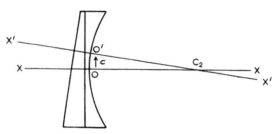

**Figure 12.10** The prism displaces the optical centre of a minus lens towards the apex of the prism.

In both cases, the distance $c$ through which the optical centre has been displaced by incorporating the prism is in accordance with Prentice's rule when written in the transposed form

$$c = \frac{P}{F}$$

Although these diagrams have used plano-convex and plano-concave lens forms, the same principle applies to curved lenses. In effect, a prescribed prism can be incorporated in any lens by working the two surfaces at the appropriate angle to each other. One method of control during manufacture is by checking the prism thickness difference as explained in Chapter 13. This technique is not restricted to plano prisms in isolation.

The position of the centration point of a lens – normally the standard optical centre position – is affected only by any prescribed decentration. For example, if 2 mm inward decentration is ordered, the centration point moves 2 mm inwards from the standard optical centre position.

In the absence of any prescribed prism, the optical centre of the lens is intended to be located at the centration point. In other words the prismatic effect at the centration point should be zero.

The position of the centration point is not altered by the mere inclusion of a prism in the prescription. It is either the standard optical centre position or as indicated by any decentration specified. In either case the prismatic effect exerted by the lens at the centration point is intended to be as prescribed. It follows from this that if the prescribed prism were neutralised by a prism of the same power but with its base in the opposite direction, the optical centre of the combination should then coincide with the centration point. This is one method of checking the accuracy with which the finished lens has been made.

## Prism by decentration: spherical lenses

One reason for decentring a lens is to place its optical centre in the desired position relative to the wearer's pupil. In some cases decentration may be used to obtain the effect of a prescribed prism without the necessity for working the lens specially.

Take, for example, the prescription

R + 5.00 DS $2^\Delta$ base down

Assume for the purpose of this example that no decentration has been specified. Therefore, the optical centre of the lens is to be positioned at the boxed centre of the eyeshape (standard optical centre position). It is at this point that the prismatic effect of the lens is required to be $2^\Delta$ base down.

As previously seen, the prismatic effect of a spherical lens is proportional to the distance from the optical centre. Also, in the case of a plus lens, the direction of the base is towards its optical centre, as in *Figure 12.5a*. Consequently, there can be only one point on this lens at which the prismatic effect is the specified $2^\Delta$ base down. In this case, it is immediately above the optical centre. Therefore to obtain this effect at the standard optical centre position, the lens – together with its optical centre – must be moved downwards by the necessary amount.

This can be found from Prentice's rule in the form of

$$c = \frac{P}{F}$$

Applied to the above example

$$c = \frac{2}{5} = 0.4 \, \text{cm} = 4.00 \, \text{mm}$$

The decentration required is therefore 4 mm down.

The general principle is illustrated in *Figure 12.11* in which G represents the centration point and O the optical centre of the lens after a downward

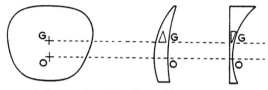

**Figure 12.11** Downward decentration of a spherical lens. The prismatic effect at the centration point G is base down on a plus lens and base up on a minus lens.

decentration. The base direction of the resulting prismatic effect at G is shown for both plus and minus lenses. From this diagram it is possible to deduce the general rule as follows:

> To obtain a prescribed prism, decentre a plus lens in the same direction as the base of the prism and a minus lens in the opposite direction.

In practice, the scope for decentration is limited by the size and shape of the required finished lens in relation to blank size available. It is also only possible to decentre to obtain prism on single vision lenses as multifocals have intermediate and reading areas to be considered where it is not acceptable to move the whole lens bodily.

## Decentration by prism: spherical lenses

In the previous section it was seen that it is possible to decentre a single vision lens to obtain a prismatic effect but the converse is also true – prism can be worked on to a lens to obtain decentration.

If the lens cannot be bodily moved, the optical centre within the lens can be moved. The situation whereby this would become necessary would be when a blank size is not large enough to obtain the decentration required bodily.

Certain lens types are not suitable for working prism for decentration, normally shaped segment (D segment and curve top segments), multifocals and progressives. This is due to the fact that when a prism is worked to move the optical centre across the lens, the reading area must also be moved proportionally to keep it narrower than the distance. With single vision lenses this is not necessary and round segment multifocals can have the segments rotated to compensate but shaped segments and progressives, due to design constraints, cannot.

If the lens type allows, the formula used is

$$P = c \times F$$

which was referred to earlier.

For instance, a +6.00 DS lens that needs to be decentred 3 mm in but blank size is not large enough to allow this. Use the formula

$$P = c \times F$$
$$P = 0.3 \times 6$$
$$P = 1.8^\Delta \text{ in}$$

(Remember that any decentration has to be converted to centimetres.) If $1.8^\Delta$ of prism is incorporated into the lens this will give the equivalent result as if it had been bodily decentred by 3 mm.

If the lens had been a −6.00 DS the same formula would have been used resulting in the same amount of prism. However, the prism direction would have been OUT.

The general rule is as follows:

When working prism for decentration on a plus lens, the prism base direction is the same as the direction of the decentration. On a minus lens it is opposite.

## Prism by decentration: sphero-cylinders

Size permitting, sphero-cylinders can also be decentred to produce a prescribed prismatic effect. If the base–apex line coincides with one of the principal meridians of the lens, the calculation is quite simple. Proceed as with a spherical lens in the meridian concerned. As an example, consider the prescription

L + 1.00 DS − 5.00 DC × 90 $1^\Delta$ base in

The principal meridians of the lens are vertical and horizontal, the latter coinciding with the base–apex line of the prescribed prism. In this meridian, the principal power of the lens is −4.00 D. Consequently, the decentration must be out – opposite to the base of the prism – and the amount follows from the formula

$$c = P/F = 1/4 = 0.25 \text{ cm} = 2.5 \text{ mm}$$

If the base–apex line does not coincide with one of the principal meridians the problem becomes more complicated. Even so, the graphical method about to be described affords a relatively simple means of solution. There are three essential steps as follows.

1 The prescribed prism is resolved into two components corresponding in direction to the two principal meridians of the lens.
2 By applying Prentice's rule, the required decentration is found for each meridian separately.
3 The resultant of the two decentrations is found and resolved into horizontal and vertical components.

This method will now be explained by reference to the example

R −2.00 DS −1.00 DC × 60

dec. for 1<sup>△</sup> base up 2<sup>△</sup> base in

The complete construction is shown in *Figure 12.12* and the steps are as follows:

1 Draw a pair of perpendicular lines HH and VV to represent the horizontal and vertical meridians, the point of intersection G being taken as the centration point. On this framework, lines at 60 degrees and 150 degrees can now be inserted to show the principal meridians of the lens. In the axis meridian, which is at 60 degrees, the principal power is that of the sphere alone, namely, −2.00 D. The other principal power, in the 150 degree meridian, is that of the sphere and cylinder combined, −3.00 D. These powers should be entered on the diagram as shown, with a bold letter R to indicate a right lens.

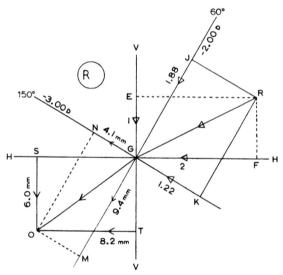

**Figure 12.12** Example of graphical construction for finding required decentration of an astigmatic lens.

2 Choose a suitable scale for prisms, say 40 mm = 1<sup>△</sup>. Then mark off, along the upper part of VV, a length GE of 40 mm to represent the prescribed 1<sup>△</sup> base up, and along the nasalward part of HH a length GF of 80 mm representing the prescribed 2<sup>△</sup> base in.
3 Complete the rectangle GERF. Its diagonal GR represents the resultant single prism equivalent to the combination of prescribed prisms.
4 From R drop the perpendiculars RJ to the 60 degree meridian and RK to the 150 degree meridian. The lengths GJ and GK represent another pair of prisms, equivalent to the prescribed pair because both sets have the same resultant GR, but aligned with the principal meridians of the

lens. It is helpful to insert the small triangles indicating the base directions.

5 Measure the lengths GJ and GK. On the scale employed they will be found to represent $1.88^\Delta$ base 60 up and $1.22^\Delta$ base 150 down.

6 Work out the decentration required along the 60 degrees meridian in which $F = 2.00$ D and $P = 1.88^\Delta$ base 60 up. Prentice's rule gives

$$c = P/F = 1.88/2 = 0.94\,cm = 9.4\,mm$$

Since the lens power is minus, the decentration must be in the opposite direction to the prism base, that is to say downwards along 60 degrees. Accordingly, mark off the downward length GM along the 60 degree meridian to represent 9.4 mm on any convenient scale, say 8 or 10 times.

7 Repeat this process for the 150 degree meridian in which $F = 3.00$ D and $P = 1.22^\Delta$ base 150 down. The decentration must again be in the opposite direction to the prism base, that is to say, upwards along the 150 degree meridian, the amount being

$$c = 1.22/3 = 0.41\,cm = 4.1\,mm$$

Mark off GN to represent this length on the scale chosen.

8 Complete the rectangle GMON. Its diagonal GO represents the oblique decentration needed, the point O thus indicating the displaced position of the optical centre. It is, however, more convenient in practice to specify oblique decentrations in terms of their vertical and horizontal components, in that order. Consequently, from O drop the perpendiculars OS to HH and OT to VV. On the chosen scale their lengths will be found to indicate

6.0 mm down and 8.2 mm out

which is the required decentration.

The necessity for constructing the resultant prism GR does not arise, of course, unless the prescription includes both vertical and horizontal prisms.

Appendix 4 gives a purely mathematical solution along with a useful calculation table.

## Decentration by prism: sphero-cylinders

The following is a good approximate method of calculating the prism required to obtain a specified amount of decentration on a sphero-cylinder lens. Prentice's rule will be used but before this can be implemented the power in the meridian in which we are decentring must be calculated. If the axis of the prescription is 90 or 180 then this is easy (see Chapters 9 and 10). If the axis is other than this, a little more thought is required. For example

R +4.00 DS −2.00 DC × 25
decentre 6 mm in

Assume that the blank will now allow this decentration to be obtained bodily.

From the example above it is known what the power is at 25 (+4.00 D and at 115 (+2.00 D) but what is really needed is the power at 180 – the direction of the decentration.

Find the sine of the axis, so the sine of 25 = .4226. Then square it which equals 0.1785, which when rounded becomes 0.18. Therefore, for every one dioptre of cylinder power 0.18 of a dioptre is effective at 180. Consequently the value of a cylinder power of –2.00 D must be multiplied by 2.

$$(0.18 \text{ D}) \times (-2.00 \text{ D}) = -0.36 \text{ D}$$

This is added to the sphere power (which of course is effective in all meridians) remembering to obey signs. Therefore

$$(+4.00 \text{ D}) + (-0.36 \text{ D}) = +3.64 \text{ D}$$

The power of the lens in the horizontal meridian for prismatic purposes is +3.64 D.

Using

$$P = c \times F$$
$$P = 0.\bar{6} \times 3.64 = 2.18$$
$$P = 2.18^{\Delta}$$

In practice, this would probably be rounded to $2.25^{\Delta}$. The direction, because the power is plus, would be prism base in.

If the requirement had been

R +4.00 DS –2.00 DC × 25
decentre 6 mm up

Then, exactly the same procedure would be followed up to the point whereby for every dioptre of cylinder power, 0.18 of a dioptre is effective at 180 but because the power of the vertical is now required, 0.18 must be subtracted from 1.00.

$$(1.00 \text{ D}) - (0.18 \text{ D}) = 0.82 \text{ D}$$

Therefore, for every dioptre of cylinder power, 0.82 of a dioptre is effective at 90. Using a cylinder power of –2.00 D the value must now be multiplied by 2.

$$(0.82 \text{ D}) \times (-2.00 \text{ D}) = -1.64 \text{ D}$$

This is added to the sphere power (which of course is effective in all meridians) remembering to obey signs. Therefore

$$(+4.00 \text{ D}) + (-1.64 \text{ D}) = +2.36 \text{ D}$$

The power of the lens in the vertical meridian is +2.36 D.
Using

$$P = c \times F$$

$$P = 0.6 \times 2.36 = 1.42$$

$$P = 1.42^\Delta$$

In practice this would probably be rounded to $1.50^\Delta$. The direction, because the power is plus, would be prism base up.

# Chapter 13

# Ophthalmic prisms

This chapter is a natural follow-on from the previous one, where the concept of optical centres and prisms was first introduced.

## Definitions

A plano prism can be defined in simple terms as a wedge of transparent material (*Figure 13.1*). The surfaces are both plane and so the prism is without focal power, or plano; but they are not parallel, being ground at an angle to each other. The sharp edge AA' at which they meet, or would meet if extended, is termed the refracting edge; and the refracting or apical angle *a* is the angle contained in a principal section, that is to say, a straight slice through the prism perpendicular to the refracting edge (*Figure 13.1b*).

For ease of illustration, the prism shown diagrammatically in *Figure 13.1a* has been drawn rectangular, but it could obviously be reduced to any desired shape. The thin edge is loosely termed the apex and the thick edge the base.

It is possible to have a plano prism in meniscus form, that is to say with one convex and one concave surface as in *Figure 13.1c*. The two surfaces combined are substantially without focal power but are ground at an angle to each other so as to produce the desired prismatic effect.

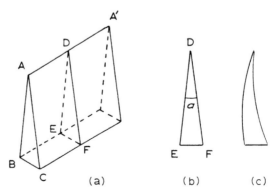

**Figure 13.1** (a) A plano prism; (b) a principal section; (c) principal section of a meniscus plano prism.

# Deviation

The essential property of a plano prism is that it deviates or changes the direction of light passing through it. An object viewed through a plano prism is therefore seen in a different direction from that in which it would appear to the naked eye.

This effect is illustrated in *Figure 13.2*. A typical ray PQ is deviated towards the base of the prism, from which it emerges in the direction RS. To an eye placed at S, any point K on the line PQ would be seen in the direction SR, as though it were at K'. It will be noted from the diagram that the displacement of the image (KK') is towards the apex of the prism.

The angle *d* through which the light is deviated by the prism is termed the angle of deviation, or more simply the deviation.

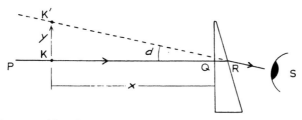

**Figure 13.2** Deviation (*d*) and apparent displacement (*y*) produced by a plano prism.

# Use of prisms

An object engaging one's attention is seen most clearly when both eyes are turned so as to gaze at it directly – resulting in what is termed binocular fixation. Normally, the ocular movements required for binocular fixation are carried out with remarkable speed and precision. With some individuals, however, binocular fixation can be made easier or more comfortable if the ocular rotations required are deliberately modified by a prism before one or both eyes.

Prisms are rarely prescribed on their own. Usually, they are ordered in conjunction with a prescription for lenses. Fortunately, this does not mean that a separate prism has to be worn in front of the lens. The desired effect can be incorporated in the lens by one of the methods described in Chapter 12.

# Units of angle

There are many units of angle. For most practical purposes the unit employed is the degree, based on the division of a circle into 360 equal sectors.

For mathematical and scientific analysis a different system of angular measurement is employed which does not depend on any arbitrary division of a circle. According to this system – sometimes known as circular measure – an angle is defined in terms of a pure number, the ratio of two lengths. In *Figure 13.3*, OA is a straight line pivoted at O.

If this line is rotated about O so that it takes up the position OA', the angle $\theta$ through which it has turned would be expressed in circular measure as the ratio of the length of arc AA' to the radius OA. The unit of angle, termed a radian, is therefore that angle in which the length of arc is equal to the radius.

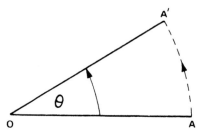

**Figure 13.3** Basis of 'circular measure'.

To convert radians into degrees, imagine the line OA in *Figure 13.3* to have made a complete revolution, equal to 360 degrees. In this case, the length of arc is the complete circumference of the circle which is equal to $2\pi$ times the radius. Hence

$$2\pi \text{ rad} = 360°$$

whence

$$1 \text{ rad} = 180/\pi \text{ degrees} = 57° \ 18' \text{ approx}$$

and

$$1 \text{ degree} = 0.01745 \text{ rad}$$

According to the modern metric system known as SI (Système Internationale) the only angle recognised for scientific use is the radian and its one-thousandth part, the milliradian (mrad). At one time, however, the hundredth part of a radian – termed a centrad and denoted by the symbol $\nabla$ – was used as a unit of prismatic deviation. It is now obsolete.

For use in ophthalmic optics, a special unit of angle termed the prism dioptre (symbol$^\triangle$) has been devised. Despite its unfortunate and confusing name, it is so convenient that it has now gained universal acceptance. An angle $\theta$ is expressed in prism dioptres simply by multiplying its tangent by 100. For example, if $\theta$ is 10 degrees, then

$$\theta \text{ in}^\triangle = 100 \times \tan 10°$$

$$= 100 \times 0.1763 = 17.63^\triangle$$

One of the advantages of this system is that it lends itself readily to the practical determination of prismatic deviation by measuring the apparent displacement $y$ of an object viewed through the lens at a distance $x$. In *Figure 13.2*, for example, the tangent of the angle of deviation $d$ is $y/x$ so that

$$d \text{ in}^{\Delta} = \frac{100y}{x}$$

A minor disadvantage of the prism dioptre is that it is not strictly a unit because the tangents of angles increase at a faster rate than the angles themselves, as shown by the following values.

| Angle in degrees | Tangent of angle | Angle in prism dioptres |
|---|---|---|
| 2 | 0.0349 | 3.49 |
| 4 | 0.0699 | 6.99 |
| 6 | 0.1051 | 10.51 |
| 8 | 0.1405 | 14.05 |
| 10 | 0.1763 | 17.63 |
| 12 | 0.2126 | 21.26 |
| 14 | 0.2493 | 24.93 |
| 16 | 0.2868 | 28.68 |
| 18 | 0.3249 | 32.49 |
| 20 | 0.3640 | 36.40 |

Nevertheless, up to about 6 degrees the relationship between angles in degrees and their equivalents in prism dioptres is seen to be reasonably uniform and most of the angles with which we are concerned in ophthalmic lenses fall within this range.

## Prism power

The deviation $d$ undergone by a ray passing through a plano prism of apical angle $a$ is affected by:

1 the angle of incidence;
2 the apical angle of the prism;
3 the refractive index $n$ of the material, which itself varies with the wavelength of the light.

The power of an ophthalmic plano prism is defined as the deviation it produces, expressed in prism dioptres on a ray incident normally at one surface.

An assortment of flat plano prisms is normally included in every ophthalmic trial case and refracting unit used for testing sight. In practice, very few prisms over $8^{\Delta}$ are prescribed but in most refracting units and the larger trial lens sets the range may extend up to $15^{\Delta}$ or even $20^{\Delta}$.

When a prism is of low power the relationship between deviation and the apical angle is given to a sufficient degree of accuracy by the approximate formula

$$d = (n - 1)a$$

which can also be written as

$$\tan a = \frac{\tan d}{(n - 1)} = \frac{P}{100(n - 1)}$$

where $P$ is the power of the prism.

Suppose, for example, that a flat plano prism of power $15^\Delta$ is to be made from glass of refractive index 1.523 and that the apical angle needed to produce this result is to be found.

The approximate formula would give

$$\tan a = \frac{15}{52.3} = 0.2866$$

so that

$$a = 16° \, 0'$$

Unfortunately, this is not quite accurate enough in all cases. The accurate formula is as follows:

$$\tan a = \frac{\sin d}{n - \cos d}$$

Before applying, the deviation ($d$) must be determined. This is found from

$$\tan d = \frac{P}{100}$$

$$\tan d = \frac{15}{100} = 0.15$$

$$\tan d = 8° \, 32'$$

The following formula can now be applied

$$\tan a = \frac{\sin d}{n - \cos d}$$

$$\tan a = \frac{0.1484}{1.523 - 0.9889} = 0.2780$$

Whence

$$a = 15° 32'$$

By dint of some mathematical manipulation, the above expression can be put in the more convenient form

$$\tan a = \frac{P}{100(n - 1) + nP^2/200}$$

Although this is now an approximation, the resulting errors are negligible. For instance, applied to the example just worked through, it would give

$$\tan a = \frac{15}{52.30 + 1.714} = 0.2776$$

whence

$$a = 15° 31'$$

## Prism thickness difference

*Figure 13.4* shows a principal section through a flat plano prism. The difference between the edge thickness $p$ at the apex of the prism and the edge thickness $q$ at the base of the prism is termed the prism thickness

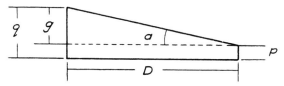

**Figure 13.4** Prism thickness difference: $p$ = edge thickness at apex; $q$ = edge thickness at base; $g$ = prism thickness difference = $q - p$.

difference. In the diagram it is denoted by $g$. For a given apical angle there is clearly a relationship between the prism thickness difference and the diameter over which it is measured. Hence, when grinding a prism the apical angle can be controlled by working to a predetermined thickness difference over a specified diameter. The base–apex line is marked on the underside of the blank and the edge thickness is calipered at each end to ensure that the necessary prism thickness difference has been observed. The power of the prism can thus be checked before it is removed from its button or holder.

Although strictly an approximation, the following formula is useful for the calculation of prism thickness difference

$$g = \frac{D \times P}{100(n-1) + \dfrac{nP^2}{200}}$$

where

$g$ = prism thickness difference in mm
$D$ = diameter
$n$ = refractive index
$P$ = prism.

As an example, a prism of $3^\Delta$, 50 mm diameter made in crown glass (1.523 index).

$$g = \frac{50 \times 3}{100(1.523 - 1) + \dfrac{1.523 \times 3^2}{200}}$$

$$g = \frac{150}{52.3 + \dfrac{13.71}{200}}$$

$$g = \frac{150}{52.3 + 0.07}$$

$$g = \frac{150}{52.37}$$

$$g = 2.86$$

In practice the prescription house would normally have a set of charts calculated for different prism amounts but only for one diameter! Although many different diameter lenses are processed in a prescription house the blocks on to which they are mounted are generally one size. Therefore, when checking prism thickness difference, the callipers are pushed up to the side of this block and measurements taken at the apex and the base. The difference between the two readings should be equal to the prism thickness difference over that block diameter (*Figure 13.5*).

The reader may also encounter a slightly easier approximate formula for the calculation of prism thickness difference

$$g = \frac{D \times P}{100(n-1)}$$

## Prism base setting

If any point on the refracting edge of a plano prism were taken as the apex, a principal section through that point would determine a straight

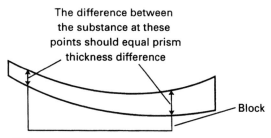

Figure 13.5 Prism thickness difference.

line on each surface. Any of such possible lines is a base–apex line. The importance of the base–apex line is that it fixes the direction of the plane in which the deviation produced by the prism takes place.

The object of an ophthalmic prism is to produce a displacement, in a specified desired direction, of the images seen through it. As we have already noted, the direction of image displacement is always towards the apex of the prism or away from the base. Hence, to produce a displacement upward, any base–apex line must be vertical, with the base of the prism below the apex, that is, down. It has become an accepted standard in ophthalmic practice to use the base of the prism to specify its setting in relation to the eye. This is known as the base setting and can be defined as the direction from apex to base.

Several methods can be used for specifying the base setting of an ophthalmic prism.

The two possible vertical settings are *base up* and *base down*, the meanings of which are obvious. The two possible horizontal settings are *base in* and *base out*, the word *in* meaning towards the nose.

Oblique settings can be specified by the use of standard axis notation followed by 'up' or 'down' as intended. For example, 'base 150 up' means that the base–apex line lies along the 150 degree axis meridian, the direction from apex to base being upwards along this line. Similarly, 'base 150 down' means that the base–apex line lies along the 150 degree meridian, the direction from apex to base being downwards along this line.

Another method is based on the 0–360 degrees protractor illustrated in *Figure 13.6*. This protractor incorporates standard axis notation (0–180°) in its upper half but the numbering is completed round the lower half of the circle from 180 to 360 degrees. One of the advantages of this system is its brevity. For example, 'base 150' and 'base 330' denote, respectively, 'base 150 up' and 'base 150 down' in the notation used previously.

This system can also be used for non-oblique prisms. Base up becomes 'base 90', base down becomes 'base 270', base in or out becomes 'base 0' or 'base 180', depending on whether referring to a right or left lens.

A base–apex line can be easily marked on a plano prism by means of a focimeter equipped with a marking device. It is merely necessary to rotate the prism until the displacement of the image seen in the eyepiece is exactly horizontal. The marking device then places on the prism three

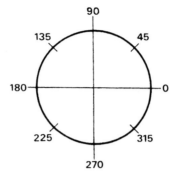

**Figure 13.6** The 360 degrees protractor.

dots which lie on a base–apex line. The direction (right or left) in which the image is displaced also indicates the side on which the base of the prism is situated. A scale in the eyepiece records the displacement of the image directly in terms of prism dioptres, thus giving the power of the prism as well.

Another method of finding the base–apex direction is to view a crossline chart through the prism, rotating the latter until one of the limbs appears unbroken, as in *Figure 13.7*. Two dots marked on the prism as shown then determine a base–apex line. The other limb of the crossline would be seen displaced towards the apex, appearing slightly curved if the prism were of high power. In this event, noticeable colour fringes would be seen, because the deviation varies with refractive index and hence with the wavelength of the incident light.

## Dividing prisms

Even if a prescription specifies a prism for one eye only, the same effect can be obtained by dividing the prism between the two eyes. This

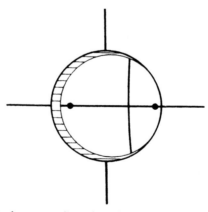

**Figure 13.7** Marking the base–apex line of a prism with the aid of a crossline chart.

expedient is sometimes advantageous. For example, it reduces the various image defects such as colour fringes and distortion which are noticeable with strong prisms. It also leads to a better match for weight and thickness.

That part of the original prism which is transferred to the other eye must always have its base direction reversed, bearing in mind that base out for one eye is opposite in direction to base out for the other eye, and similarly with base in. For example, $R4^\Delta$ *base out* would become, when equally divided

    $R2^\Delta$ base out
    $L2^\Delta$ base out

On the other hand, $R4^\Delta$ *base up* would become, when equally divided

    $R2^\Delta$ base up
    $L2^\Delta$ base down

Although an equal division is usual, it is by no means essential.

The above is sometimes referred to as 'splitting' or 'split' prisms. It should be performed only after seeking permission from the prescriber.

## Compounding and resolving prisms

Prescriptions occasionally call for a vertical prism in conjunction with a horizontal one, for example

    $L3^\Delta$ base down $4^\Delta$ base out

Or indeed, the above could be as a result of splitting prisms. The original order might have specified

    $R6^\Delta$ up
    $L8^\Delta$ out

A more balanced appearance would be obtained by splitting the prisms into

    $R3^\Delta$ up $4^\Delta$ out
    $L3^\Delta$ down $4^\Delta$ out

Taking our example (L), it is fairly evident that the combined effect could be produced by a single prism of appropriate power with its base in some oblique setting.

To find this resultant prism, draw an accurate diagram, remembering to work in standard notation. *Figure 13.8* reminds the reader of what was

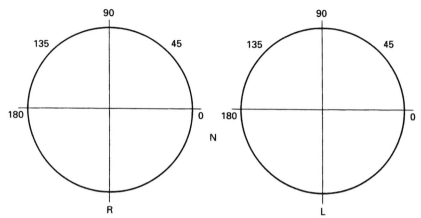

**Figure 13.8** Standard notation. N = nasal.

demonstrated in Chapter 7 with regard to this. Measurements are taken from an observer's point of view and the axis starts at zero on the right-hand side of each eye and goes around anti-clockwise.

Draw a set of lines at right-angles to one another and mark the nasal area along with the primary directions based on this (*Figure 13.9*).

Picking a suitable scale, i.e. 1 cm = 1 dioptre, mark a point equivalent to $3^\Delta$ down (*Figure 13.10*).

Now, mark a point equivalent to $4^\Delta$ out (*Figure 13.11*).

Construct a rectangle based on this and draw in a diagonal from the centre of the crosslines to the corner of the rectangle just drawn (*Figure 13.12*). This line represents both the magnitude and the base setting of the resultant prism. The line measures 5 units and therefore equals $5^\Delta$

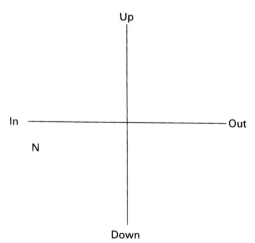

**Figure 13.9** Left eye representation showing principal directions.

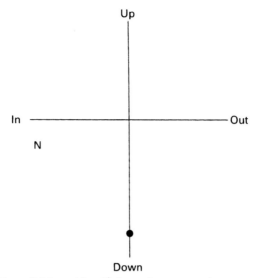

**Figure 13.10** As *Figure 13.9* but with a 3$^\Delta$ down drawn to 'scale'.

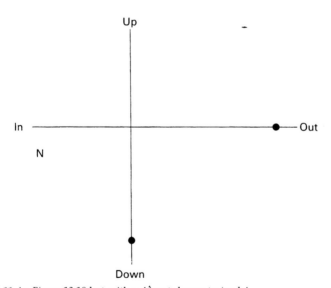

**Figure 13.11** As *Figure 13.10* but with a 4$^\Delta$ out drawn to 'scale'.

dioptres. The direction in relation to the centre of the crosslines and nasal area is down and out. Expressed in terms of a 360° notation the base direction is 323 (see *Figure 13.6*).

If a 180° notation is required the diagonal line needs to be extended so that it lies above the horizontal; measure the axis indicated (*Figure 13.13*).

Therefore, the answer to compounding the prisms in the example is either

$5^\Delta$ base 323

or

$5^\Delta$ base 143 down (or $5^\Delta$ base 143 out)

There is a mathematical solution to compounding prisms.

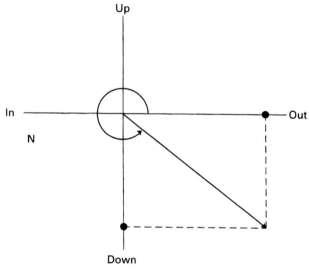

**Figure 13.12** As *Figure 13.11* but construction completed to show magnitude and angle of oblique prism.

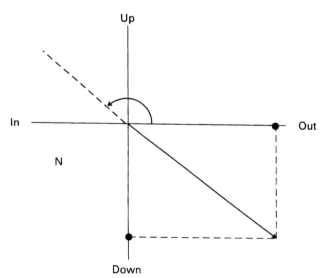

**Figure 13.13** As *Figure 13.12* but showing angle of prism in standard notation.

To find the magnitude of the single prism to replace the two separate prisms the following should be used:

$$P_R = \sqrt{P^2{}_V + P^2{}_H}$$

where

$P_R$ = the single resultant prism
$P_V$ = prism vertical
$P_H$ = prism horizontal

Remaining with the example the expression looks like this:

$$P_R = \sqrt{3^2 + 4^2}$$
$$P_R = \sqrt{9 + 16}$$
$$P_R = \sqrt{25}$$
$$P_R = 5^\Delta$$

To obtain the base setting use

$$\tan \theta = \frac{P_V}{P_H}$$

$$\tan \theta = \frac{3}{4}$$

$$\tan \theta = 37$$

A 'rough' diagram shows the prisms fall below the horizontal line (*Figure 13.14*). Therefore, the 37° must be where marked. This needs

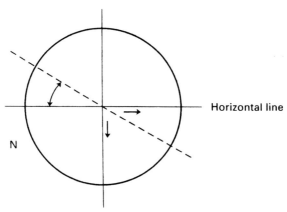

**Figure 13.14** A 'rough' diagram to ascertain if allowance has to be made to axis to bring into standard notation.

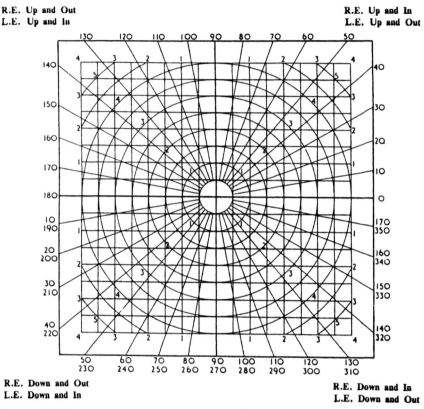

**R.E. Up and Out**
**L.E. Up and In**

**R.E. Up and In**
**L.E. Up and Out**

**R.E. Down and Out**
**L.E. Down and In**

**R.E. Down and In**
**L.E. Down and Out**

**Figure 13.15** Compounding and resolving prisms. The concentric circles give the magnitude of the resultant prism, while the protractor scaling shows the prism base setting for both the 180 and 360 degrees systems.

to be converted to standard notation by subtracting from 180 (180 − 37 = 143).

A compromise between the graphical and mathematical method is to use a chart as shown in *Figure 13.15*. The squares represent individual prisms with the resultant being based on the number of concentric circles (including the distances between them where the vertical and horizontal elements do not fall directly on a circle). The axis can be determined in either 180 or 360 degree notation.

*Figure 13.16* shows the chart as it should be used for our example, $3^\Delta$ down $4^\Delta$ out left eye. The small dots (•) represent 3 squares down, 4 squares out. The large dot (●) represents the completion of the 'rectangle'. It lies on the 5th circle out from the centre and therefore the magnitude of the prism is $5^\Delta$. The axis can be determined by the line drawn through the large dot and the centre of the chart (143°).

The process of finding the single prism which replaces two given prisms with different base settings is termed *compounding*. The reverse process, known as *resolving*, consists of finding the vertical and horizontal

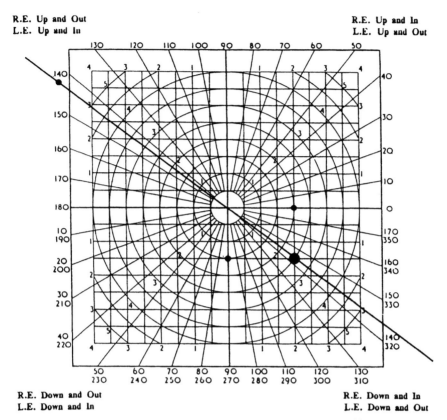

**Figure 13.16** Chart with vertical and horizontal prism values represented by • a magnitude of combined effect (●).

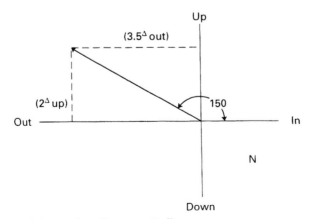

**Figure 13.17** Resolving a prism diagrammatically.

components which when combined would be equivalent to a single oblique prism, an example of which is shown below:

R4$^\Delta$ base 150 up

Draw a set of lines at right-angles to one another and mark the nasal area along with the primary directions based on this, and construct the prism at the required angle (*Figure 13.17*). Then complete the rectangle and measure the vertical and horizontal components. These are equivalent to the separate prisms

R2$^\Delta$ up 3.5$^\Delta$ out.

# Chapter 14

# Neutralisation

## Basic principle

Neutralisation is a simple, quick and surprisingly accurate method of checking or determining the power of a lens. It is carried out with the aid of a trial lens case or neutralising set, the only other piece of equipment needed being a crossline chart with its limbs horizontal and vertical. In default of such a chart, a window frame or other vertical and horizontal intersections can be used. It needs to be stated that the following is very rarely used today, except at educational establishments in an effort to help students understand certain basic optical elements.

Neutralisation is a process akin to weighing an article on a pair of scales. The article is placed in one pan and its weight is neutralised by placing standard weights in the other pan until the beam is level. In a similar way, lenses of known power are placed in contact with the lens under test until the power of the combination is reduced to zero. The lenses are then said to neutralise. Although the method is essentially one of trial and error, speed and confidence grow with practice and experience.

If the effects of lens thicknesses and other complications are ignored, it can be assumed that a lens under test will be neutralised by another lens or combination of lenses of equal but opposite power. For example, a +1.00 D lens is neutralised by a −1.00 D lens, the combined power being zero, and so on.

How do we know when a state of neutralisation has been achieved? The test is a simple yet sensitive one and is explained in the next section.

## Transverse and scissors movements

If a crossline chart or other suitable target is viewed through a parallel sheet of glass with plane surfaces free from defects, such as waviness, and the glass is then moved at right-angles to the line of sight – up and down or from side to side – there will be no apparent movement of the target. If however, the experiment is repeated with any minus spherical lens, it will be noted that in whatever direction the lens is moved transversely, the target appears to move in the same direction. This is termed a *with movement.* On the other hand, plus lenses give rise to an *against movement,* the target always appearing to move in the direction opposite to that of the lens. It is on the observation of these transverse movements that neutralisation depends: neutralisation is judged to occur when no such movements are detectable.

There is an apparent exception to the rule that plus lenses cause an against movement. If a medium or high-powered plus lens is held at a sufficient distance from the eye, the against movement will change to a with movement. When this occurs, it will also be seen that the image is inverted. In practice, no confusion can be caused because it is quite impossible to mistake a strong plus lens for a minus lens; and as neutralisation proceeds, the power of the combination becomes too weak for this reversal of movement to occur. *Figures 14.1* and *14.2* demonstrate transverse movements.

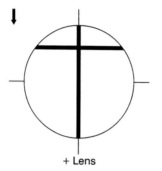

+ Lens

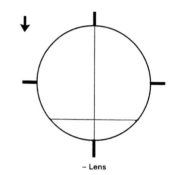

– Lens

**Figure 14.1** The effect of a plus lens when the 'transverse test' is applied. (Notice how the plus lens magnifies the limbs of the crossline.)

**Figure 14.2** The effect of a minus lens when the 'transverse test' is applied. (Notice how the minus lens minifies the limbs of the crossline.)

One also has the consideration that a plus lens will always be thicker at the centre than at the edge, whilst a minus will be thinner at the centre than at the edge.

When there is no displacement of the limbs, the point of intersection is the optical centre (*Figure 14.3*).

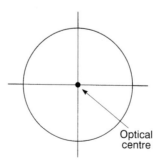

Optical centre

**Figure 14.3** How to find the optical centre of a lens.

Image movements of a quite different kind are utilised to determine at the outset whether a lens of unknown prescription is spherical or astigmatic. In the rotation test, the crossline chart is viewed while the lens is being rotated about the line of sight in a clockwise or anticlockwise direction. If the limbs of the crossline appear to remain horizontal and vertical, then the lens is of spherical power only. Astigmatic lenses behave very differently. As these are rotated, the intersecting lines comprising the crossline target appear to rotate in different directions from each other (*Figure 14.4b*) giving rise to what is aptly termed a scissors movement.

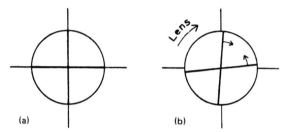

**Figure 14.4** 'Scissors' movement.

Scissors movement is also turned to good account to locate the principal meridians of an astigmatic lens: only when these meridians are exactly parallel to the crosslines does the scissors effect disappear (*Figure 14.4a*).

## Some general rules

A few general rules should be borne in mind:

1  *Always place the target at the furthest convenient distance.* A detailed study of the optics of neutralisation shows that significant errors creep in if a near target is employed.
2  *Always hold the lenses at arm's length.* By this means, small transverse movements are accentuated and made more visible.
3  *Use the fewest neutralising lenses possible to obtain the desired power and place the strongest of them next to the lens under test.* The reason for this rule is that errors due to lens thicknesses and separations are thereby reduced.

It goes without saying that the greatest care needs to be taken to avoid the lenses coming into contact with each other, which causes surface scratches.

A common mistake is to write down the powers of the neutralising lenses and forget to change their sign. The utmost vigilance is needed to avoid this pitfall.

## Neutralising spherical lenses

This is a very straightforward procedure. If the power of the lens is not known, a good idea can be obtained by noting the magnification it gives and the extent of the transverse movement.

Suppose that a first estimate is −5.00 D. Accordingly one selects a +5.00 D neutralising lens and, holding the two together at arm's length, look at the distant crossline and note whether the movement is 'with' or 'against'. If it is a with movement, the power of the combination is still minus, which means that the unknown lens is stronger than −5.00 D. On the other hand, if an against movement is seen, the +5.00 D neutralising lens must be the stronger of the two, and so the unknown lens must be weaker than −5.00 D. In either case the amount of movement will give an indication how close we are to neutralisation.

The next trial can now be made. If, for example, a moderate with movement was found at the first trial, one should try again with a stronger neutralising lens, say, +6.00 D. An against movement would now indicate a balance of plus power and would prove the lens to be weaker than −6.00 D. The field would hence be narrowed down considerably and only one or two more trials should be necessary to determine the power with some accuracy.

## Neutralising astigmatic lenses

The neutralisation of astigmatic lenses depends on exactly the same principles but naturally requires more steps. Two different methods are available.

*Method 1.* Only spherical neutralising lenses are used, the procedure being to neutralise each of the two principal meridians independently. The first step is to square up the lens under test with the crosslines until no scissors effect is seen. Its principal meridians are then horizontal and vertical.

The vertical meridian may now be neutralised by the procedure already described, the lens being moved up and down and attention confined to transverse movements of the horizontal limb of the crossline chart. If there is no apparent vertical movement when, say, a +1.50 D sphere is held in contact with the lens under test, then the principal power of the latter in the vertical meridian is −1.50 D.

The horizontal meridian may now be neutralised in a similar manner, attention being confined to transverse movements of the vertical line. In this way the principal power of the lens in the horizontal meridian may be determined.

Assume the horizontal meridian to be +2.00 D. Knowing the principal powers of the lens the prescription in either transposition can now be written down. In the example given it would be

−1.50 DS +3.50 DC

or

+2.00 DS −3.50 DC

The following rule may be useful. If the two principal powers are $A$ and $B$, then the two alternative transpositions are:

$A$ sphere combined with $(B − A)$ cylinder

or

$B$ sphere combined with $(A − B)$ cylinder.

It is, of course, essential to take signs into account when subtracting one principal power from the other. To subtract a negative quantity, change its sign to positive and add.


*Method 2.* In this method both spherical and plano-cylindrical neutralising lenses are used, the aim being to secure neutralisation of the lens as a whole.

As in Method 1, the first step is to square up the principal meridians of the lens under test with the crosslines by rotating it until the scissors effect disappears.

Also as in Method 1, the next step is to neutralise the vertical meridian with a spherical lens. Assume that a −1.00 D neutralising sphere is needed for this purpose.

It is at this point that the two methods diverge. Neutralisation has been achieved in the vertical meridian but there will still be transverse movement in the horizontal meridian due to the cylinder power of the lens. This movement would be neutralised by adding to the neutralising sphere a plano cylinder of the requisite power with its axis vertical.

One accordingly proceeds as follows:

A first estimate of the cylinder power can be made by noting the residual horizontal movement of the vertical line when the lens under test is moved from side to side with the neutralising sphere held in contact with it. For example, a small against movement might suggest a cylinder power of +0.50 D. The next trial would hence be made with a −0.50 D cylinder from the neutralising set, held with its axis vertical in contact with the −1.00 D neutralising sphere previously found. In practice it will be found convenient to hold the lens under test in one hand and the neutralising lenses in the other, keeping the three as close together as possible. It is very important that the axis of the neutralising cylinder should be accurately aligned: any error can easily be detected because it will give rise to scissors effect. A transverse test in the horizontal meridian is now made with the whole combination and the process repeated until the correct neutralising cylinder has been found. All transverse movements should now have disappeared, in which case the prescription of the lens can be written down by merely reversing the signs of the neutralising lenses. For example, if they are −1.00 D sphere and −0.25 D cylinder, the prescription of the lens is +1.00 DS +0.25 DC. Each of the methods described above has points in its favour. The first is probably the more accurate but the second is often preferred.

It is important to realise that neutralisation by itself gives no information as to how the total power of the lens under test is divided between the two surfaces. In other words, it tells us nothing about the form of the lens. This can be ascertained with the aid of a lens measure.

## Neutralisation of curved lenses

The neutralisation of curved lenses presents a point of difficulty. To check the back vertex power of a lens, the neutralising lenses should be placed in contact with the back surface – a requirement which cannot be fulfilled. In practice there would be an air space of some 3–6 mm which would affect the accuracy of the result. In order to obtain closer contact the usual procedure is to hold the neutralising lenses next to the front surface. Unfortunately, the result thus obtained is the front vertex power – sometimes known as the *neutralising power* – and this is not the same as the back vertex power, being invariably weaker.

With minus lenses the difference is usually small enough to ignore but with plus lenses the difference does become significant. For example, a regular meniscus of average thickness with a back vertex power of +5.00 D would neutralise at the front surface as +4.75 D. Unless a carefully calculated allowance is made, it must be admitted that neutralisation fails as a method of checking the power of curved plus lenses over about +2.00 D. A focimeter – an instrument to be described in the next chapter – is needed for this purpose.

When neutralising curved lenses, attention must be confined to a small central portion of the crosslines. Even when the lens is accurately neutralised the ends of the crosslines may show some movement. This is not a true transverse movement but is due to aberration and should be ignored. A good idea is to make a 'mask' – a small piece of paper with a hole – to ensure that the aberrations at the lens edge are not picked up. This allows for concentrated gaze to be obtained through a small central portion of the lens. Simply hold the mask up to the lenses being neutralised.

# Chapter 15

# The focimeter (lens analyser or lensmeter)

The focimeter is probably the one instrument that is most used throughout optics – in the consulting room, dispensing area, workshop and prescription house. Without a focimeter, it would be very difficult to check accurately the large volume of lenses which are produced and sold today.

The conventional type of focimeter originating around 1910 employs an optical system which depends on the skill and experience of the operator in judging the position of best focus, adjusted by a manual control. During recent years, a radically different type of instrument has appeared in which visual judgement is replaced by photosensors and electronic circuitry. In short, it is automated.

A practice uses the focimeter when the patient's old spectacle lenses need to be verified and when their new spectacles are complete, and need to be checked for accuracy before being issued. The laboratory uses the instrument to check lens powers and prisms, set axes, before glazing and then to give a final check to the finished spectacles before despatch.

To carry out all of these tasks, an accurate instrument is required. After all, it would be of little point producing perfect lenses if there were no instrument to match this accuracy when checking the final product. To be effective, the design should be correct, the mechanical stability of the instrument must be guaranteed and there should be no possibility of wear and tear allowing inaccuracies to creep in after prolonged use.

A focimeter can be used to check:

> spherical lens power
> cylindrical lens power
> axis
> reading addition
> prismatic correction – power and direction
> optical centre of the lens.

It can also be used to mark:

> actual optical centre
> required optical centre when prism is present
> axis direction.

Suitably designed focimeters will also measure contact lens powers.

The more sophisticated machines (and these are the ones generally referred to as lens analysers or lensmeters) offer additional features. Some can produce transmission graphs of tinted or ultra-violet-treated lenses, normally between 290 and 700 nm. Not only can the graph be printed, but the amount of visible light transmitted along with ultra-violet trans- mittance is indicated on the printout. A very useful tool for checking the integrity of any tint or ultra-violet treatment. Other lens analysers allow determination of distance between optical centres without having to align the lenses central in the device. They can even determine any vertical prismatic imbalance that might exist between a pair of glazed lenses. Others have programs especially designed so that checking of pro- gressive lenses becomes easier. The analyser directs the operator to the strategic points on the lens where measurements should be taken. In addition, some can produce contour plots of progressives to allow comparison of different types or help in identification.

Most have printers incorporated so that a 'hard copy' of what is seen on the screen can be produced. Needless to say, many have facilities for linking to a computer system. Once the computer has been programmed with relevant standards it is possible for the analyser and computer working in conjunction to deem whether a particular lens is a pass or fail!

Some have attachments that allow blocking of single vision lenses for glazing so that laying off operatives can position the lens correctly with regard to the patients requirements and apply a glazing block at the same time, thereby removing the need for a separate operation.

Most recent developments have been the ability of the analyser to determine the refractive index of the lens being assessed. This is very useful with the ever-increasing number of higher index materials on the market.

Over the years there have been many designs of focimeter, but they have all been produced from two basic designs:

1 Ocular or eyepiece (*Figure 15.1*), where an image is viewed through an optical system, similar to a telescope or microscope eyepiece.
2 Projection, where an image is projected on to a screen which the operator then views.

Nowadays, projection models can be further subdivided into those where the results are viewed 'optically' and those that are displayed electron- ically (digitally) on an output screen – either LED, LCD or VDU. Whichever system is used, the same basic principles apply. A measuring system is set up and calibrated in its 'zero' state, so that the target image is correctly focused or the electronic circuit is balanced. When the lens to be measured is introduced, the system becomes unbalanced. By various means the focimeter is then brought back into 'focus' or balance and the results read from the scale or screen.

The use of LEDs to take the readings automatically necessitates the use of red light. For lens materials with lower Abbe numbers (normally higher index) this can cause inaccuracies, hence the facility on most analysers to adjust the Abbe number to that of the material being

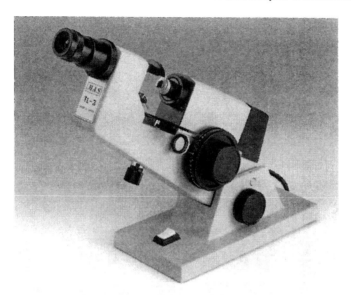

**Figure 15.1** A conventional eyepiece focimeter.

checked. Failure to do this will produce inaccurate power readings. Traditionally 'manual' focimeters work on a different wavelength and will give accurate readings across a range of Abbe numbers.

## Eyepiece design

A basic layout for an optical eyepiece instrument is shown in *Figure 15.2*. This shows:

T   = illuminated target
C   = collimating lens system
LR = lens rest
O   = objective
G   = graticule
E   = eyepiece.

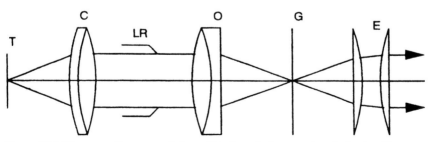

**Figure 15.2** Diagrammatic representation of the layout of an eyepiece focimeter. (From Jarratt, A. J., by permission.)

Light from the target, which is at the focal point of the collimator, is passed as a parallel beam through the lens rest, towards the objective. This, in turn, brings the light to a focus at the graticule. The sharp image is then viewed by means of the eyepiece telescopic system.

If an unknown lens is now introduced into the beam path, with its back surface against the lens rest, the light will no longer emerge parallel and the image at G will be out of focus (*Figure 15.3*). By moving the target towards or away from the collimator, the light can be brought back into focus. As the lens rest is at the other focal point of the collimator, the movement of the target is directly proportional to the power of the unknown lens. This means that the size of the image seen in the eyepiece remains constant for any power under test and a linear scale can be used for measurement.

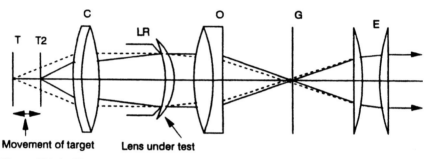

**Figure 15.3** As *Figure 15.2* but with a 'lens' introduced to the system. (From Jarrett, A. J., by permission.)

The measuring scale can either be engraved around the handwheel, used to move the target into focus, or directly attached to the target. The former method is cheaper to produce but can lead to inaccuracies due to mechanical wear. The wheel has to be linked to the target by means of gearing and this gearing wears. This in turn produces 'backlash' or slack in the system. This slack means that the measuring wheel can turn before the target is moved, introducing an error.

It is best to attach the scale to the target and to view this scale through an independent magnifying system, either on a separate screen or in the eyepiece. With this method, any wear that is present does not affect the accuracy, as the reading is taken directly from the target.

The target can be in the form of a ring of dots. When a spherical lens is being measured, the dots will remain in a ring shape, but a cylindrical lens will show the dots as a series of lines. It will be possible to bring these into focus along the two principal meridians of the lens (i.e. at right-angles to each other). These two positions will give the spherical and combined powers – the difference between the two being the cylindrical power (*Figure 15.4*).

This ring target provides the easiest method of focusing but for low cylinders (say 0.25 D), the lengths of the lines produced are very short and look very much like slightly distorted dots. In these circumstances it is

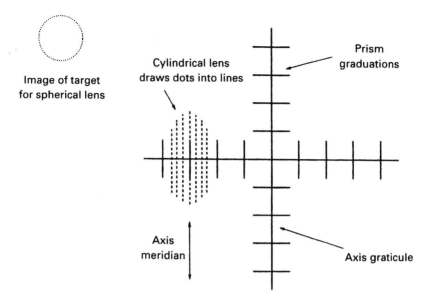

**Figure 15.4** Ring target demonstrated. (From Jarratt, A. J., by permission.)

difficult to determine the axis direction. A more accurate method for these low cylinders is to provide a crossline target or perhaps a combination of both.

By providing a rotatable crossline graticule, which can be viewed in the eyepiece, the axis can be determined. The crossline is rotated so that it aligns with the target lines and the axis is then read from a protractor scale.

## Projection instruments

Projection focimeters work on similar lines, i.e. the lens to be measured is introduced into the optical beam path of the system and the system is then brought back to zero and the lens power read from the scale or screen.

A typical design for such an instrument is shown in *Figure 15.5*. Here the parts are the same as *Figure 15.2*, except

$$
\begin{aligned}
\text{M1 to M5} &= \text{front silvered mirrors} \\
\text{S1} &= \text{image viewing screen} \\
\text{S2} &= \text{power reading screen} \\
\text{PS} &= \text{power scale.}
\end{aligned}
$$

An image of the target T is formed by the optical system on screen S1. If a lens is introduced at the lens rest (LR), the system again becomes out of focus and a blurred image is formed. By moving the target, towards or away from the collimator, the image can be brought back into focus. The movement of the target T is projected via the mirror M5 on to a small

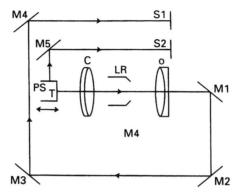

**Figure 15.5** Diagrammatic representation of the layout of a projection focimeter. (From Jarratt, A. J., by permission.)

viewing screen S2, the amount of movement relating to the power of the lens under test.

Apart from one or two differences, the choice between the designs is basically one of cost and preference. The eyepiece designs are always cheaper than a projection type but are no less accurate. There are certain advantages in a projection design – there is no requirement for the operator to adjust the eyepiece for his or her ocular correction and several viewers can see the results at the same time – this cannot be done with an eyepiece design.

## Preliminary adjustment

Eyepiece designs depend for their final accuracy, on the accuracy with which the operator sets the eyepiece adjustment. The user's eye becomes part of the optical system and this must be taken into account. Any uncorrected ocular error in the eye will affect the actual measurement of the lens power.

Therefore, before use the machine must be set to zero. If this is not done, or is not carried out accurately, the results will always be wrong. The setting must also be carried out correctly; if it is adjusted to a setting which is too minus, the user can accommodate to bring the target image back into focus. In this condition, the machine will not be set at 'zero' and could be out by a significant amount. To ensure an accurate setting, the eyepiece adjustment ring should always be racked outwards so that the setting is to the plus side; this will overcome any latent accommodation that might be exerted. The ring is then turned towards the minus direction, until the target becomes clearly focused. The machine will then be set to zero, without any accommodation error. This resetting should always be carried out before the machine is used. Someone else with an uncorrected ocular condition may have used the focimeter in the meantime. If a check is not made, an error will occur.

A similar check should also be carried out at regular intervals during the working day. If an operator uses the machine for long periods, fatigue may affect the user's ocular condition and a correction to the setting may be required to overcome this. These problems do not occur with a projection model, as the image is projected on to a screen and therefore the operator's eye is not then a part of an optical system; accommodation or fatigue will not affect the actual measurement of the lens power. This, and the fact that several viewers can see the results at the same time, is the main advantage of projection models.

It is essential that all focimeters are calibrated on a regular basis. This is normally facilitated by the use of a calibration gauge, specially made for the purpose. Calibration is different from preliminary adjustment in that it checks the integrity of the focimeter, not the operator.

If a company is a holder of a ISO 9000 certificate or equivalent, then part of its regular regime is to recalibrate all of its measuring equipment.

## Preliminary overview

Lenses are normally positioned with their back (or concave) surface against the lens rest. This ensures that the focimeter reads the back vertex power of the lens, which relates to the prescribed power required by the patient. Strictly speaking this only holds good for distance Rx read directly through the optical centre of the lens. Near powers in multifocals and progressives do not relate directly to the prescribed power, due to difference between the beam path of the focimeter and the optical path for the wearer. This subject is, however, outside the scope of this overview.

The only time when a lens is measured with its convex surface against the lens rest is when it has a front surface segment or addition. Here, it is correct to read the front vertex power for the distance and near portions and to take the difference between the two as being the correct reading addition. If this is not done, the reading power will appear to be too high, as it is affected by the lens thickness – in these cases the back vertex reading power will always be higher than the true prescribed power.

Current designs now make extensive use of micro-electronics, for both measurement and display. Using these, it is now possible to determine lens powers automatically and to have the results displayed on a digital screen (*Figure 15.6*). This does not necessarily ensure a higher degree of accuracy over purely optical designs but it can allow a less experienced operator to take readings, particularly useful within a practice where a trainee or receptionist can easily check lens powers and axes. For higher volume work within the manufacturing industry, a careful choice has to be made. Some of the present designs are too sensitive for very fast work; a slight movement of the lens can swing an axis or alter a power reading quite alarmingly.

These digital focimeters can be obtained in two basic versions. The first still allows the operator to focus a target on a screen and a power is then read off from a digital screen. As an alternative, the whole operation can be fully automatic. The lens under test is placed in the lens clamp and the machine automatically resets and then displays the results on the screen. With this type, no operator intervention is required, other than putting the lens in place and adjusting one or two controls.

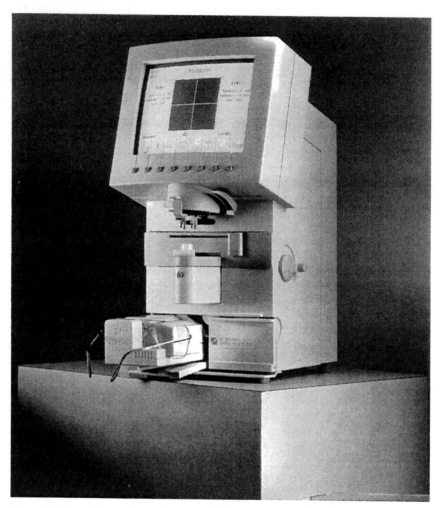

**Figure 15.6** A modern automatic lensmeter. (Picture courtesy of Carl Zeiss.)

One other advantage of the modern digital machine is its ability to display the sphere and cylinder powers, rather than the cross cyl form (e.g. individual powers for each meridian). One of the easiest mistakes to make when using a normal optical design is incorrect mental arithmetic to arrive at the sphere/cyl powers.

It should be made clear that whilst the more advanced types of focimeters allow less experienced people to obtain a power reading, there is far more to checking a lens than just its power. The axis, prism, vertical imbalance and insets all have to be assessed for conformity to the relevant standard. Skill is required to determine that even though a lens may not be 100% correct, it may still be within specified tolerances. Without a doubt, the newer breeds of focimeter do make the task of training easier.

## To determine lens power

The following notes describe the routine to be followed when verifying the power of finished spectacles. It will be assumed that the focimeter is of the non-automated type.

A focimeter measures the vertex power corresponding to the surface in contact with the lens rest. Hence, to measure the back vertex power the back vertex of the lens should be placed against the rest. Before final focusing adjustment is made, the platform and position of the spectacles should be adjusted so as to centralise the target with reference to the eyepiece graticule or projection screen. When checking a lens in uncut form it is normal to drop the platform down out of the way as its main function is to support spectacle frames in the correct horizontal position.

Spherical lenses should present no difficulty because the target is in focus in only one position and the power is given directly by the reading on a dioptre scale.

Astigmatic lenses are not quite so easy to check because the instrument does not record the prescription as written but the principal powers of the lens. However, the following simple scheme should remove all difficulties.

| **Power recorded** | **Direction of focal lines** |
|---|---|
| | *First reading* |
| Sphere alone | Rt angles to cyl axis |
| | *Second reading* |
| Sphere + cyl | Parallel to cyl axis |

Suppose, for example, that the perscription is

+2.00 DS −3.50 DC × 40

The first reading should be that of the sphere alone (+2.00 D) with the focal lines at 130 degrees. The second reading should be the algebraic sum of sphere and cylinder (−1.50 D) with the focal lines at 40 degrees.

It is perhaps worth mentioning that when the target consists of dots, the length of each focal line is proportional to the cylinder power of the lens under test. When the cylinder power is 0.25 D or less, the focal lines are very short and it is difficult to judge when they are exactly parallel to the index line on the eyepiece graticule.

To determine the power of an astigmatic lens when its prescription is unknown, the following routine should be adopted:

1 Bring either set of lines into focus and record the first reading as the spherical power, e.g. +1.75 D.
2 Focus the other set of lines, this time recording their direction as well as the power reading, e.g. +1.25 D at 30 degrees. The latter figure gives the axis direction.
3 To find the cylinder power, subtract the first reading from the second, taking signs into account. In this instance it should be (+1.25 D) − (+1.75 D) = −0.50 D.

The prescription is therefore

+1.75 DS –0.50 DC × 30

If the +1.25 D reading had been taken first, the result would have been

+1.25 DS +0.50 DC × 120

which is, of course, the plus cylinder transposition of the first prescription.


## Centration and prismatic effects

Presume that a plano prism is under test. The target should be seen in sharp focus when the power scale records zero but it will appear displaced from the centre of the eyepiece graticule. As expected, the amount of displacement is a measure of the prism power, which can be read from a scale in the eyepiece graticule. The direction in which the target image is displaced gives the direction of the prism base. For example, an upward displacement indicates prism base up and so on.

Assume that a plus spherical lens is under test. If the optical centre falls on the optical axis of the instrument, no prismatic effect is introduced and the target when focused should therefore be seen in the centre of the eyepiece graticule. On the other hand, if the lens is decentred with respect to the instrument, it will give rise to a prismatic effect as though by decentration and the target image will be displaced accordingly.

The focimeter can thus be used to locate the optical centre of a lens; alternatively, it will measure the prismatic effect at a given point on a lens, provided that the given point can be accurately positioned on the optical axis of the instrument. The optical axis should, of course, pass through the centre of the aperture of the lens rest.

All focimeters have a marking device used for checking the accuracy of optical centration. It places three dots in a horizontal line on the lens, the centre dot lying on the optical axis of the instrument. Consequently, when the lenses are so positioned that there is no displacement of the target image, the central dot marks the position of the optical centre of the lens under test. After each lens has been 'dotted' (assuming a completed pair of spectacles has been checked at this stage, as against individual separate lenses), the spectacles can be transferred to a suitable frame rule to check whether the optical centres are in the correct position relative to the lens shape, that is at the centration points.

Checking is also very simple when the prescription incorporates a prism, for example, $1^\Delta$ base down. In this case the height of the individual lens or pair of spectacles can be adjusted so as to displace the target image downwards with its centre exactly on the $1^\Delta$ graduation of the prism dioptre scale. The marking device would then be operated, the central dot showing the position of the optical centre when the prescribed prism is neutralised. If the lens has been correctly made, the central dot will coincide with the centration point.

# Verification procedures

## Procedure for checking high power prisms

A prismatic lens will move the target image across the screen and if the prismatic power is too high the image can disappear from the screen entirely. To overcome this, many focimeters can be fitted (some come as standard) with a prism compensator, or separate supplementary prisms. They, in effect, will realign the beam path through the instrument so as to bring the target back into view.

## Procedure for checking high powers

As with prismatic supplementary lenses, some focimeters can be fitted with a lens to increase the power range to that normally achievable. For example, assume that a focimeter has a maximum plus power range of +25.00 dioptres and a +28.00 DS lens needs to be checked. A supplementary −5.00 D lens may be available which is then slotted into the special holder. Effectively, this decreases all readings through the focimeter by −5.00 dioptres. If the +28.00 DS lens is placed into the focimeter it should read, because of the supplementary lens, +23.00 DS ((28.00) + (−5.00)).

As with supplementary prism lenses, do not forget to remove them when they are finished with, otherwise problems will occur!

## Procedure for checking differential prism (vertical imbalance)

Ideally, unless instructions to the contrary, it would be expected that both optical centres of a pair of spectacles should be on the same horizontal plane (level with each other). If they are not then what is termed 'vertical imbalance' can be induced. On lower powers a small difference between the heights of the optical centres will not cause a great prismatic error; however, as the power increases so does the vertical prismatic error.

It is important when checking a pair of lenses that the 'high to low' rule is used, that is to say, when checking to ascertain what prism has been induced due to the optical centres not being level, the lens that is the highest power in the vertical meridian must always be checked first. For example, the following Rx:

R+ +2.00 DS +1.00 DC × 90

L+ +0.25 DS +3.00 DC × 180

The right lens is +2.00 D in the vertical, the left is +3.25 D, and therefore the left eye is checked and 'dotted' before checking the right eye. Any prism exhibited should then be compared to allowed tolerances.

## Procedure for checking add powers

As indicated earlier in this chapter, most lenses are checked at the back vertex. However, a special procedure needs to be adopted for checking the addition on lenses that have the segment or progressive surface incorporated into the front. In fact most multifocal and progressive lenses are of this design, with very few having the segment incorporated into the back surface.

The procedure for checking lenses with front surface additions should be as follows:

1 Check distance Rx in the normal manner – back vertex power.
2 Turn lens around in focimeter so that the front of the lens is resting against the lens rest (*Figure 15.7*). Bring any set of focimeter lines into focus and note the power reading (it will not necessarily be exactly the distance power).

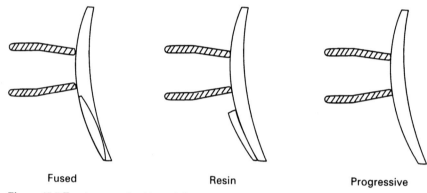

Fused                    Resin                    Progressive

**Figure 15.7** Front vertex checking of distance portion.

3 Remaining with the lens with its front towards the lens rest, move it so that the segment or reading area is positioned over the focimeter (*Figure 15.8*). Bring into focus the same set of lines applicable in step 2. The addition is equal to the difference between the two readings obtained from steps 2 and 3.

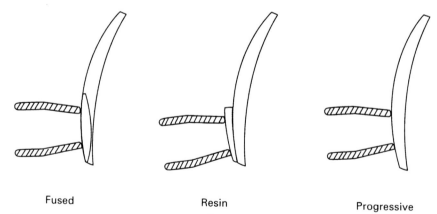

Fused                    Resin                    Progressive

**Figure 15.8** Front vertex checking of reading portion. The difference between the power in the distance (*Figure 15.7*) and the power in the reading is equivalent to the addition.

It may be applicable to use a supplementary prism when checking in the reading area due to the fact that often the image is very low down in the focimeter target area or indeed, in some instances, off the target completely.

Why check addition in this 'strange' way? The patient looks through the lens from the other side! The answer is simple. When the semi-finished manufacturer is producing a lens with a front surface addition they do not know exactly what prescription or thickness the finished lens will be. For this reason they can only ensure that the relationship between the distance and reading areas are correct for the surfaces they are producing, which as stated, are on the front. If one takes the middle lens in *Figure 15.8* and assume that the front surface of the distance portion is +6.00 D, then to create a +2.00 reading addition the curvature on the segment would be +8.00, the difference between the distance and reading curvature creating the required +2.00 addition. However, this +6.00 D base lens could be used for a range of powers between plano and +4.00, the higher powers would have a greater finished lens thickness than the lower powers which in turn will have the effect of placing the addition farther away from the patient. This will affect the power perceived by the patient in the reading area. As this is beyond the semi-finished manufacturers control, the addition is checked on the surfaces they do control – the front.

Most lens analysers have a facility to calculate the addition automatically based on measurements taken in the distance and reading areas.

## In conclusion

This chapter by way of an introduction to the focimeter and its uses cannot replace practical tuition given by an experienced operative. It is not possible to use a focimeter just by reading about it. 'Hands on' experience is needed which can only be achieved by sitting down with a focimeter and 'having a go'.

# Chapter 16

# Glazing

The operation of fitting lenses to a spectacle frame or mount is known variously as mounting, fitting or glazing. The term is usually understood to include the previous process of cutting and edging. Nevertheless, it is the frame which is glazed, not the lenses.

Edging is the name given to the process of grinding away the lens edge to produce the finished size and shape required, at the same time imparting the desired edge form. The insertion of lenses into rimmed plastic frames is known as *springing in* or *pushing in* and the glazing of rimless mounts as *rimless fitting*.

## Laying off

Before a lens can be edged it must be marked so that its cylinder axis (if any) is set as specified by the prescription and its optical centre is in the correct position relative to the lens shape. For bifocals and trifocals the segment top position relative to the horizontal centre line, along with the horizontal positioning of the segments, have to be taken into consideration. Progressives, whilst not having a segment, have to have their fitting cross positioned as per the patient's requirements. This process is known as *laying off*. It is performed with the aid of a focimeter and its marking device – often as a sequel to checking the power of the lens.

In using the focimeter for laying off there are several sources of inaccuracy which are apt to be overlooked or ignored. In the first place, the focimeter target should itself be accurately centred with respect to the eyepiece graticule. This, unfortunately, is not always the case. Secondly, the marking attachment may not be correctly positioned or may develop excessive play through wear. The 'three points' should lie on a line which is parallel to the 180 degree meridian of the axis protractor and the centre point should, of course, be accurately positioned on the optical axis of the instrument. Neither of these assumptions can be taken for granted and the instrument should therefore be checked from time to time with a calibration gauge as suggested in Chapter 15.

As referred to earlier, laying off is normally a sequel to the actual checking of the lens for its optical properties. As part of this process the lens will have been 'dotted' by the marking device of the focimeter, thus indicating the optical centre position and the horizontal meridian. It should be appreciated that whilst a focimeter can actually dot the cylinder axis, it would normally be used to dot the horizontal meridian when the axis has been set to the patient's requirements. The aim of the prescription house throughout the subsequent procedures is to keep the dots horizontal, for then it is clear that the lens is set at the correct axis.

The laying off of the lens is normally performed by a machine but it can be performed by hand. Although an outdated system, laying off by hand can still be a useful skill. High powered lenses are often handled this way because, when placed under the viewer of a marking/laying off machine, the image is distorted due to the power.

The following is a brief description of laying off by hand. A protractor (*Figure 16.1*), focimeter and felt pen are necessary to perform the task.

The focimeter is used to mark the optical centre and horizontal meridian, as outlined above, by means of three 'dots'. If no decentration is called for, the uncut lens is merely placed on the protractor with the marked optical centre directly over the centre of the protractor. At the same time the dots indicating the horizontal direction must be made to lie on the horizontal line of the protractor. If a decentration has been

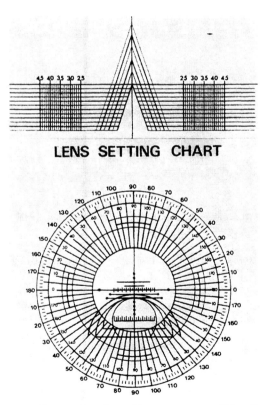

**Figure 16.1** A protractor/lens setting chart. (Picture courtesy of Norville Optical, Gloucester, England.)

specified, the lens must be placed on the protractor so that the marked centre is correspondingly displaced.

In either case, when the lens has been correctly set, a horizontal line is marked across its front surface immediately over the horizontal line of the protractor, and a short vertical stroke is made immediately over the vertical line of the protractor.

*Figure 16.2* shows a lens with its axis at 70 degrees laid off for the right eye so as to give a decentration of 2 mm down and 3 mm in. It is customary to indicate the nasal extremity of the horizontal line by means of an arrow head, as illustrated, and to mark the lens R or L to indicate right or left. Some companies prefer to mark up the lens on the front surface, whilst others will mark the back.

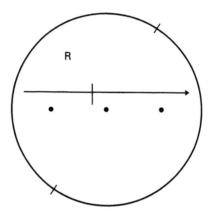

**Figure 16.2** Lens laid off for the R eye to give a decentration of 2 mm down and 3 mm in (marked up on front).

In laying off a lens, accuracy and neatness go hand in hand. Thick, wavy lines create a poor impression and make it impossible for the glazing staff to attain a high degree of accuracy. There is no reason why a low standard of artistry should be accepted as inevitable. A good deal of practice is required but it is possible to draw freehand, with a felt pen, a remarkably straight yet thin line.

Bifocals, trifocals and progressives deserve a special mention, for of course they have the additional consideration of segment position, both vertically and horizontally, or fitting cross position.

If the distance optical centre and cylinder axis have been correctly worked in relation to the segment height and insetting specified, no special treatment should be required. In practice, however, especially with low powers, it is extremely difficult to control these surfacing details with all the accuracy desired. In order that the segments of a pair should reasonably match for height and insetting, it may hence be necessary to make some small compromises in relation to distance optical centres and cylinder axes, taking advantage of the permitted tolerances.

There are many devices designed to replace the hand marking procedure just described. One is the projection marker. The lens with its focimeter dots is viewed against the protractor and positioned to give any decentration required. The marking device is then actuated.

A further development renders this second marking unnecessary. When the lens is correctly positioned in relation to the protractor, the device for holding the lens in the automatic edger – either a suction cup or pad with double-sided adhesive tape – is pressed straight on to the lens.

Some edging systems, due to previous input of information will display visually where such items as optical centres, segment tops or fitting crosses should be placed, the operative only having to match the lens position shown on screen.

## Lens cutting

Having now layed-off the lens it must now be cut to the correct shape. Today, this is achieved by the use of automatic edgers (*Figure 16.3*). However, many years ago before resin lenses, this process was done by hand. The eyeshape was drawn on to the lens and a wheel cutter was subsequently used to score the surface. Cribbing pliers were then used to reduce the glass lens to its approximate shape. Alternatively, shanking tongs could be used to crumble the edge away until it roughly resembled the eyeshape. The lens would then be hand edged on an abrasive wheel to obtain the final fit and finish. Designs of automatic flat edging and bevel edging machines have improved over the years. In all these machines the

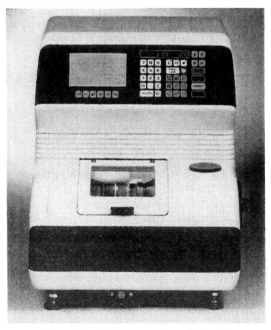

Figure 16.3 An automatic lens edger. (Picture courtesy of Weco.)

lens is mounted on a rotating spindle and held against the grinding surface of an abrasive wheel by gravity or spring pressure (*Figure 16.4*). Traditionally, the shape was controlled by a template or former.

Developments in automatic edging machinery have followed several interesting lines. The first was the introduction of diamond impregnated wheels which removed material very quickly. A later development was the introduction of various ingenious systems for controlling the rotation of the spindle so as to eliminate unproductive time. Instead of revolving at uniform speed, the spindle is allowed to dwell in one position as long as material is being removed. Another notable innovation is the idea of combining flat edging and bevelling in one machine. A diamond impregnated wheel is used to flat edge the uncut lens to the desired shape and virtually to size, whereupon it is automatically transferred to other wheels within the machine to either put the final flat edge or bevels on it.

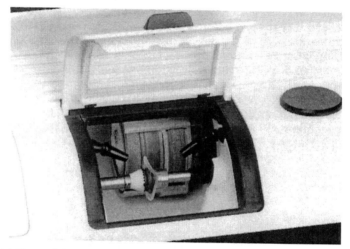

**Figure 16.4** Lens edging in progress. (Picture courtesy of Weco.)

Today's modern edging machines can be set to run in conjunction with a robotic unit. The lenses are loaded automatically and information regarding shape, bevel style, etc. is determined from a bar code on the front of the job tray. Many have the facilities to apply all types of bevels, grooves or flat edges along with safety chamfers and polished edges, all in one operation of the machine. They can perform 'double-checks' to ensure sizing is precisely to the pre-determined requirements. Operatives can control the bevel/groove position to satisfy any special requests on the order or to enable a difficult order to be fulfilled. This can be on the basis of a one-off or can be pre-programmed into the machine for continued use under specific circumstances. It is beyond the scope of this brief account to describe all the various machines embodying these and other developments and refinements. They all incorporate distinctive valuable features and their designers have shown great ingenuity.

In giving this brief description of automatic lens edgers, several different relevant factors have been introduced, namely, how does the machine know what shape to cut and what finish does it put on the lens edge? Take each one in turn.

## Cutting and edging formers

The established traditional way of converting an uncut lens to the desired shape is by the use of a former. It is normally made from flat plastics material but metal plates have also been used. It is held in position on the machine by holes or slots which not only determine the horizontal line of the shape but also the standard optical centre position. In the design illustrated (*Figure 16.5*), the horizontal line passes through the centre of each hole. The centre of the middle hole, which lies on the axis of revolution of the former, is the box centre position. The size and positioning of the locating holes may vary.

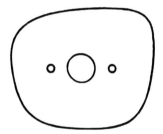

**Figure 16.5** A former with three holes for location.

A prescription house would normally keep in stock formers for all the most popular frames it handles. As frames are available in three, four or more different eyesizes, a former for each would have to be held. For those frames where a former is not available from stock a former cutting machine is used. The frame is mounted on the machine and a 'feeler' arm is inserted into the groove and is traced around the inner rim. A cutter placed elsewhere on the machine mirrors the feeler's movements on to a blank flat plate of plastics to create a former. These formers are then either used once and discarded or labelled and put into stock for future use. It is not hard to imagine all the problems of keeping and indexing all of these! Problems also occur unless several formers of the same size are kept, in that when the former required is out in the workshop on another order, a decision has to be made as to whether to allow the job to wait for the former to be returned or to make another on the former or pattern making machine.

Today's more efficient method is to use electronic formers. The frame is still traced around the inner rim, but the shape is stored in a computer memory and can be recalled at any time. Various systems are available, the main difference between these and the traditional former method being that the former does not actually exist with the computer-assisted principle, except in its memory!

Technology such as this facilitates what could be termed 'distance edging', allowing the frame to be traced at one location and the lenses edged to precisely the correct size and shape at another. The edged lenses can then be sent to the location holding the frame, for insertion into it. This way, no valuable time is lost whilst the frame is sent in the post to the prescription house. It gives all concerned greater control of the situation and a speedier outcome for the patient.

## Edge forms and finishes

### Flat edge

Illustrated in *Figure 16.6a* is the simplest form of edge. It is used mainly for lenses fitted to rimless mounts or as an intermediate stage in the production of other edge forms.

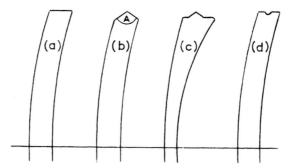

**Figure 16.6** Common edge forms: (a) flat edge; (b) bevel edge; (c) minibevel; (d) grooved edge.

### Bevel edged

The bevel edge form illustrated in *Figure 16.6b* is used for lenses to be fitted into rimmed frames, the bevel being inserted into a groove on the inside of the rim. The included angle of the bevel, shown as A in the diagram, is usually in the neighbourhood of 115–120 degrees. To avoid pressure on the peak of the bevel and the attendant risk of chipping the lens, the groove in the rim is made with a smaller included angle, usually 90–100 degrees. This gives clearance at the apex, the pressure being exerted on the shoulders of the bevel as shown in *Figure 16.7*.

It will be apparent from this diagram that there is a relationship between the angle of the bevel and the size of the lens that will fit a given rim, assuming that the latter cannot be stretched. If the angle of the bevel is decreased, the peak is able to penetrate further into the groove. Therefore, to facilitate the standardisation of lens sizes in the case of metal frames, it is widely accepted that the stated lens size applies to a bevel with an included angle of 115 degrees.

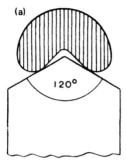 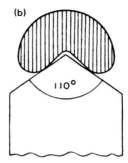

**Figure 16.7** Two eyewires of identical cross-section, showing how the lens size may be affected by the included angle of the bevel.

## Minibevel

The peak of a normal bevel lies approximately midway between the two surfaces. With strong minus lenses and high cylinder powers, a centrally placed bevel leaves too much of the lens protruding in front of the rim. By using a minibevel (*Figure 16.6c*) the peak may be moved forward as shown so as to produce a more pleasing appearance.

## Grooved edge

A grooved edge is simply a flat edge with a central groove (*Figure 16.6d*) used mainly on lenses fitted to spectacles of the nylon supra type.

Sometimes only the lower part of the lens is grooved to accommodate the nylon cord, the upper part that fits into the rim of the mount being bevelled accordingly. Some styles of supras have what is termed a *gallery nylon* inserted into the rim of the mount allowing the prescription house to groove the lens all the way around, with no additional application of bevels required. A word of caution. Some supras have a 'metal' gallery incorporated into the top rim instead of a nylon one. If one attempts to glaze glass lenses into such a supra it will be very prone to chipping, if not during the glazing operation, certainly when being worn by the patient. Unlike the nylon type, there is no 'give' hence, the most brittle part, the glass lens, will in most instances chip.

Some plastics rimmed frames have what can perhaps be termed a *'reversed groove'*, which is not a groove at all. It can be best visualised by imagining the frames as having a bevel instead of the groove and the lens as having a groove instead of a bevel. The two factors still hold the lens in position but in a 'reversed' sort of way. It should be noted that whilst flat edge, bevel edge and minibevel edge finishes are put on to a lens by automatic lens edgers, grooving is normally performed on a separate machine designated specifically for that purpose.

## Milled edge

A milled edge is sufficiently described by saying that it resembles the milled edge of a coin. Its use is confined to rimless monocles, the purpose of the milling to afford a surer grip. This operation is normally performed manually with the aid of an edging wheel.

### Scalloped edge

Also termed a 'facetted edge', this is a decoration formed on a flat edged lens by a series of small scallops around its periphery. It is illustrated in its various forms in *Figures 16.8* and *16.9*. This again is a procedure carried out on a specific machine, not the automatic lens edger. Facetting is

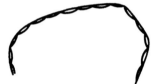

**Figure 16.8** Upper half of a lens with a scalloped edge.

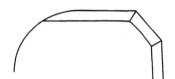

**Figure 16.9** Upper half of a lens with a facetted edge.

normally restricted to resin lenses. Scalloped or facet edges should not be applied to Transition (resin photochromic) or AR-coated lenses. As the photochromic elements are imbibed into the front surface, application of facetting will remove them leaving a lens that is non-photochromic in this area. As the majority of lenses requiring an AR coating and/or hard coating are treated whilst in uncut form, the application of scalloped or facetted edge will remove the coating in this area.

### Polished edge

The surfaces left by edge grinding are grey or dull. To improve their appearance when they are not concealed by rims, the edges of the lenses are sometimes polished but this can give rise to increased reflections.

### Safety chamfers

It is very important that any sharp edges or corners left after edging should be removed by a neat safety chamfer, as illustrated in *Figure 16.10*.

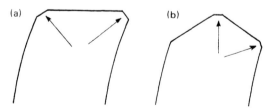

**Figure 16.10** Safety chamfers (indicated by the arrows): (a) flat edged lens; (b) bevel edged lens.

A safety chamfer is certainly required at the peak of a bevel and on the concave surface of the 'curved' lenses, though less frequently on the front surface of bevel edged lenses.

Safety chamfers can be applied by hand, running the lens lightly around a hand edging wheel to create a neat chamfer. Machines referred to as *pin bevellers* can also be employed to obtain the same result automatically or the process can be incorporated into the edging machine operation.

## Hand edgers

A hand edger (*Figure 16.11*) is still an indispensable piece of equipment even though most of the work may be performed by automatic machines. It will be used by a skilled technician to achieve a final good fit of a lens to a frame or to apply a safety chamfer.

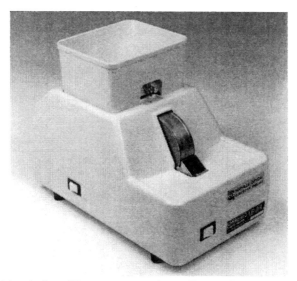

**Figure 16.11** A hand edger. (Picture courtesy of Norville Autoflow, Gloucester, England.)

As with automatic lens edgers, hand edgers would normally have a method whereby coolant can be applied during edging processes. It also helps to keep the dust content to a minimum.

## Other considerations

Some edging machines have no cooling liquid whatsoever and are referred to as dry cut edgers. An efficient vacuum system is therefore required to remove the subsequent dust. Polycarbonate, for example, is a material that lends itself to the dry cut system.

It should be realised that different lens materials cannot be edged on the same wheel, due to their different characteristics. A modern prescription house would normally have some machines set up to cut glass, some for resin and some even subdivided for different types of glass or resin, or indeed different edge finishes.

Before moving on to the actual glazing of different types of frames, a mention should be made here of two special methods of holding lenses for automatic edging. The first is to mount the lens on a rubber suction pad fitted with a location key or block by which it is held accurately in position on the machine. The second, a development of the first, replaces the suction part of the holder with double-sided sticky tape. Both methods allow the lens to be put back on the machine with the knowledge that its location will be accurately repeated. This then enables the lens to be checked in the frame and then returned to the edger if the fit is not correct.

Before leaving this subject a word or two should be mentioned regarding the care and maintenance of machinery. No machine will perform at its best if not properly treated or if the manufacturer's instructions are ignored. Routine truing or 'dressing' of the grinding wheels following the makers' recommendations is of particular importance. Likewise, recalibration of the machine on a regular basis is essential.

## Glazing of plastics frames

The characteristics of different plastics frames are covered in Chapter 3, which should be read in conjunction with this particular section.

From the standpoint of glazing, rimmed spectacle frames are divided into 'metal' or 'plastics' according to the material used for the rims. It would be generally agreed that plastics frames are the easier to glaze. One reason is that the lens size is not so critical since the rims are capable of being slightly stretched or shrunk.

In glazing a plastics frame, heat is required to soften the rims so that they can be eased over the edge of the lens, allowing the bevel to enter the groove. A higher temperature is needed for acrylic materials (such as Perspex) than for the commoner cellulosic plastics. Although bunsen gas burners can be used it is more common for an electric frame heater to be employed, the bunsens being reserved for where localised heat is required or where the frame material is thicker than average. Bunsens are also used to manipulate parts of plastics frames to help achieve correct set up. Obviously, care and skill is needed to ensure that the frame is heated sufficiently to manipulate but not enough to burn.

The simplest form of frame heater is built round a suitable electric heating element or an infra-red bulb. Other types incorporate a blower directing a stream of hot (or cold) air on to the frame. Another form of heater consists essentially of a small tank filled with minute glass beads, the temperature of which is thermostatically controlled. Whatever the source of heat employed it is essential that the frame should be softened sufficiently without becoming scorched or blistered.

The process of fitting the lens into the rim is often referred to as *pushing in* or *springing in*. When the frame is cooled after glazing it should not be possible to rotate the lens in the rim by finger pressure alone. Nevertheless, it is sometimes necessary to correct a misalignment or small error in the axis setting. In such cases removal and reinsertion of the lens can be avoided by the use of special pliers incorporating two rubber pads, between which the lens can be firmly gripped and turned.

## Glazing of metal frames

The traditional type of joint fitted to metal frames serves a double purpose: to close the rim about the lens and to provide a means of attachment of the side. The latter should be able to pivot freely but should not be so loose that it can fall under its own weight. Although this type of joint is small and neat, it does require the lens size to be very exact. If the lens is only slightly oversize the two halves of the joint will be forced apart as shown in *Figure 16.12*, thus throwing an undue strain on the joint screw and tending to make the side loose. On the other hand, the lens should not be made undersize because it could then be rotated in the rim or even dislodged. No gap should be visible at any point between the edge of the lens and the metal eyewire.

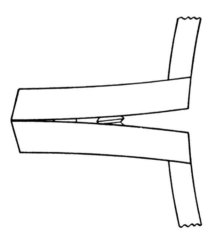

**Figure 16.12** Traditional type of joint used in metal frames, showing the effect of an oversize lens.

This traditional type of joint is now used very infrequently and its place has largely been taken by other designs. One consists of a short tube or barrel attached to each frame end of the eyewire. The joint screw passes through a clearance hole in one tube and engages in the other which is threaded. Since the purpose of this construction is merely to close the rim, the spectacle sides require a separate means of attachment.

The block joint now in common use is attached to the upper end of the rim and has a recess which accommodates a short threaded tube or barrel soldered to the lower end of the rim. The block also provides a means of pivoting the side, which can be removed without opening the rim (*Figure 16.13*).

Another operation which may be necessary before inserting the lens is to bow the eyewire to follow the peak of the bevel on the lens. The more the shape of a curved (meniscus or toric) lens departs from a circle, the more its edge wanders backwards and forwards from a frontal plane. The presence of a high cylinder, whatever the shape, may have the same effect if the peak of the bevel remains in the middle of the edge all the way round. Bowing of eyewires can be greatly facilitated by the use of specially designed pliers.

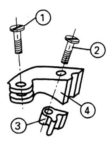

**Figure 16.13** Block joint: (1) dowel screw; (2) closing block screw; (3) threaded barrel; (4) closing block joint.

To counter the general tendency of joint screws to work loose, various expedients have been devised. For example, the barrel joint may have a second (grub) screw set at right-angles into the side of the barrel so as to lock into the thread of the main screw. Sometimes a lock nut is fitted to the screw. Dimpling the end of the screw and splaying it after glazing is another expedient. A simple alternative to these methods is to apply a solution such as Loctite to the screw thread before insertion.

Though the point may seem too elementary to mention, care should be taken to see that the blade of the screwdriver matches the slot in the screw head; much damage to the latter would thereby be prevented.

## Glazing of nylon supra mounts

The glazing of nylon supra mounts calls for a means of grooving the edge of a lens. The type of machine devised for this purpose uses a thin wheel with a diamond-impregnated edge and incorporates a mechanical device for steering the lens so that the groove remains central despite variations in edge thickness. Some glazers nevertheless scorn such contrivances, preferring to guide the lens by hand. This calls for a good eye, a steady hand, and a remarkable nervous system!

Once the length of the nylon cord has been adjusted and the end sealed up, the mount is ready to receive the lens. The bevelled upper edge is inserted into the groove in the rim of the mount and all that remains is to manoeuvre the nylon cord into the groove. The trick is to use a length of woven tape, about 1 cm wide, looped round the nylon cord to pull it taut and guide it into the groove, starting at one end and working round. When the last piece of cord falls into position, the tape can be pulled out. A strip of thin plastics material can be used instead of woven tape.

A variation on the above is a design of frame that has very thin metal rims that are intended to fit into the groove in the lenses.

## Rimless fitting

In rimless mounts which are of various styles the lens is held in position by a screw or screws passing through it or by claws engaging in small slots cut in the edge. Glass lenses are obviously more difficult to drill and fit than resin, due to their brittle nature, more so certain types such as high index or photochromic.

Some of the more fashionable rimless mounts have four holes per lens, requiring a high degree of skill to ensure accurate drilling and machining of the holes. It would be inadvisable to attempt to fit glass lenses into such multi-holed rimless mounts.

A few points of general interest. Experience has shown that drilling a hole in one operation is too risky because of the probability of fracturing the lens when the drill breaks through the second surface. It is consequently standard practice to drill in two stages. The hole is started on one side and the drill allowed to penetrate just over halfway. The lens is then turned round and the drilling completed from the other side. Alternatively, devices are available that drill through the lens from above and below simultaneously.

After drilling, the edges of the holes should be chamfered. Those parts of the mount that will be in contact with the lens may need to be carefully shaped to avoid uneven pressure. Small plastic washers and tubes are sometimes employed. Another important operation may be to file down and neatly finish off the ends of screws without damaging the gold skin of the mount.

More recent developments include drilling holes in the *edge* of the lens to take small prongs which are fitted to the mount. Holes are also being replaced with slots to match special fittings on the mount to give an alternative to the traditional rimless hole.

## Testing for strain

As a matter of routine all lenses fitted to metal rimmed frames or rimless mounts should be examined for strain in a polariscope or strain tester.

In its current form this simple instrument consists essentially of an evenly illuminated screen viewed through two separated polarising filters between which the work to be examined is held. The filters are 'crossed' so that light from the screen, polarised by the first filter, is largely extinguished by the second. As a result, the screen appears uniformly dark. If an unmounted lens is placed between the filters it will be seen clearly through the filter nearer the observer's eye but will appear to be uniformly dark like the screen behind it. If, however, the lens is subjected to mechanical pressure – gripped in a pair of pliers, for example, though this experiment should not be tried on a new lens – the resulting strain is revealed by what appears as a bright patch of light flaring out from the point of pressure. This should always be treated as a danger signal when seen on finished work.

A lens fitted to a metal-rimmed frame should not be expected to be completely free from strain. If it is, it is undoubtedly too small! On the other hand, isolated patches of severe strain demand investigation as they indicate excessive pressure at these points. For example, it may be found that there is some irregularity in the groove, a slight kink in the eyewire or perhaps a 'high spot' on the lens. Whatever the fault it should be remedied because it may cause the lens to chip.

Rimless work should be examined with particular care because excessive pressure in the neighbourhood of the hole will almost certainly lead to a breakage.

Some experience is needed in judging the true significance of the visible indication of strain described above.

## Faults and defects

These may be divided into defects of shape, incorrect size and miscellaneous faults of workmanship.

Defects of shape include wrong shape (which may be due to an error in the selection of the template or former), poor shape and bad match (between right and left). Although rare, errors caused by electronic tracing cannot be dismissed. It should also be realised that the appearance of wrong shapes or mismatch between the two eyeshapes can be caused by the lenses being inserted off axis, the remedy being to simply re-insert correctly.

Errors of size require little comment. If a lens can be turned in the rim by hand pressure alone it is obviously too small. The importance of correct size when glazing metal frames has already been stressed.

Errors in sizing can cause problems with lens retention within the frame. Since man first inserted lenses into a frame the conventional way to check that they are secure and not about to fall out has been to apply a slight pressure to the glazed lenses. In these 'technological' days it was felt this method was insufficient and a method had to be devised that would apply a consistent pressure and not rely on the varying strengths of the glazers thumb!

BS 7394 Part 2 (1994) specifies apparatus and how to go about checking lens retention. It applies to all spectacles with the exception of rimless and semi-rimless mounts.

The device is shown in *Figure 16.14*.

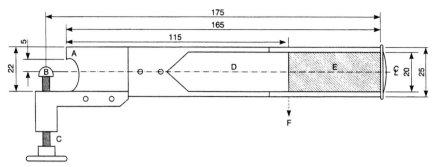

**Figure 16.14** Test lever. (A) Nib. (B) Pressure pad. (C) Adjuster screw. (D) Lever. (E) Lead mass. (F) Centre of mass. All dimensions in millimetres. (From BSI with permission.)

It consists of a lever acting under gravitational forces. The important points here are that the lever has to have a total mass of 250 g (±3 g) and that the position of the centre of the mass from the 'nib' that rests on the rim (see *Figure 16.15*) is 115 mm (±3 mm).

With the test lever in position, the retention test is considered satisfactory if the lever can be left for 5 seconds (±1 second) without displacing the lens.

In an everyday working situation it is not practical to test every single lens that has been glazed, but it makes good sense to test samples at random.

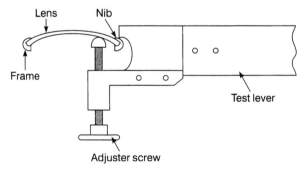

**Figure 16.15** Location of the test lever on the test specimen. With the frame horizontal, the nib rests securely on the frame, not on the lens nor at the interface between the lens and the frame. (From BSI with permission.)

Among common faults of workmanship one could mention is omission of safety chamfers and excessive safety chamfers. The latter are sometimes the result of an attempt to edge out a chip at the edge of the lens. A shallow chip at the edge if sometimes termed a *flake* and if it is very small, a *spark*. Automatic edging machines sometimes leave a series of sparks all round each edge of the lens. This effect is known as *starring*. It is unimportant if the sparks are small enough to be removed by the normal safety chamfer.

When a lens is neatly bevel edged by hand, each shoulder of the bevel should present a smooth and regular surface. The presence of numerous facets, a term which is self-explanatory, betrays workmanship needing improvement.

Whenever water is used as a lubricant in edging, the lens should be carefully dried as soon as the operation has been completed. If water is allowed to dry on the surface of a lens it leaves a deposit known as a water stain which is very difficult to remove.

In Chapter 2 the importance of standards was stressed. At various points throughout this publication mention is made with regard to the use of them. All those working within the optical sector should have access to them for they provide clear guidance and help prevent misunderstandings. They can be referred to and used to ensure we are all working from the same 'rule book'. All workshops and practices should have copies.

An extract from BS 7394 Part 2 (1994) is shown below. It is only an extract and the reader is urged to obtain the full copy (and indeed other standards), but it does clearly define what is required and expected of a good glazed frame.

## Glazing

### Bevelled lenses

The bevel should be smooth, regular, free from chips and starring and reasonably free from facets, with a safety chamfer at the peak and at each edge where necessary.

When mounted, the lenses should be free from excessive strain caused in mounting, but should be securely held in position so that movement or rotation in the frame cannot occur under any normal condition of use. Lenses after mounting should not depart significantly from the strain pattern of the edged lens. No gaps should be visible between the edge of the lens and the rim. The halves of joints should close properly without undue force and without leaving a noticeable gap at the joint.

### Rimless and other lenses

Flat-edged lenses should present a smooth finish with a neat safety chamfer at each edge. Holes for rimless should be drilled at the correct distance from the edge according to the type of mounting. Slots and grooves, when required should be accurately positioned. Brow-bars should be carefully adjusted to follow the edge of the lens. The ends of screws should be neatly finished.

All lenses should be neatly and carefully fitted to ensure that they are securely held in position yet show no significant strain when examined in a polariscope or strainviewer.

### Effect of glazing on frames

Care should be exercised to ensure that the dimensions of the spectacle front, after glazing, do not differ substantially from the corresponding dimensions before glazing. It should be borne in mind that significant alterations to rim shape, aperture size or bridge dimensions may considerably shorten the useful life of finished spectacles. When glazing metal frames, care should be taken not to damage any protective coating on the metal.

## Setting up

At the conclusion of glazing it is normal practice to adjust the frame, i.e. *set it up* to the requirements stated on the prescription order. That is to say ensuring that side angles, temple widths, head widths, angle of let-back (see Chapter 5), etc. are as requested. More often than not these details, or some of them, have not been completed on the order form; in this instance the glazer will 'set up' the frame so that it has a balanced, symmetrical appearance.

It would be prudent on alterations requiring anything other than minor adjustments to remove the lenses to avoid any possible chipping. The performance of this task can be facilitated by the use of special pliers and tools designed for the purpose. Any major adjustments such as shortening sides, etc. can be performed either by the glazer or more likely by a repair/alterations section within the prescription house. Illustrated in *Figure 16.16* are some of the various tools a glazer or repairer may use.

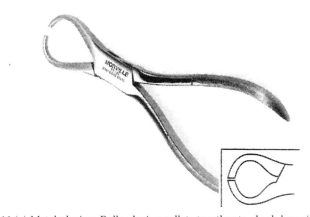

**Figure 16.16** (a) Metal glazing. Pulls glazing collets together to check lens size.

**Figure 16.16** Tools used by a glazer or repairer.

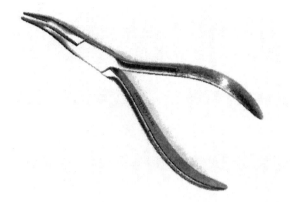

**Figure 16.16** (b) Bendsnipe. For those awkward places.

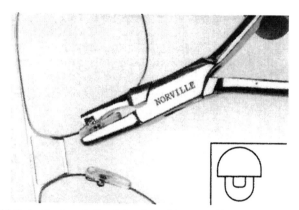

**Figure 16.16** (c) Pad adjustment. Specially shaped jaws enable pads to be adjusted without damage.

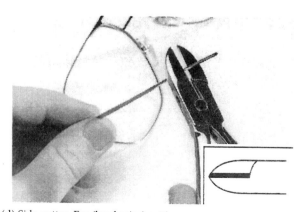

**Figure 16.16** (d) Side cutter. For 'hard wire' cutting.

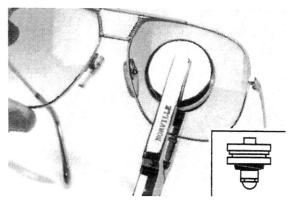

**Figure 16.16** (e) Lens adjustment.

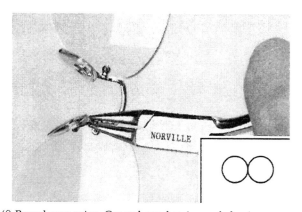

**Figure 16.16** (f) Round nose snipe. General use, bracing and shaping.

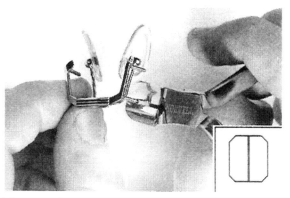

**Figure 16.16** (g) Screw cutting.

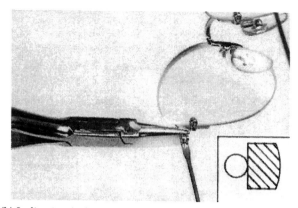

**Figure 16.16** (h) Inclination (nylon jaw). Temple adjustment (metal frames).

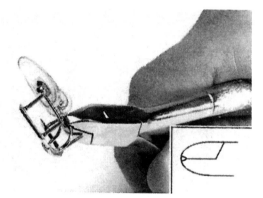

**Figure 16.16** (i) Strap. Precise holding and adjusting of metal rims.

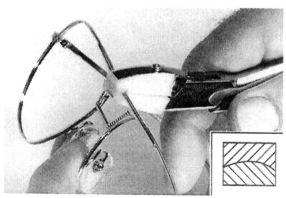

**Figure 16.16** (j) Curved holding slotted nylon. For holding metal sides during adjustments.

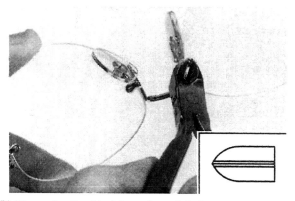

**Figure 16.16** (k) Diagonal cutter. Ideal for awkward rimless screws.

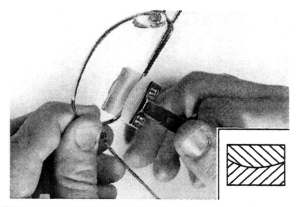

**Figure 16.16** (l) Rim curving. With plastic jaws for adjusting metal eyerims to follow lens curvature.

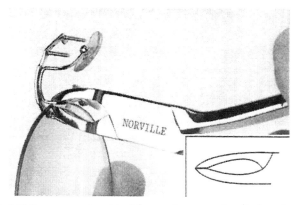

**Figure 16.16** (m) Hollow nose snipe. Ideal for precise, accurate adjustments.

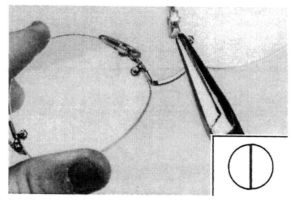

**Figure 16.16** (n) Half round long nose snipe. All purpose plier with extra long nose for difficult-to-get-at places.

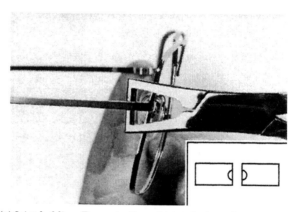

**Figure 16.16** (o) Joint holding. Firm retention of joint during adjustment.

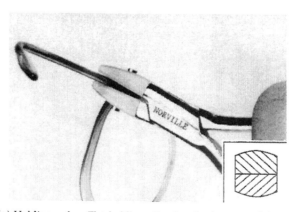

**Figure 16.16** (p) Holding nylon. Flat holding plier for plastic or metal frames.

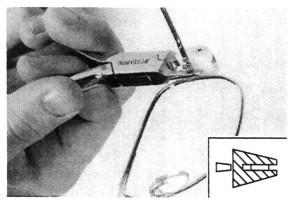

**Figure 16.16** (q) Joint angling. Firm holding of side joints during adjustments.

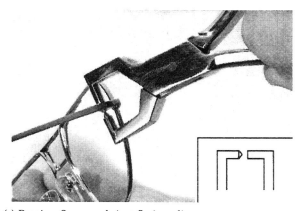

**Figure 16.16** (r) Peening. Screw and rivet flaring plier.

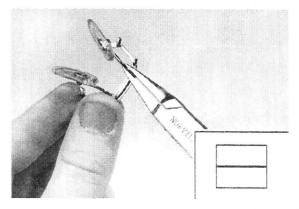

**Figure 16.16** (s) Flat nose 4 mm. Used for general purposes; particularly useful for holding temples on thin metal frames.

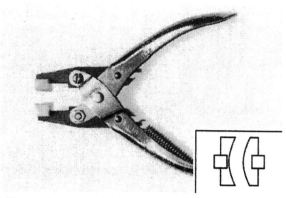

**Figure 16.16** (t) Rim curving spring. With nylon jaws for shaping metal eyerims to follow lens contour. (Pictures courtesy of Norville Optical, Gloucester, England.)

# Chapter 17

# Inspection/final verification

Before despatching a completed pair of spectacles the prescription house will have applied a series of quality assurance checks at various stages of manufacture culminating with what is termed final checking or verification, the 'last chance' to ensure the product conforms to and is within applicable standards. Similarly, before the spectacles are given to the patient the optician will also ensure that they correspond to the requirement.

Both manufacturers and the profession have a duty of care to ensure that the product supplied to the patient is correct within permitted tolerances.

A suggested checklist for final verification of a completed pair of spectacles follows.

## Checklist for final verification

1 Check frame is as requested for style, colour and size.
2 Check side lengths and angles (if specified).
3 Check tightness of fit – lenses and hinges.
4 Check general set-up and presentation of frame.
5 Check that lens type and material is correct.
6 If multifocal or progressive, check segment top/fitting cross position against requirements.
7 Check cosmetic finish of both lenses and frame, e.g. burns, file marks, odd or oversize shapes, buckled rims, gaps, starring, stress, incorrect screws, surface/lens faults, thickness (not too thick or thin), etc.
8 Check that any tint, coating or anti-reflection request has been supplied correctly.
9 Check any special instructions have been adhered to.
10 Having completed the above series of visual/cosmetic checks it is necessary with the aid of a focimeter to check:
   (a) power
   (b) axis
   (c) distance/reading centres
   (d) prisms
   (e) additions.

Whenever checking as above it is important to ensure that if an error is found, checking is not just stopped at that point of the checklist and the order rejected accordingly, as there may be other errors. For example, if rejection occurs due to the lenses being loose (step 3) and the rest of the checklist is not completed, then the order would go back to the glazer for correction. It takes time to correct the fault, but how frustrating and a waste of valuable time if, after all this, the checker then finds the powers incorrect and rejects the lenses that someone has just spent costly time ensuring are a good fit!

Once all the above checks have been completed it would then be prudent to clean the lenses and frames and ensure that there are no scratches or other blemishes that detract from the overall appearance or would cause problems to the patient. This check is normally performed at the end. It is quite possible if extreme care is not exercised, to scratch or mark lenses when performing the above checks and it is therefore logical to inspect for scratches after all the other checks have been completed.

The checklist refers to surface/lens faults (point 7) and this deserves further clarification. Most prescription houses have special desks or tables given over to the task of final inspection, namely having a black background illuminated by some form of light (bulb or fluorescent tube) mounted just above and in front of the black background. There is normally some form of shield to prevent uncomfortable glare to the observer's eye. The black background and the high illumination facilitate easy inspection of the lenses for various faults. It can be used in several different ways. Inspection may entail looking directly through the lens. For best results it should be positioned approximately 12" in front of the eye, directly between the light source and the observer. It may have to be moved around and even tilted so that each area of the lens can be carefully examined. *Figure 17.1* features an extract from BS 2738 Part 1 (1998) and illustrates the recommended method for lens inspection.

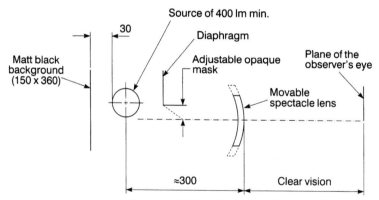

**Figure 17.1** An extract from BS 2738 Part 1 (1998) illustrating the recommended method for lens inspection. *Note*: the diaphragm is adjusted to shield the eye from the light source and allow the lens to be illuminated by the light. Dimensions in millimetres. (From BSI with permission.)

Another method is to reflect light. This involves holding the lens literally right next to the light source and viewing the area which is brightly illuminated by the reflected image of the source.

There is also a technique known as shadowing. By flaring the light through the lens it is possible to detect errors either on the surface or within the material.

It may also be appropriate at this stage to mention a device referred to as a shadowscope. Whilst it is unlikely that this would be in the final checking/verification area, a comprehensive prescription house will have access to one. In essence, it consists of a small but intense source of light such as a 6 volt 30 watt projector lamp, a narrow beam from which passes through an aperture to form an even patch of light on a white screen. If necessary, a condensing lens can be used to increase the brightness. The lens to be examined is held in the path of the beam. If it is free from defects, the patch of light on the screen will still be even and clear though it may have changed its size and shape. Alternatively, any defect in the lens material or on either of the surfaces will reveal its presence by casting a shadow indicating its exact location and extent.

So what faults are there likely to be? There are those in the lens caused during the original manufacturing and those on the surfaces caused by subsequent processing.

## Faults in the lens

Due to technological advances and improved methods of manufacture and quality control, such errors are rare. However, it is necessary to mention them here for the sake of the odd occasion when they may be encountered.

*Colour.* In optics a lens is referred to as being 'white' when no tint or coating has been requested, therefore lenses should exhibit a high degree of clearness and transparency. Any trace of iron oxide in the silica used to manufacture glass will cause an unwanted green tinge in it. Certain high index glass materials exhibit a slight yellowness which has to be accepted and is a bi-product of the chemicals used to increase the indices.

CR39 resin lenses when they were first introduced had a tendency to be slightly yellow in colour. This is no longer a problem. However, some high index resins, similar to glass, have a very slight yellow tinge to them. Very slight yellowness can also be caused by treating resin lenses with an ultraviolet inhibitor. Colouration in polycarbonate lenses can also be expected, and exhibits itself in the form of a light grey appearance.

*Strain.* When glass is being manufactured it is important that it is allowed to cool gradually back to room temperature. This process is referred to as annealing. Failure to do so can result in the outer surfaces cooling before the inner portion, thus resulting in strain. It should be noted that strain can also be caused by glazing both glass and plastics lenses too tightly in the frame (see Chapter 16).

*Bad metal.* Sometimes also referred to as bad stock or stones, it is the name given to any foreign particles that may appear in a glass lens. They can be caused by undissolved batch materials or impurities from the manufacturing process itself.

*Bubbles.* During the manufacture of glass a large volume of gas is given off during the melting process. It is important that the glass is kept fluid enough to allow these bubbles to work their way through the surface. Extremely small bubbles are referred to as seeds. It is rare to find bubbles or seeds in today's ophthalmic glass.

A form of bubble will sometimes occur towards the very edge of resin lenses caused during the original mould filling. However, they rarely cause problems as being at the extreme edge, they are removed during the glazing process.

*Feather.* A cluster of bubbles or seeds in the glass is often referred to as feathers.

*Veins.* Can be best described as a fine thread or streak in the material, normally caused by insufficient mixing of the batch materials. If they are pronounced in appearance they are sometimes referred to as cords and if extremely faint, stria. All have the appearance of what can only be described as a thin, empty tube running through the material.

All of the above covers faults that can occur, within the lens.

## Surface faults

*Tarnish.* High index glasses are particularly prone to this defect, caused by some form of chemical reaction due to one or more of the chemicals used in the manufacture oxidising at the surface, causing stains to appear.

*Crazing.* A series of criss-cross cracks in the surface of the lens. In glass it can be caused by sudden chilling but with resin it is more likely to be from solvent action or stress. Polycarbonate is particularly prone to attack from acetone. Whilst the hardcoat will normally protect the lens, if acetone comes into contact with the uncoated edges or the area around drill holes, if a rimless, then crazing will result.

Another form of crazing can occur when a combination of AR coat and resin materials come into contact with excessive heat, perhaps during the heating of a plastic frame during the glazing or setting up procedure. High index resins are more prone to this phenomenon.

Crazing is a common reason for laboratory returns caused by patients leaving their AR-coated spectacles in a hot place, normally the dashboard of their car!

Crazing can also occur if resin lenses are glazed too tight. It starts from localised hairlines radiating inward from the overly stressed area of the edge of the lens or from an overly tightened screw mount. Occasionally if the lens is evenly oversized, the equal stress will result in the centre area crazing or even cracking.

*Hole.* Normally caused by insufficient smoothing, the thickness of the material being removed being less than the depth of the deepest pit of the generated surface. It can also be caused by breaking into a bubble. It can sometimes lead to drag marks (see explanation below).

*Grey.* Caused by incomplete polishing, the appearance being grey.

There are a multitude of situations or combination of situations that can cause the lens surface to be grey. Inaccuracy in the generated curve on the lens or the tool will be certain to cause problems. If the generated surface is not smooth enough (too rough) this can cause greyness. Other reasons could be either the generator or the smoothing/polishing machines being off axis. Even the incorrect set up of the smoothing/polishing machines could create problems i.e. incorrect stroke, lack of lubrication of bearings, incorrect pressures, etc. If pad application on the tool is not correct, i.e. wrinkles or polishing slurry is insufficiently mixed or is not flowing correctly, this too will cause greyness.

*Polishing burn.* If the lens surface is allowed to get too hot during the polishing process by lack of lubrication between the polishing pad and the lens, a polishing burn or blister can occur.

*Waves.* A wave is an undulation or ripple in the lens surface. It produces a noticeable 'kick' when viewing a straight line. It can take many forms depending upon the geometry of the lens surface and how it has been produced.

To ascertain if a wave exists, hold the lens at arm's length and look at something horizontal and straight such as a window ledge or the edge of a table through the lens. Many will use a lit fluorescent tube as the 'straight line'. Now move the lens up and down whilst continuing to look through it and watch for any 'kick' in the straight line, as this represents a wave. Generally speaking the lower the power of the lens, the easier it is to detect a wave.

With regard to resin lenses, heat or pressure at any point in the surfacing process can cause waves. If the air in the area of the blocking process is too humid or the least bit of moisture is allowed to rest on the surface to be blocked, then the process of taping/varnishing can cause a form of wave referred to as 'orange peel', so named because of its appearance.

Another form of wave can be caused by a wrinkle in the tape applied prior to blocking, which under the pressure of the blocking process is impressed into the lens. Sometimes both 'orange peel' and tape creases can be removed by heating in boiling water.

Generating is another process that can wave a lens. Too large or too fast a cut creates both heat and pressure sufficient to cause a wave. Hot coolant or poor coolant distribution can also lead to waves.

In general, any mechanical imbalance that disrupts the intended motion of the equipment can wave a lens. Over polishing, to compensate for such errors, can itself lead to waves due to wear on the pad.

A form of circular wave around the edge of the lens can be produced by blocking (see 'Blocking or pressure distortion' below). A form of circular wave in the centre of the lens can be caused by a mismatch between the generated curves on the lens and the smoothing/polishing tool. All too often the wrong tool is selected, noticed by the operator who then substitutes the correct one but because of initial error, an area in the centre remains uncorrected and is perceived as a wave or ripple, normally in the central area.

So what of waves on glass lenses? With the majority of lenses now being manufactured from some form of resin material, it has become less of a problem. In addition, improved machinery and manufacturing techniques have reduced the instances of waves even further.

Unlike resin lenses that generally have a moulded front surface and, in the case of stock lenses, a moulded back surface as well, most glass lenses be they semi-finished or finished have to be surfaced both sides. The semi-finished lens manufacturers will surface the front, leaving the prescription house to complete the back, and in the case of the finished stock lens manufacturers, they surface both sides, unlike their counterparts in resin lens manufacture who will mould their lenses without the need for any surfacing. Because of this, glass semi-finished and stock lenses are prone to particular waves seldom seen on resin. A singly produced spherical surface can have waves similar to those depicted in Figure 17.2, sometimes referred to as rings. However, if it is a mass-produced spherical surface such as on stock lenses or semi-finished blanks, only portions of the wave can be seen (*Figure 17.3*). If a lens has an edge chip then a wave referred to as a *drag mark* can be caused, starting at the chip, following the machine motion.

*Scratch.* Reasonably self-explanatory and caused by penetration of the surface, characterised by jagged edges. Usually caused by incorrect handling or by contamination of polishing liquid.

*Dig.* Essentially a short scratch caused by incorrect handling such as striking or dropping the lens.

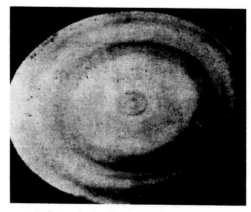

**Figure 17.2** Waves on a singly worked spherical surface.

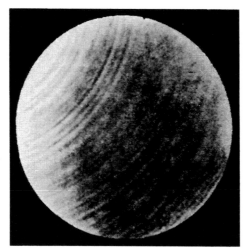

**Figure 17.3** Waves on a block-worked spherical surface.

*Sleek.* A very fine type of scratch, the difference being the absence of jagged edges. They can be caused, especially on resin lenses, by simply cleaning or wiping with a dirty cloth.

*Bruise check.* This takes the form of a crescent shaped mark on the lens, which is a result of it having been subjected to some form of impact.

*Chip.* A reasonably self-explanatory term, normally occurring during the surfacing of the lens (especially plus prescriptions) or during glazing. Very shallow chips are referred to as flakes. Very small ones around the lens edge caused during edging are referred to as *sparks* and are collectively known as *starring* or *brights*.

*Abuse marks.* This covers a 'multitude of sins' simply due to bad handling.

*Blocking or pressure distortion.* Excessive temperature or pressure can cause circular distortions on the finished surface of semi-finished resin lenses, usually equal in diameter to that of the block used to hold and position the lens during surfacing.

*Bead marks.* Where a bead bath has been used to assist in the glazing of a plastics frame, it is not unusual if the beads are too hot or the lens is allowed to be immersed too long, for the beads to make an impression on resin lenses. They form a 'pitted' appearance across the surface of the lenses. Warming the lens can sometimes remove them.

Ensuring the product is suitable for the purpose for which it was intended and at the same time is cosmetically acceptable, is an important task. Unlike some industries, a 100% check of all products is implemented.

# Chapter 18

# Chapter revision

Having completed Part 2 it may be as well to review and check understanding by answering the following questions. (Answers begin on next page.)

1 If the distance between the boxed centres of a frame are 72 mm and the patient has monocular pupillary measurements of R 30, L 32.5, express this as decentration values for each eye.

2 Calculate the prismatic effect at a point 4.5 mm from the optical centre of a −3.75 DS lens.

3 Given the prescription L −8.75 DS, what amount of prism would have to be incorporated to obtain the equivalent of 2.5 mm decentration in? Also state prism direction.

4 Given the prescription R +4.25 DS 1.5$^\Delta$ UP, how much decentration would be required to obtain the equivalent of the prism stated? Also state in what direction the decentration would have to be.

5 With the aid of diagrams illustrate what happens to an object being viewed through a prism.

6 Calculate the prism thickness difference of a 4$^\Delta$ prism made in standard resin material over a diameter of 62 mm.

7 A prescription is received where the prismatic requirements are R 4.5$^\Delta$ UP, L 6$^\Delta$ IN. 'Split' these prisms equally between the two lenses. (You are not required to calculate the resultant prism; just state the split prism values.)

8 Compound the following prisms into a single resultant prism: L 3$^\Delta$ UP 2$^\Delta$ IN, clearly stating the resultant angle.

9 Describe how to check an addition that is incorporated into the front surface of a lens.

10 Why can you not facet a resin Transitions lens?

11 How can you check for strain in a lens?

12 Imagine you are conducting final verification of a completed pair of spectacles. List all the points to be checked.

**Finally – an experiment**

13 Draw a crossline chart on card as shown in *Figure 18.1*. Obtain three stock lenses

+2.00 DS, −2.00 DS and +2.00 DS +1.00 DC

(two meniscus and one toric).

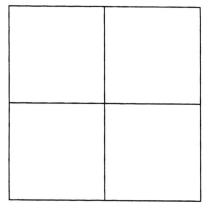

**Figure 18.1** Crossline chart.

Stand the crossline chart up and hold the +2.00 DS approximately 20 cm in front of and level with it. Look through the lens at the crossline. Move the lens slowly down and keep looking through it.

(a) What happens to the horizontal line on the chart?
(b) Start again; this time move the lens sideways to the left. What happens to the vertical line on the chart?
(c) Repeat both experiments with the −2.00 DS lens. What is noticeable?
(d) Take either the +2.00 DS or −2.00 DS, hold it level with the chart and approximately 20 cm away as before. Hold it as steadily as possible but turn it like a steering wheel. What happens?
(e) Now take the +2.00 DS +1.00 DC lens and repeat the experiment. What is noticeable?
(f) Select the +2.00 DS lens again; hold it level and approximately 20 cm from the chart. Do not move the lens, just observe through it. What is noticeable regarding the vertical and horizontal limbs of the crossline?
(g) Repeat the experiment but this time with the −2.00 DS lens. Again, what is noticeable?

## Answers

1 R 6 mm IN; L 3.5 mm IN
2 1.69$^{\Delta}$

3  2.19$^\Delta$ base out
4  3.5 mm UP
5  Object P will appear displaced towards the apex of the prism (P')
   (*Figure 18.2*).

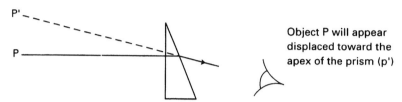

Object P will appear
displaced toward the
apex of the prism (p')

**Figure 18.2** Object being viewed through a prism.

6  4.97 mm
7  R 2.25$^\Delta$ UP 3$^\Delta$ IN L 2.25$^\Delta$ DOWN; 3$^\Delta$ IN
8  3.6$^\Delta$ UP and IN at 124
9  With the *front* of the lens resting against the focimeter measure the
   power in the distance portion. Then still with the front of the lens
   against the focimeter, measure the power in the reading area. The
   difference between the two measurements is equal to the addition.
10 The photochromic elements are only imbibed into the front surface
   and do not penetrate very deeply into the material. Applying a facet
   would remove the photochromic elements.
11 Between a set of cross polarised filters with their axes at right-angles
   to one another.
12 Checklist for final verification

   (a) Check frame is as requested for style, colour and size.
   (b) Check side lengths and angles (if specified).
   (c) Check tightness of fit – lenses and hinges.
   (d) Check general set-up and presentation of frame.
   (e) Check that lens type and material is correct.
   (f) If multifocal or progressive, check segment top/fitting cross
       position against requirements.
   (g) Check cosmetic finish of both lenses and frame, e.g. burns, file
       marks, odd or oversize shapes, buckled rims, gaps, starring, stress,
       incorrect screws, surface/lens faults, thickness (not too thick or
       thin), etc.
   (h) Check that any tint, coating or anti-reflection has been supplied
       correctly.
   (i) Check any special instructions have been adhered to.
   (j) Having completed the above series of visual/cosmetic checks it is
       necessary with the aid of a focimeter to check:
       (i)   power axis
       (ii)  distance/reading centres
       (iii) prisms
       (iv)  additions.

13 (a) It moves in the opposite direction, i.e. upwards.
   (b) It moves in the opposite direction, i.e. sideways to the right.
   (c) It moves in the same direction, i.e. downwards and sideways to the left.

   With reference to (a), (b), (c) – this illustrates that plus lenses give 'against' movement and minus lenses give 'with' movement. Therefore it is possible to identify a lens without the use of a focimeter. The test is referred to as the transverse test.

   (d) Nothing.
   (e) A phenomenon referred to as *scissors movement*. The test itself is referred to as the *rotation test (Figure 18.3)*.

   With reference to (d) and (e) – this illustrates that because spherical lenses are the same power in each meridian, nothing happens when they are rotated. The toric lens produces scissors movement because the power changes across it from one principal meridian to the other. Identification can therefore be made without a focimeter as to whether a lens is spherical or astigmatic.

   (f) The limbs are thicker because a plus lens magnifies.
   (g) The limbs are thinner because a minus lens minifies.

## Additionally

If any lens is held in front of the crossline chart so that the limbs are not displaced, then the optical centre position can also be found (*Figure 18.4*).

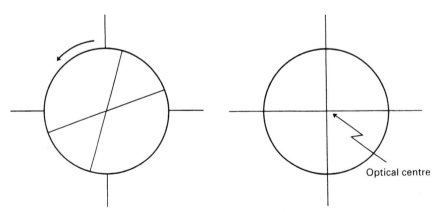

**Figure 18.3** Scissors movement.    **Figure 18.4** Finding optical centre position.

# Part Three

# Chapter 19

# Fused multifocals

## Basic construction and properties

Fused multifocals function on the principle that a curve of given radius produces a stronger focal power on glass of relatively high refractive index than on the 'crown' glass normally used for spectacle lenses.

The construction of a round segment is illustrated in *Figure 19.1* in which (a) is the front view of a finished lens and (b) is a vertical section. Although the lens has two continuous surfaces, it is really made up of two separate lenses of different materials, one implanted in the other. The main lens is of spectacle crown glass but the reading segment, shaded in *Figure 19.1b*, is made of glass of a higher refractive index.

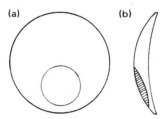

**Figure 19.1** Construction of fused bifocals: (a) front view; (b) vertical section.

Whilst the majority of fused multifocals are based on and around crown glass, high index multifocals are available. To accommodate the segment a spherical depression curve is worked in the lower part of the blank used for the main lens. The curve on the contact surface of the segment button is deliberately made 0.25–0.50 steeper than the depression curve on the main lens so that initially contact is only made at the centre. The buttons that will form the segments and the main lenses will be thoroughly cleaned before passing into the air-conditioned assembly room, where an operative will assemble the components ready for the fusing process. To ensure there is no dust between the two surfaces the operative uses a carefully illuminated inspection booth. A soft brush is used to clean the contact surfaces. The two components are put together and because the curve on the segment button is slightly steeper than that of the depression curve on the main lens, an interference spot is visible at the contact point.

By pressing down the top surface of the button with a pair of tweezers, if all is well the interference spot moves in a straight line to the point where the pressure is being employed. If, however, there is dust present the spot will be deflected and will follow a course around the dust particle. In this instance the components are separated, brushed and the operative tries again. The process of applying pressure is repeated in a number of positions until no deflection of the interference spot is observed.

The operative then places two short pieces of wire, first dipped in gum, about 1 cm apart to support the segment button at the bottom. Alternatively, special 'feelers' are used instead of wire.

Placed on a carborumdum block the assembled components are pre-heated in a combined furnace and annealing lehr before being brought to a temperature of around 640°C at which point fusion of the components take place. The segment button gradually sags under its own weight, expelling air towards the feeler wires at the bottom. As the components continue their journey through the lehr the temperature reduces until they emerge from the furnace at about 100°C. They are allowed to cool to room temperature when the wire feelers are removed and the fused lenses subjected to rigorous inspection.

Care must be exercised in the choice of glass used for both the main section and the segment. Although different, they must be compatible in that their coefficient of expansion must be as near as possible so that they heat and cool at about the same rate.

To facilitate handling and provide a margin for safety, the button is initially left much thicker than required. After fusing, the button may project several millimetres from the main surface of the blank. This surplus material is subsequently removed when a continuous surface is worked on the segment side of the lens, the resulting segment in some instances being less than 0.3 mm at its centre.

The production of a fused multifocal calls for a high degree of care and technical skill. Extreme precautions are necessary to ensure that the contact surfaces are perfectly clean and do not entrap any particles of dust. Another great difficulty is to prevent distortion of the contact surfaces under the very high temperature necessary for fusing (approximately 650°C). It is possible, though unusual, to produce fused multifocals with the segment on the concave surface of the lens.

Fused bifocals were invented by John L. Borsch Jr, of the USA. His father, John Borsch Sr had developed a lens similar to a fused (*Figure 19.2*). It consisted of a main lens with a depression cut in it. A higher refracting index button was placed in the depression and sealed in by cementing a cover lens to the back surface. He called the lens *Kryptok*, a Greek term meaning 'hidden' or 'secret'. John Borsch Jr took his father's idea one stage further, using a heat fusing technique instead of a cover plate.

After their introduction at the beginning of the present century, fused bifocals quickly displaced the cemented type. Their barely noticeable

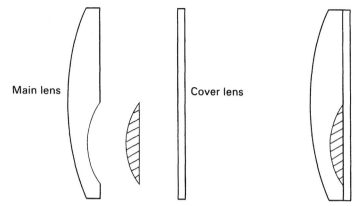

**Figure 19.2** Construction of a Kryptok bifocal. (After Jalie, M. *Principles of Ophthalmic Lenses*, ADO, by permission.)

dividing line, mechanical stability, and moderate cost gave them enormous advantage.

One technical drawback must now be mentioned. Because refractive index varies with wavelength, the power of prisms and lenses is a minimum for red light at one end of the visible spectrum, increasing to a maximum for violet light at the other end. The resulting differences in the deviation undergone when 'white' light passes through a prism or a non-central area of a lens is termed dispersion. In spectacle lenses, it is the cause of the coloured fringes which may be noticed near the edges of the field of view. Unfortunately, the higher index glass used for the segments has a much higher dispersive effect than the hard crown glass used for the main lens. In some cases it can give rise to disturbing colour fringes in the reading portion, especially in the area just below the dividing line. As a rule, this defect becomes worse with increasing segment diameters and additions.

Another factor that needs to be taken into account is that the segment is of a softer glass than that used for the main lens and therefore may scratch more easily than the surrounding surfaces. All patients should be instructed never to place their spectacles face down on a desk or table, be they fused or any other type of lens.

Although solid tinted fused are comparatively rare these days, photochromics are very popular. In these instances the main lens will be made out of photochromic glass whilst the segment would normally be 'white'. Because of the depression curve in the main lens, this does mean that there is less coloured material behind the segment, resulting in a lighter tint in the reading area. The higher the addition and the larger the segment, the more noticeable the difference becomes. *Figure 19.3* illustrates this particular phenomenon.

From *Figure 19.3* one can also appreciate that, with regard to minus powered multifocals (where the lens is thinner at the centre than at the edge), sufficient thickness of lens is left to ensure the depression curve is not cut into from the back. The higher the addition, generally, the deeper

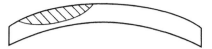

**Figure 19.3** Illustration to demonstrate how tint will be lighter behind the segment due to the depression curve. (After Jalie, M. *Principles of Ophthalmic Lenses*, ADO, by permission.)

the depression. This could mean that some fused multifocals are slightly thicker at the centre than, say their (solid) counterparts.

All of the above however, does not detract from the very useful function that fused lenses perform. The majority of glass multifocals are supplied in this form. The factors illustrated are not faults but points to be taken into account before the lens is dispensed.

## Shaped (non-circular) segments

Fused bifocals with shaped segments were first produced by United Kingdom Optical Co. Ltd. In the 1920s they were marketed under the trade name *Univis*, a contraction of 'universal visibility'.

Two of their original shapes, which they denoted by the letters B and D respectively, are illustrated in *Figure 19.4*. Though the patents have long since expired and shaped segments are in general production in many countries, the letters B and D are widely used to indicate the two shapes in question, as indeed the name 'univis' has been adopted to describe a shaped segment, not necessarily made by United Kingdom Optical Co.

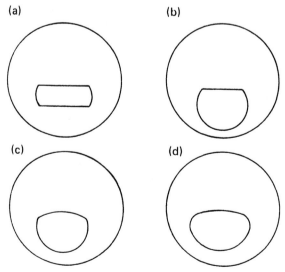

**Figure 19.4** Shaped segments of fused bifocals: (a) B shape; (b) D shape; (c) C shape; (d) P(anto) shape.

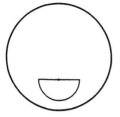

**Figure 19.5** 'Old' Univis C.

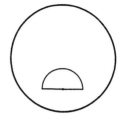

**Figure 19.6** 'Old' Univis A.

The original Univis series included a shape C, which was the lower half of a circle, its diameter forming the upper boundary (*Figure 19.5*). A modified form of this shape with a curved top (*Figure 19.4c*) was introduced by American Optical Company and is called shape C by some manufacturers now producing it. There also used to be a Univis A which was an 'old' Univis C upside down (*Figure 19.6*). Another variant, introduced by Bausch & Lomb under the trade name *Panoptik*, is shown in *Figure 19.4d*. Today the shape is referred to as 'panto' (an abbreviation for pantoscopic) or simply 'P' and it is available from several manufacturers.

The manufacture of shaped segments calls for a preliminary fusing operation to produce a composite button. As shown in *Figure 19.7*, shape

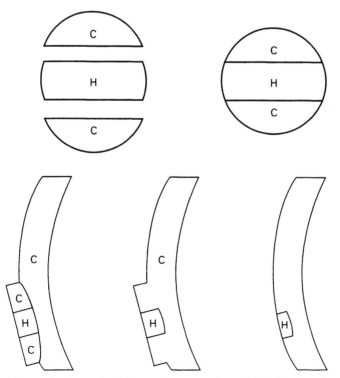

**Figure 19.7** Composite button for B shape: C = crown glass; H = high index glass. (After Jalie, M. *Principles of Ophthalmic Lenses*, ADO, by permission.)

B requires a three-piece button, the two outer components being made from the same crown glass as the main lens. The crown glass used for the composite button must have exactly the same refractive index as the main lens as any slight difference will readily be seen in the form of a circular ring between the two glasses. To prevent this the tolerance on the refractive index is a mere ±0.0003. The interfaces are all plane and need to be optically worked to ensure a satisfactory fusing. Some manufacturers angle the two flat contact surfaces to deflect the reflections that occur at the dividing line. Some also coat the contact surfaces to reduce the intensity of the reflection at the line.

When the components of the composite button have been prepared they are carefully cleaned and clamped together with an asbestos strip to hold them together during the initial fusing process performed in a furnace that will produce the composite button. With the asbestos strip removed, the button is now prepared in a similar manner to that described for round segments. Fusing takes place at a slightly higher temperature of around 680°C.

When the composite button is itself fused to the main lens, the crown glass portions merge into it and disappear. The same principle is used to supply other types of shaped segments, including trifocals (*Figure 19.8*).

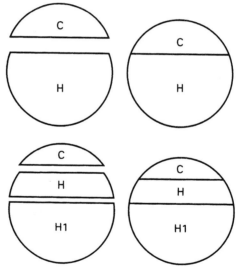

**Figure 19.8** Shaped segments. C = Crown glass; H = high index; H1 = higher index.

Shaped segments have two important optical advantages. First, since the segment top is only a short distance above the centre of the segment circle, the amount of image jump is considerably reduced. For the same reason, chromatic aberration near the segment top is also reduced. Thanks to this, some of the shaped segments illustrated have become available in a range of segment diameters up to 40 mm.

# Fused blanks

The term blank is widely used to denote a piece of glass from which a lens can be made, at any stage of completion before the surfacing of the second side. After that it becomes an uncut.

Apart from a few common spherical prescriptions, it is clearly impossible for fused bifocals to be stocked in uncut form. Instead, they are worked individually to prescription from suitable blanks.

Traditionally, fused blanks were offered by their manufacturers in several stages of completion after fusing. The earliest is what is often termed a rough blank in which the segment button is left projecting. Within limits, any spherical curve can be ground on the segment side of the blank while it is in this stage.

Next comes the roughed blank, in which the surplus segment material has been removed and the segment side ground to approximately the curve intended on the finished lens. Bifocal blanks with shaped segments are sometimes supplied in this form.

Finally, we have the semi-finished blank in which the segment side has been not only ground but smoothed and polished, leaving only the second side of the lens to be worked. This is the form in which the great majority of fused blanks are supplied to prescription laboratories.

The front surface curve of a semi-finished lens blank normally incorporates a vertex power allowance made by the manufacturer. This allowance is based on an estimate of the average finished thickness of the range of lenses for which the blank is likely to be used. For example, a blank with a nominal front surface power of +8.00 D may have an actual surface power of +7.80 D, representing a vertex power allowance of 0.20 D. Reference to this requirement/allowance has already been made in Chapter 8. It is very important for prescription laboratories to know the actual front surface power. Fused multifocal blanks are generally available in a wide range of front surface powers, so that the finished lens can be given surface curvatures appropriate to the given distance prescription.

It will be evident from *Figure 19.1* that once the segment surface has been finished, any subsequent removal of material will inevitably reduce the segment diameter. This explains the difficulty in making fused bifocals with very low reading additions: in such cases the segments are then so thin that precise control of the surfacing operation on the segment side becomes exceptionally critical to achieve specified segment diameter.

# The reading addition

Although the power of the distance portion of a fused bifocal is not determined until the second side has been worked, the reading addition is fixed as soon as the segment side has been finished. The way in which the reading addition comes into being can be explained quite simply.

The relationship between the focal power ($F$) in dioptres of a surface, its radius of curvature ($r$) in millimetres and the refractive index ($n$) of the material is expressed by the formula

$$F = \frac{1000(n-1)}{r}$$

Let us apply this expression to the front surface of a fused bifocal, assuming the refractive indices of the two glasses to be 1.523 (main lens) and 1.654 (segment). Let us also suppose that the radius of curvature of the convex surface worked on the segment side of the blank is 100 mm. According to the above formula, the distance portion will have a surface power of

$$\frac{1000(1.523-1)}{100} = +5.23 \text{ D}$$

whereas the power of the segment surface will be

$$\frac{1000(1.654-1)}{100} = +6.54 \text{ D}$$

Thus, the mere change in the refractive index of the glass will have increased the surface power from +5.23 D to +6.54 D: an addition of +1.31 D.

Similarly, if the distance portion had been worked with a surface power of +10.00 D, calculation shows that the power of the segment surface would have been +12.50 D, giving an addition of +2.50 D.

These two examples illustrate a general rule: for any pair of refractive indices there is a fixed ratio – sometimes termed the blank ratio – between the surface power worked on the main lens and the addition thereby produced. For indices of 1.523 and 1.654 the ratio is almost exactly 4. Therefore, as we have seen, a surface power of +5.23 D gave an addition of +1.31 D and +10.00 D gave an addition of +2.50 D.

It should not be inferred from the above that the reading addition of a fused bifocal is provided only by the segment side of the lens. Unless it is plane, the fused contact surface also contributes to the total reading addition, and the same ratio law applies, subject to a change of sign. For example, presume that the front surface of the lens provides an addition of +1.50 D whereas a (total) reading addition of +2.50 D is required. Another +1.00 D is needed and this is obtained by working a contact surface of –4.00 D on the main lens. The matching convex surface on the segment button would have a surface power of +5.00 D, owing to the higher index, and the two together in contact would have a combined power of +1.00 D.

Although it is possible to obtain a full range of reading additions by the use of one refractive index button and varying the contact (depression) curve, it is more common these days to have standardised depression curves and a range of different index buttons. For example, a manufacturer may decide to have four depression curves across the range of lenses produced. This in turn may require the use of some 10 different indices from around 1.562 up to 1.680. By limiting the number of depression curves, production is made easier and therefore more efficient and cost effective.

It is quite possible for the addition provided by the front surface of the lens to be greater than the total required. In this event, the fused contact surface must add minus power, which means that the countersink curve worked on the main lens must be convex. The above also confirms why when checking a front surface addition, the special procedures outlined in Chapter 15 must be adopted.

## Vertical prism compensation

Patients can experience problems on any type of lens where there is a marked difference in power between the lenses, even single vision ones. It is more common for the *anisometropia*, as it is technically referred to, to cause problems on multifocal lenses when patients move their gaze down to reach the reading area.

From Chapter 12 it has already been seen that all lenses have a prismatic element. The lens on the left in *Figure 19.9* will exert more prismatic 'pull' than the one on the right when viewing through the lower portions. It is generally accepted that there should be no more than $1.5^\Delta$ of vertical imbalance between a pair of lenses. Above this, binocular vision becomes uncomfortable.

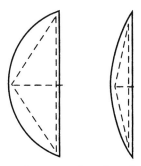

**Figure 19.9** The higher the power, the greater the prismatic effect.

Straight top fused multifocals lend themselves to a process termed *bi-prism*. At the outset it should be stated that it is the prescriber who initiates any action to reduce or eliminate vertical imbalance, not the prescription house. If the prescriber wants imbalance eliminated, it should be clearly stated so on the order. As an example

R – 0.50 DS
L – 3.25 DS
Add 2.00

As the addition is equal for both eyes it can be ignored as the segments will exert the same prismatic 'pull' for each eye.

Using Prentice's formula (see Chapter 12)

$$P = c \times F$$

the prismatic elements of each lens can be determined.

Assume that the NVP (near visual point) lies 8 mm below the distance optical centre. The figure is arbitrary and for ease of calculation some deem to be 10 mm.

For the right eye

$$P = 0.8 \times 0.50$$

$$P = 0.4^{\Delta} \text{ base down}$$

For the left eye

$$P = 0.8 \times 3.25$$

$$P = 2.6^{\Delta} \text{ base down}$$

The imbalance is

$2.2^{\Delta}$ base down left eye

$(2.6^{\Delta}$ base down$) - (0.4^{\Delta}$ base down$)$

The bi-prism process, sometimes referred to as *slab-off* normally removes base up prism from the upper half of the lens. So in this instance the left lens would be produced with $2.2^{\Delta}$ base up, distance and reading. Then $2.2^{\Delta}$ base up is removed from the upper distance portion of the lens by the bi-prism, slab-off technique.

The result is a pair of lenses with equal prisms ($0.4^{\Delta}$ base down) in the reading. The $2.2^{\Delta}$ base up still effective in the reading is cancelling $2.2^{\Delta}$ base down in the left eye, thereby equalising the prismatic effects at near.

Consider another example

R +2.50 DS +2.00 DC × 180
L +1.50 DS +0.50 DC × 180
Add 2.00

In Chapter 10 toric lenses and the powers in their principal meridians were discussed. Therefore, it can be ascertained that in the vertical meridian the right eye is +4.50 D and the left +2.00 D.

Applying Prentice's rule to each in turn

R   $P = c \times F$

$$P = 0.8 \times 4.50$$

$$P = 3.6^{\Delta} \text{ base up}$$

L   $P = c \times F$

$P = 0.8 \times 2$

$P = 1.6^{\Delta}$ base up

As power is plus in the vertical both prism directions are 'up'.

The vertical imbalance is therefore $2^{\Delta}$ base up right eye. In this instance the left lens would be produced with $2^{\Delta}$ base up, distance and reading. Then $2^{\Delta}$ base up is removed from the upper distance portion of the lens by the bi-prism slab-off technique. The result is a pair of lenses with equal prism ($3.6^{\Delta}$ base up) in the reading. The additional $2.0^{\Delta}$ base up in the reading of the left eye means that, combined with the prismatic element already in the lens, the values are equalled for right and left. *Figure 19.10* illustrates diagrammatically the steps involved. Actual curvatures have been exaggerated to allow appreciation of the process.

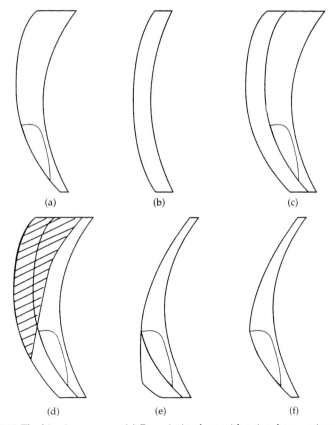

(a)                     (b)                     (c)

(d)                     (e)                     (f)

**Figure 19.10** The bi-prism process. (a) Prescription lens with prism base up incorporated. (b) A 'mask' is prepared. (c) Mask is temporarily bonded to prescription lens. (d) Lens is surfaced to remove the base up prism previously incorporated with special care being taken to ensure alignment with segment top (shaded area represents material removal). (e) The result of (d) above. (f) Remainder of mask removed leaving only the reading portion with base up prism.

The prismatic effect exerted by a cylinder is always at right-angles to its axis direction. Thus, if the axis is vertical, only a horizontal effect is exerted, equal to that of a sphere of the same power. If the cylinder axis is horizontal, only a vertical effect is contributed.

The prismatic effect of a cylinder at an oblique axis has an oblique base setting and therefore needs to be resolved into vertical and horizontal components. These components have been calculated for various cylinder powers and axes and are set out in *Table 19.1* on pages 232 and 233. The base settings given in this table apply to plus cylinders. For minus cylinders it is merely necessary to reverse both base settings, the magnitudes remaining unchanged. For example, a −2.50 D cylinder at axis 30 degrees in the left lens would exert a prismatic effect of

$1.3^\Delta$ base down $0.7^\Delta$ base out

When considered in conjunction with a sphere, Prentice's rule can be applied to the sphere element and the table used for the cylindrical element. The figures can be set out in tabular form, as in the following example

R −4.50 DS +2.50 DC × 40
L −7.00 DS +1.00 DC × 50
with a͞ segment inset of 2 mm each eye

With regard to the right sphere, the vertical prismatic value is equal to

$P = c \times F$

$P = 0.8 \times 4.50$

$P = 3.6^\Delta$ base down

With regard to the right sphere, the horizontal prismatic value is

$P = c \times F$

$P = 0.2 \times 4.50$

$P = 0.9^\Delta$ base in

By application of *Table 19.1* to the right cylindrical element the result is

$1.4^\Delta$ base up, $1.2^\Delta$ base out

Tabulate the values:

| R | Vertical effect | Horizontal effect |
|---|---|---|
| Due to sphere | $3.6^\Delta$ base down | $0.9^\Delta$ base in |
| Due to cylinder | $1.4^\Delta$ base up | $1.2^\Delta$ base out |
| Total | $2.2^\Delta$ base down | $0.3^\Delta$ base out |

The total prismatic effect at the near visual point on the right due to the distance prescription is therefore

R 2.2$^\Delta$ base down, 0.3$^\Delta$ base out

The left Rx is

L −7.00 DS +1.00 DC × 50

Tabulate the prismatic values to obtain:

| L | Vertical effect | Horizontal effect |
|---|---|---|
| Due to sphere | 5.6$^\Delta$ base down | 1.4$^\Delta$ base in |
| Due to cylinder | 0.2$^\Delta$ base up | 0.3$^\Delta$ base in |
| **Total** | 5.4$^\Delta$ base down | 1.7$^\Delta$ base in |

The total prismatic difference between the two lenses is therefore

3.2$^\Delta$ base down 1.4$^\Delta$ base in

Bi-prism allows no control over the horizontal elements therefore only the vertical imbalance can be addressed. The left lens would be produced with 3.2$^\Delta$ base up distance and reading. Then 3.2$^\Delta$ base up is removed from the upper distance portion of the lens by the bi-prism, slab-off technique. The result is a pair of lenses with equal prisms (2.2$^\Delta$ base down) in the reading.

The result of working a straight top fused multifocal with a bi-prism is what can only be described as a very light 'ridge' running across the front surface in line with the segment top. For this reason straight top segments are so suitable for this process as they already have a distinct line; the segment top and the bi-prism are made to coincide with this (*Figure 19.11*).

## Fused trifocals

As presbyopia advances the patient requires progressively stronger reading additions to obtain good near vision. The patient can reach a

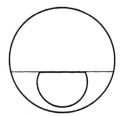

Figure 19.11 The faint 'ridge' on a bi-prism lens.

**Table 19.1** Prismatic effect (in∆) at the near visual point due to plus cylinders at various axes

| Right lens cylinder axis | Cylinder power | | | | | | | | Left lens cylinder axis |
|---|---|---|---|---|---|---|---|---|---|
| | +0.50 | +1.00 | +1.50 | +2.00 | +2.50 | +3.00 | +3.50 | +4.00 | |
| 0° | 0.4 up – | 0.8 up – | 1.2 up – | 1.6 up – | 2.0 up – | 2.4 up – | 2.8 up – | 3.2 up – | 180° |
| 10° | 0.4 up 0.1 out | 0.8 up 0.1 out | 1.2 up 0.2 out | 1.6 up 0.3 out | 2.0 up 0.4 out | 2.4 up 0.4 out | 2.8 up 0.5 out | 3.2 up 0.6 out | 170° |
| 20° | 0.4 up 0.1 out | 0.8 up 0.3 out | 1.2 up 0.4 out | 1.5 up 0.6 out | 1.9 up 0.7 out | 2.3 up 0.8 out | 2.7 up 1.0 out | 3.1 up 1.1 out | 160° |
| 30° | 0.3 up 0.2 out | 0.7 up 0.4 out | 1.0 up 0.6 out | 1.4 up 0.8 out | 1.7 up 1.0 out | 2.1 up 1.2 out | 2.4 up 1.4 out | 2.7 up 1.6 out | 150° |
| 40° | 0.3 up 0.2 out | 0.6 up 0.5 out | 0.9 up 0.7 out | 1.1 up 1.0 out | 1.4 up 1.2 out | 1.7 up 1.4 out | 2.0 up 1.7 out | 2.3 up 1.9 out | 140° |
| 50° | 0.2 up 0.3 out | 0.4 up 0.5 out | 0.6 up 0.8 out | 0.9 up 1.0 out | 1.1 up 1.3 out | 1.3 up 1.5 out | 1.5 up 1.8 out | 1.7 up 2.0 out | 130° |
| 60° | 0.1 up 0.2 out | 0.3 up 0.5 out | 0.4 up 0.7 out | 0.6 up 1.0 out | 0.7 up 1.2 out | 0.9 up 1.5 out | 1.0 up 1.7 out | 1.1 up 2.0 out | 120° |
| 70° | 0.1 up 0.2 out | 0.2 up 0.4 out | 0.2 up 0.7 out | 0.3 up 0.9 out | 0.4 up 1.1 out | 0.5 up 1.3 out | 0.6 up 1.5 out | 0.6 up 1.7 out | 110° |

| | 100° | 90° | 80° | 70° | 60° | 50° | 40° | 30° | 20° | 10° | 0° |
|---|---|---|---|---|---|---|---|---|---|---|---|
| 80° | 0.2 up / 1.3 out | 0.2 up / 1.2 out | 0.2 up / 1.0 out | 0.1 up / 0.8 out | 0.1 up / 0.7 out | 0.1 up / 0.5 out | 0.1 up / 0.3 out | – / 0.2 out | | | |
| 90° | – / 0.8 out | – / 0.7 out | – / 0.6 out | – / 0.5 out | – / 0.4 out | – / 0.3 out | – / 0.2 out | – / 0.1 out | | | |
| 100° | – / 0.2 out | – / 0.2 out | – / 0.2 out | – / 0.1 out | – / 0.1 out | – / 0.1 out | – / 0.1 out | | | | |
| 110° | 0.1 up / 0.3 in | 0.1 up / 0.2 in | 0.1 up / 0.2 in | 0.1 up / 0.2 in | 0.1 up / 0.2 in | – / 0.1 in | – / 0.1 in | – / – | | | |
| 120° | 0.5 up / 0.8 in | 0.4 up / 0.7 in | 0.3 up / 0.6 in | 0.3 up / 0.5 in | 0.2 up / 0.4 in | 0.2 up / 0.3 in | 0.1 up / 0.2 in | 0.1 up / 0.1 in | | | |
| 130° | 0.9 up / 1.1 in | 0.8 up / 1.0 in | 0.7 up / 0.8 in | 0.6 up / 0.7 in | 0.5 up / 0.6 in | 0.3 up / 0.4 in | 0.2 up / 0.3 in | 0.1 up / 0.1 in | | | |
| 140° | 1.5 up / 1.2 in | 1.3 up / 1.1 in | 1.1 up / 0.9 in | 0.9 up / 0.8 in | 0.7 up / 0.6 in | 0.6 up / 0.5 in | 0.4 up / 0.3 in | 0.2 up / 0.2 in | | | |
| 150° | 2.1 in / 1.2 in | 1.8 up / 1.0 in | 1.5 up / 0.9 in | 1.3 up / 0.7 in | 1.0 up / 0.6 in | 0.8 up / 0.4 in | 0.5 up / 0.3 in | 0.3 up / 0.1 in | | | |
| 160° | 2.6 up / 0.9 in | 2.2 up / 0.8 in | 1.9 up / 0.7 in | 1.6 up / 0.6 in | 1.3 up / 0.5 in | 1.0 up / 0.4 in | 0.6 up / 0.2 in | 0.3 up / 0.1 in | | | |
| 170° | 3.0 up / 0.5 in | 2.6 up / 0.5 in | 2.2 up / 0.4 in | 1.9 up / 0.3 in | 1.5 up / 0.3 in | 1.1 up / 0.2 in | 0.7 up / 0.1 in | 0.4 up / 0.1 in | | | |
| 180° | 3.2 up / – | 2.8 up / – | 2.4 up / – | 2.0 up / – | 1.6 up / – | 1.2 up / – | 0.8 up / – | 0.4 up / – | | | |

Minus cylinders: reverse the base settings tabulated above.

point, therefore, where their bifocals give them good distance and near vision but they have a problem focusing at intermediate, i.e. around arm's length. If they try to use the distance area of their bifocal lens for intermediate vision they find it too weak. If they tilt their head back and try to use the segment part of the lens, they find it too strong as well as uncomfortable. What is needed is an intermediate portion – trifocals.

The techniques of manufacturing fused bifocals with shaped segments lend themselves admirably to the production of trifocals. *Figure 19.12* shows three of the types in current production.

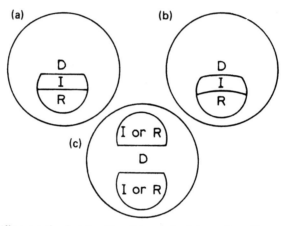

**Figure 19.12** Different trifocal styles: D = distance; I = intermediate; R = reading.

The designs shown in (a) and (b) of *Figure 19.12* are based on bifocals with shape D and C segments respectively. Trifocals of these two types are made from composite buttons such as that illustrated in *Figure 19.13*. Two different high index glasses are required for the intermediate and near portions. For any chosen pair of glasses, the resulting intermediate addition is always a fixed proportion of the near addition, often in the neighbourhood of 50%.

Segment diameters of some makes range up to 35 mm. The intermediate portion is also available in various depths. In general, the

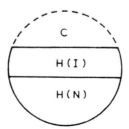

**Figure 19.13** Composite button for fused trifocal: C = crown glass; H(I) and H(N) = different high index glasses for intermediate and near portions.

preferred depth is 6 to 8 mm but the range may extend to 10 mm or more.

Trifocal design (c) in *Figure 19.12* is intended to cater for vocational or other special needs in which an area of clear vision at intermediate or near distances is also required above eye level. The two segments are quite independent and their diameters as well as their respective additions can be varied within reasonable limits.

The advancement of progressive lenses (Chapter 22) into the optical market has reduced the quantity of trifocals prescribed. However, they still occupy a very important niche in the world of optics.

# Chapter 20

# Glass solid multifocals

## Basic features

Solid multifocals, as their name implies, differ from the fused and cemented types in being made from a single piece of material. This may be either glass or one of the optical resins but the respective methods of manufacture are entirely different. In all of them, however, the addition is obtained by a change of curvature, the segment surface being more strongly convex or less deeply concave than the neighbouring surface of the distance portion. Because they do not depend on a high index material to provide the addition, solid multifocals are relatively free from the chromatic aberration associated with fused multifocals.

Although the term *solid* can be used to describe glass or resin lenses made from one piece of material, in practice it tends to be used on its own to indicate glass lenses are required. An order received by a prescription house stating 'solid 38 bifocals' would inevitably be supplied in glass.

A well-made lens of this type may be hard to distinguish from a fused bifocal except by touch, the change in curvature being detectable when the fingertip is lightly passed across the dividing line. Lenses in which the dividing line has been completely obliterated are usually referred to as seamless or blended bifocals.

Glass lenses are made from large saucer-shaped mouldings. A circular area in the centre becomes the reading portion or RP, while the surrounding zone forms the distance portion or DP. These two areas being of different curvature, are ground and polished separately. Great care and skill has to be exercised to ensure that the 'ridge' between distance and reading is kept to a minimum.

Although it has been usual for many years to produce the bifocal effect on the concave surface of the lens, the alternative construction with the segment on the convex surface has come back into use, although only in a small way, the majority still having the segment on the back surface. This has in some ways made the solid bifocal the 'odd one out' in the optical world. The majority of multifocals today (fused glass, resin multifocals, glass and resin progressives) are all supplied with the front surface finished, the prescription house working the concave side. Because solids are supplied finished on the concave side a whole range of smoothing and polishing tools have to be set aside especially for front surface working.

The basic manufacturing technique, patented by A. H. Emerson and M. Bentzon in 1906, is still in general use. There are no technical restrictions on the segment diameter. In the past, many different diameters from 12 to 60 mm have been in regular production, but the range is now reduced. Segment diameters presently available are 22, 30, 38 and 45 mm. The method and geometry of manufacture only allows the production of round, not shaped, segments. When both portions of the saucer blank have been worked the moulding is cut up into semi-finished blanks. Segments of 22 and 30 mm diameter are cut out as shown in *Figure 20.1*, the shaded areas being disposed of to leave lens as shown in *Figure 20.2*.

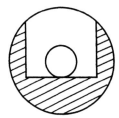

**Figure 20.1** A saucer blank worked to give a 22 or 30 mm segment. Shaded area indicates what will be cut away.

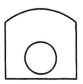

**Figure 20.2** Semi-finished 22 or 30 mm segment blank when shaded area shown in *Figure 20.1* has been removed.

On 38 and 45 mm segments, the saucer can be cut in half so two lenses can be obtained from one saucer (*Figure 20.3*). As with the 22 and 30 mm segments, the shaded areas are disposed of leaving a lens shape as depicted in *Figure 20.4*.

The above explains why generally the larger segments are cheaper as the semi-finished manufacturers can obtain two lenses from one saucer blank. It also explains why sometimes these larger segments do not allow the segment height required by the patient. It all evolves from the geometry of this lens type.

Taking as an example, a 38 mm segment bifocal – if the saucer is cut in half this means that the deepest segment possible is 19 mm (the radius of the segment). This is in fact not quite true, for there must be an allowance

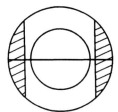

**Figure 20.3** A saucer blank worked to give a 38 or 45 mm segment. Shaded area indicates what will be cut away.

**Figure 20.4** Semi-finished 38 or 45 mm segment when shaded area from *Figure 20.3* has been removed.

made for cutting the saucer. Most prescription houses would therefore agree that 18 mm is the deepest that the segment can be set. The same principle is applied to 45 mm segments and therefore the maximum depth of 21.5 mm is reached in practice.

A way around the problem is to order an extra deep reading portion (EDRP) where the manufacturer does not cut through the middle of the saucer, but lower down. These are obviously more expensive as the manufacturer has no longer obtained two semi-finished lenses from the saucer. An additional operation referred to as 'de-pipping' has to be performed on 22, 30 mm and extra deep reading portions. Due to the symmetry of the segment and the machinery used to work the surface, a small 'pip' is formed in the centre of the segment. With 38 and 45 mm segments it is of no consequence because, as described above, the saucer is cut in half, effectively through the 'pip'. The 'pip' is created due to the fact that the smoothing/polishing tool, whilst rotating on the segment surface, is literally 'squirming' around a central point unlike at the edge where it rotates more 'freely'. This causes a very small imperfection that has to be carefully removed by subsequent polishing.

A quicker and more cost effective alternative to an extra deep reading portion is often the 30 mm segment. Whilst not as large as say a 38 or 45 mm segment it does allow high segment fitting on many frames.

The surface power of the distance portion on the segment side is popularly termed the DP curve and the power of the segment surface the RP curve. The semi-finished blanks are available in a number of standard DP curves, suitable for a wide range of prescriptions. They generally include plano, −4.00 D, −6.00 D and −8.00 D, though not necessarily in all segment diameters. Blanks with a plano DP curve are very useful for prescriptions of high power. Strong plus lenses are made in plano-convex form (segment to the rear) and strong minus lenses in plano-concave form (segment to the front).

The reading addition of a solid bifocal blank is the difference between the DP and RP curves and can hence be checked with a suitable lens measure or dial gauge spherometer, as well as by the more conventional way, the focimeter.

The finishing of solid bifocal blanks to prescription requires a very wide range of toric tools, especially if the segment is on the concave surface, in which case a plus base toroidal surface is needed on the other side. Over part of the range of tools, it is then necessary to make different vertex power allowances on the base and cross curves. A further complication is that since vertex power allowances are affected by the finished lens thickness, more than one tool of the same nominal base and cross curves may be needed.

## Upcurve solid bifocals

A variation on the lenses already featured is the upcurve bifocal. Up to now, all the lenses have been what is termed 'downcurve', a term which is self explanatory, although seldom used. The upcurve looks and feels very much like an ordinary downcurve solid bifocal except the segment is now the distance whilst the main lens area, reading, is completely opposite to the traditional downcurve. Its use is purely occupational. It is intended for those who require a large reading area with occasional use of a small distance area (the segment) at the top of the lens. In appearance it looks like a bifocal that has been put into the frame upside down!

The upcurve bifocal should not be confused with the even rarer request for an 'upside down' or reversed bifocal which is simply an ordinary downcurve turned upside down for occupational reasons.

## Seamless (blended) bifocals

The dividing line of a solid bifocal could be made to disappear if the two portions of the lens were joined by a transition zone. The principle can be seen most easily by considering a section through the segment side of a solid bifocal with a plano DP (*Figure 20.5*). A circle of suitable diameter

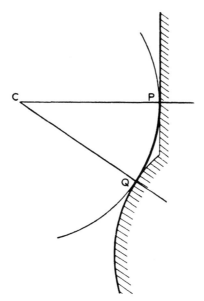

**Figure 20.5** Transition zone of seamless solid bifocal.

can clearly be positioned so as to touch both portions of the bifocal surface. At each point of contact, P and Q, there is a common normal. Hence, the circular arc PQ would blend the two curves together and eliminate the dividing line. In *Figure 20.5* the relative width of the transition zone has been greatly exaggerated for the sake of clarity. In practice, it is only a few millimetres. The zonal area is, of course, quite useless visually.

## 'Executive' (E-style) bifocals

The executive type of solid bifocal, illustrated in *Figure 20.6* was invented and produced in a one-piece construction as long ago as 1893 by the Swiss optician, H. Strubin. The trade name Executive adopted by American Optical Company has passed into general usage and the term E-style bifocal is also used as a generic term for lenses of this construction.

The E-style bifocal can be visualised as a one-piece form of the Franklin bifocal (see Chapter 23). The 'segment' is normally incorporated into the front surface and has the appearance of a straight line. If the front surface has a +7.00 D curve in the distance area and a +9.50 D curve in the near, the difference between them would create an addition of +2.50 D (see *Figure 20.6b*). Since a +9.50 D curve has a greater sag over the same diameter as a +7.00 D curve, the dividing line takes the form of a ridge with its minimum depth at the centre but becoming progressively deeper towards the periphery of the lens, as indicated in *Figure 20.6a*.

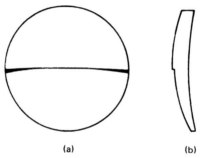

(a)                              (b)

**Figure 20.6** Construction of E-style solid bifocals.

The great optical advantage of the E-style bifocal arises from the fact that the centres of curvature of the two portions of the bifocal surface lie on a line passing through the centre of the dividing line. Consequently, there is no vertical image jump. This remains true wherever the distance optical centre is placed when the blank is finished to prescription. Moreover, the total field of view seems continuous, almost like that of a single-vision lens.

A disadvantage of this lens type is that because of its geometry it does tend to result in thicker lenses than the equivalent powered bifocal of some other design. Whilst it is possible to surface so that the lens is minimal thickness when glazed, on plus prescriptions the distance portion has to be thicker than ideally required to ensure sufficient substance for glazing is maintained in the reading area.

A process referred to as prism thinning is often employed on this lens type. Traditionally this has normally involved working an equal base down prism in both lenses, the theory being that a prism with its base down has its thinnest point at the top of the lens. Thus, from a cosmetic point of view, the lens can be produced in a thinner form.

The traditional amount of prism has been dependent upon the addition power, the prescription house normally incorporating a base down prism amount equivalent to two-thirds of the addition power. For example, an addition of +3.00 would have $2^\Delta$ down incorporated whereas a +1.50 addition would have $1^\Delta$ down.

Unfortunately, this across the board approach is not very scientific and can actually result in lenses being thicker! For any system to work successfully, factors such as segment height, depth of frame and distance power must be taken into account.

The Norville Optical Company (Gloucester) was the first to introduce what they term Intelligent Prism Thinning (IPT). It breaks away from the traditional method, in that it takes many more factors into account and no longer adopts an across the board approach. The end result is lenses with prism thinning base up, down or indeed none at all – whatever will give the most balanced and minimum substance lens, top and bottom.

Because the prescription requirements for both eyes are seldom identical, the system also has to take into account this factor. Whether prism base up, down or none at all is worked, it must be the same for both lenses otherwise an unwanted vertical prismatic imbalance will be created.

## Vertical prism compensation

In the previous chapter the consequences of a variation between the powers in the vertical meridian were examined. In cases of anisometropia, a limited degree of prism compensation can be obtained by using different segment diameters for the right and left lenses. The amount of compensation is half the difference in the segment diameters multiplied by the near addition. The large segment diameter is used for the lens requiring base down prism to reduce the imbalance at the near visual points.

Solid bifocals lends themselves very much to this because unlike fused round segments that tend to be in the region of 22–26 mm in diameter, solids offer a greater range: 22, 30, 38 and 45 mm.

The imbalance can be calculated by the method described in the previous chapter. Assume that the imbalance is $1.6^\Delta$ dioptres. The formula is

$$\frac{20 \times \text{diff prism}}{\text{add}}$$

Assume a 2.00 addition

$$\frac{20 \times 1.6}{2.00} = 16\,\text{mm}$$

Effectively this results in a requirement of 16 mm between the segment diameters to eliminate the imbalance. A 22 mm segment could be used for one eye and a 38 mm for the other. If the lenses are minus, the larger segment would be used for the lower powered lens and if plus, the higher powered lens. The above method of correcting imbalance does, however, have the cosmetic disadvantage of different segment sizes in the same frame which some patients may find unacceptable.

The E-style featured earlier in this chapter lends itself to the bi-prism technique described in Chapter 19. Because the dividing line extends completely across an E-style there is no immediate evidence that the technique has been applied.

## Prism controlled solid bifocals

In finishing a bifocal blank to prescription it is possible, given due care, to place the distance optical centre in any desired position. In the absence of instructions to the contrary, it is normally placed a few millimetres above the top of the segment. This distance is known as the segment drop.

One optical disadvantage of fused and solid bifocals alike is that very little control can be exercised over the position of the near optical centre. In fact, given the segment size and insetting, the position of the near optical centre is entirely dependent on the prescription. If the distance power is positive, the near optical centre will usually be situated somewhere between the distance optical centre and the geometrical centre of the segment. On the other hand, if the distance power is negative the near optical centre may not even be situated on the lens at all.

Nevertheless, with most prescriptions the near optical centration is adequate even though it may be imperfect. Only with certain uncommon types of prescription would any difficulty arise. For example, if there is a marked difference in power between the right and left lenses (anisometropia), the vertical prismatic effects at the near visual points might be unequal to an extent that would trouble the wearer. If a patient needing a strong minus correction insisted on a wide reading field, he/she might find invisible solid bifocals with large segments uncomfortable to wear because of the strong base down prismatic effect in the reading portions – an effect inevitably resulting from the combination of a high minus distance prescription and a large segment size. It is sometimes desired to incorporate base in prism in the reading portions only, or indeed to have prescribed prism in the distance only, an arrangement which is usually beyond the scope of fused or solid bifocals.

A special type of bifocal permitting some degree of control over optical centration or prism in the near portion is given the descriptive name of *prism controlled*. It is made by substantially the same process as conventional solids, but the moulding is tilted at a pre-determined angle when the reading portion is being worked. The result is that the segment incorporates a prism, the dividing line taking the form of a ridge of varying depth which reduces almost to zero at the base of the prism. The segment prism may be used to improve the optical centration of the reading portion, or it may be called for by the prescription.

At present, this type of bifocal is made only in the 30 mm segment size and with segment prism in $0.5^{\Delta}$ (dioptre) intervals up to $8.00^{\Delta}$ (dioptres). The base of the segment prism can be set in any desired direction

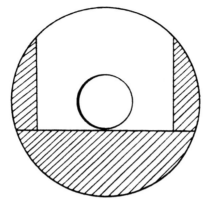

**Figure 20.7** Prism-segment bifocal blank, cut from the circular moulding.

according to the manner in which the semi-finished blank is cut from the circular moulding. By way of illustration, *Figure 20.7* shows a blank cut so as to set the base of the segment prism horizontal and to the right. Prism controlled bifocals are only available in glass material.

## Solid trifocals

Solid trifocals can be traced back to the year 1826 in which an English engineer and inventor, Isaac Hawkins, published a description of a pair which he had designed for his own use and had persuaded an optician to make. They were of the Franklin construction but with each lens in three separate pieces, each with the optical centre appropriately positioned for the viewing distance.

An array of different solid trifocal designs were available at one time but have now become virtually unobtainable.

# Chapter 21

# Resin multifocals

A distinction was made in the previous chapter between solid multi-focals in glass and solid multifocals in resin. Indeed, they are both formed from one solid piece of material, but by an entirely different process. It was also indicated that although resin multifocals are solids, the term in practice is normally used to indicate glass.

The majority of resin lenses are made from a material called allyl diglycol carbonate, or Columbia Resin 39 (CR39) and was referred to in Chapter 2.

Unlike glass solid multifocals which have the segment incorporated by physically cutting curves on to the surface, a resin multifocal is moulded.

Resin multifocals are available in an array of different shape and size segments. The segment is normally on the front surface. By running a finger lightly across the lens surface the change of curvature in the segment area can be felt. Any straight or curve top segments appear as though the upper part of a complete circular segment has been removed, leaving a narrow ledge with its maximum depth in the middle. In effect, the same kind of ledge is formed in shaped fused bifocals, but is internal and merely forms the boundary between the different types of glass.

The choice of segments is limited only by the designer's imagination. Round segments with diameters of 22, 24, 25, 28, 38, 40 and 45 mm are available. D-shaped segments range from D22 up to D45. Curve tops and a proliferation of trifocals are also available.

Many lenses have the cosmetic appearance of their glass counterparts described in Chapters 19 and 20 but as outlined, the method of manufacture is very different.

A range of multifocals is shown below in *Figure 21.1*, and it is by no means comprehensive, simply representative. Those with an asterisk are often referred to as occupational lenses, giving either wider inter-mediate portions than the average trifocal lens, or segment position more suitably placed for either occupational or recreational purposes. It was mentioned earlier that on average the intermediate addition is 50% of the near. Occupational lenses give the opportunity to substitute different values.

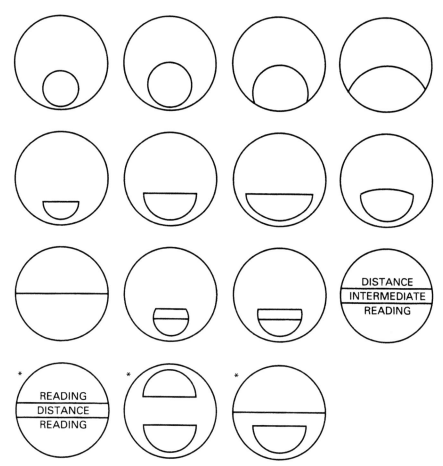

**Figure 21.1** A selection of segment sizes and shapes available in resin multifocals.
*Occupational lenses.

## Vertical prism compensation

It has been shown in Chapters 19 and 20 how to calculate vertical
imbalance and how the various lens types can be compensated to allow
for correction of this phenomenon. Resin lenses are no different. Odd size
segments as described in Chapter 20 can be used or bi-prism as described
in Chapter 19. There is, however, no lens presently on the market in resin
that is equivalent to the glass solid prism controlled.

Whilst D-shaped and E-style resin lenses are suitable for bi-prism the
techniques employed vary slightly from that of glass. In the case of resin
multifocals it is possible to obtain blanks where the bi-prism has been
incorporated into the mould, to facilitate easier manufacture by the
prescription house. There is one very radical difference from that of the
traditional bi-prism where the usual effect is to diminish base down
prism by always creating a base up bi-prism and at the same time

reducing both the imbalance and image jump. With a precast, exactly the opposite occurs, for there can only be base down in the reading, hence a base down half pair moulded bi-prism is used in the eye of lesser segment prism to equal the greater base down of the other lens, although, for plus lenses there is the opposite and more beneficial effect.

In Chapter 19 the following Rx was used as an example:

R −0.50 DS
L −3.25 DS
Add 2.00

It was calculated that the imbalance between the two lenses was $2.2^\Delta$ base down, left eye.

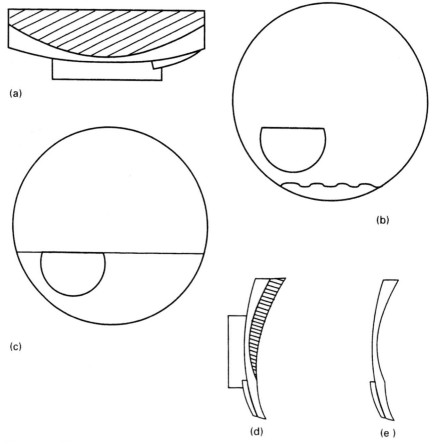

**Figure 21.2** Vertical prism compensation using bi-prism slab. (a) Whilst still on block, a mask is applied to the inside of the lens (represented by shaded area). (b) The line referred to in the text begins to appear. (c) The line is now level with segment top. (d) A side view of when the line is level with segment top. (e) The remaining mask is removed resulting in only the bottom part of the lens having a prism incorporated.

In the case of resin lenses a precast right lens would be selected with $2^\Delta$ base down (the prisms are only available in 0.50 steps with base down prism in the reading only). This would have the effect of creating a total prism amount of $2.4^\Delta$ base down in the right. The left, as seen from Chapter 19 has $2.6^\Delta$ base down prismatic effect. The end result is a pair of lenses with only $0.2^\Delta$ imbalance between them.

If for one reason or another the precast prism is not used, it is possible to work a bi-prism slab-off in a similar manner to that described for glass, with a few important differences. Remaining with the example above, a pair of resin D segments will be produced as per normal with no prism incorporated. Whilst the left lens is still on the surfacing block a resin mask would be applied to the back surface. A $2.2^\Delta$ prism base up blocking ring is fitted to the block and the inside surface regenerated until a 'line' starts appearing at the bottom of the lens, indicating a commencement of breaking through the mask previously applied.

At this stage the lens surface would be carefully smoothed until the line is within approximately 1 mm of the segment top. The lens is polished, the final stock removal bringing the line of the mask up level with the segment top. The lens is deblocked in the normal manner, the mask softening, allowing it to be peeled off. Only the bottom of the lens has had the prism worked on it and therefore the prismatic effect of both segments is now equal to $0.4^\Delta$ base down. *Figure 21.2* illustrates diagramatically the steps involved.

The major difference between glass and resin bi-prism, is that the 'ridge' coincidental with the top of the segment is on the back surface.

Using a variation of this technique it is possible to bi-prism E-style resin lenses in a similar way.

## Higher index resin lenses

An ever increasing number of multifocals are becoming available in higher index resins. The choice of segment size and shape tends to be more limited in comparison with standard resin. The method of manufacture is similar to that of CR39 in that they are thermal setting, the primary difference being in the chemical structure of the monomers and the varying resulting refractive indices such as 1.506, 1.60 and even 1.7.

The foremost benefit of higher refractive index polymers is that thinner lenses can result.

# Chapter 22

# Progressive lenses (PALs – progressive addition lenses)

A young eye can vary its power smoothly from about +60 to +70 D, enabling it to remain in focus up to a very short distance. By middle age, this range of adjustment will drop to about 4 D and it then continues to dwindle at a faster rate until there is virtually none left. (Presbyopia.)

Bifocals help matters by providing one fixed amount of extra power, while trifocals provide two, usually in steps of one dioptre or more. This is no match for what the eye was once able to do. Numerous attempts have therefore been made to devise a practicable lens that will give good clear vision at all distances and have an enhanced cosmetic appearance, hence the introduction of what is termed *progressive lenses*. Bifocals and trifocals suffer from a great disadvantage in the cosmetic arena – they have noticeable dividing lines between the distance and near portions of the lens. The line(s) mars the cosmetic appearance of the lens and is a 'give away' to the wearers age! Although these factors are cosmetically based rather than optical, to the end user, the patient, they are extremely important.

Unlike bifocals or trifocals there is no sudden fluctuation in accommodative demand. There is no 'jump' which occurs with most multifocal lenses. In simplistic terms the lenses consist of a distance portion, intermediate channel and a reading area (*Figure 22.1*). Around these are areas of the lens not intended for clear vision, but designed simply for awareness of objects and movements in the intermediate area. These areas are unavoidable and are due to the linking of distance, into intermediate, into reading. Progressive designs vary from one another by how these 'no go' areas of the lens are distributed across it. The intermediate 'corridor' of a progressive is quite narrow, measuring less than 4 mm on average. A consequence of this is a restriction of the intermediate field of view in comparison to a conventional trifocal. At the lower end of the 'corridor' which is now at or near the full reading power the intermediate power does not reach fully across the lens. This means that the reading field is narrower than for most conventional bifocals or trifocals.

Due to these restrictions, the first time wearer of progressives can normally expect to experience a 'swim' effect, where objects appear to rock slightly when coming into the field of view. In practice, this phenomenon ceases once the patient has had the opportunity to adapt to the lens design as the eye/brain combination becomes accustomed to the

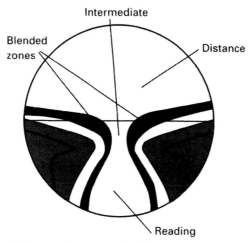

**Figure 22.1** The main elements of a progressive lens.

effect and compensates for it. This period of adaptation is applicable to all progressives and can be experienced when a patient has a change of Rx or indeed, changes the type of progressive.

It should also be noted that due to the design characteristics, the reading area of a progressive becomes smaller as the addition increases. For this reason it is advisable to dispense progressives at the early stages of presbyopia, when addition requirements are perhaps in the region of +0.75 or +1.00. The reading areas of these lenses are at their widest which allows easier adaption to the lens design. Having become accustomed, the patient then finds it easier to adapt when eventually higher additions are required.

Whilst many different designs of progressive are available they all have four main aims:

1 A stable (or nearly stable) distance vision area in the top part of the lens.
2 A intermediate progressive area to provide a transition from distance to near vision.
3 A reasonably stable near vision area.
4 Complete 'invisibility' giving single vision-type appearance.

A few lenses have tried to escape from this general purpose formula by having an intermediate segment incorporated at the top of the lens or by being specially constructed to give intermediate and near vision only, or to give preference to intermediate and reading with some vision in the distance (such as a lens designed for work with visual display units).

When thinking of progressives it tends to be in the context that this is a comparatively modern idea and it is easy to imagine lens designers in front of computers, seeking to achieve the 'perfect' design. In fact progressives are generally accepted as going back to 1907 and are attributed to Owen Aves, a leading English (Yorkshireman actually) optometrist of his day. It is worthy of a mention as it is the first progressive power lens on record. Although Aves patented his design in 1907 and produced some prototype lenses, they never became commercially available. A serious drawback was that a combination of two special surfaces was needed to produce the progressive power effect (*Figure 22.2*). It would thus have been impossible to incorporate a prescribed cylinder. Included in his patent was the machinery required to produce such surfaces. Lenses of more recent design obviate this difficulty by employing only one 'special' front surface.

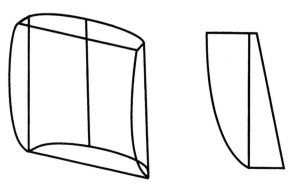

**Figure 22.2** Diagrammatic representation of Owen Aves' design for a lens using two aspheric plano-cylinders. Front surface: aspheric cylinder axis 180. Rear surface: aspheric cylinder axis 90.

A design patented in 1909 and 1914 by Henry Orford Gowlland was the basis of the first range of progressive power lenses to reach the market. They were manufactured in Canada under the trade name *Ultifo*. As shown in *Figure 22.3*, the back surface was part of a paraboloid, the surface produced by rotating a parabola (the curve PAQ) about its axis of symmetry YY. The front surface was spherical or toroidal according to the

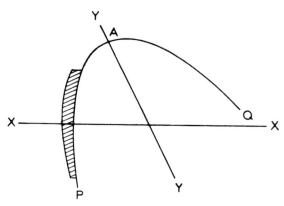

**Figure 22.3** The Gowlland lens: YY = axis of revolution of parabola; XX = optical axis of lens.

prescription. Unlike the circle, the parabola is a figure of a continuously varying curvature – steepest at its vertex A and becoming progressively flatter at increasing distances from the vertex. For example, in the lens illustrated the back surface power in the vertical meridian might vary, say, from –7.00 D at the top of the lens to –5.00 D at the bottom, giving a maximum addition of +2.00 D. Even down the middle of the lens, however, there would be a noticeable astigmatic effect arising from the geometry of the paraboloidal surface.

The introduction in 1959 of Essel's (now referred to as Essilor) *Varilux* lens, designed by Bernard Maitenaz, marked a decisive breakthrough for the progressive power concept. The design not only proved to be a commercial success but set the direction for later developments in this field.

Its main features can be summarised with the aid of *Figure 22.4* in which the dotted lines merely indicate areas of the lens. As in other progressive power designs, the varifocal surface is continuous and therefore free from dividing lines and image jump. The uncut lens is circular, its upper half D having the power of the distance prescription. A transition 'corridor' P of progressive power, reasonably free from astigmatism, blends smoothly into a small area R having the full power of the reading addition. Because of the geometry of the progressive surface, vision within the shaded lateral areas is noticeably of a lower standard than would normally be acceptable.

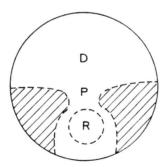

**Figure 22.4** The Maitenaz design (right lens, front view).

The original Varilux was to be superseded by a modified design termed Varilux 2 (now simply Varilux), which aimed at reducing aberration in the lateral areas by using horizontal aspheric sections.

Earlier designs of progressives have become known as 'first generation' lenses. They were what could be termed symmetrical designs, that is a lens designed around the intermediate corridor that could be used for either the right or left lens. The prescription house had only to rotate each lens about 10 degrees upwards on the nasal side to provide the necessary inset to the corridor. This meant that prescription houses only had to stock one lens in each add and base curve rather than in right and lefts.

There was one major drawback in this principal. When viewing through areas that are not central to the lens, patients were not achieving

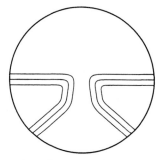

**Figure 22.5** A simple representation of a symmetrical design progressive. (From A. J. Jarratt by permission.)

identical viewing conditions for each eye. *Figure 22.5* shows a simple representation of a symmetrical design progressive. The contour lines represent the unwanted astigmatism/distortion, but the distance, intermediate and reading areas can clearly be distinguished.

*Figure 22.6* shows the symmetrical design (viewed from the front) with both lenses inset towards the nasal, achieved by swinging the lens some 10 degrees. The black circles represent the area of the lens a patient would view through if they gazed to the left.

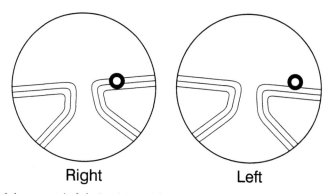

Right                    Left

**Figure 22.6** A symmetrical design (viewed from the front) with both lenses inset towards the nasal, achieved by swinging the lens some 10 degrees. The black circles represent the area of the lens a patient would view through if they gazed to the left. (From A. J. Jarratt by permission.)

As can be seen, the left eye views through an area with very little astigmatism whilst the right eye encounters a 'blurred' area.

The situation is similar if the patient gazes through the reading area at an object towards their left (*Figure 22.7*).

In this instance the left eye encounters 'blurring' in comparison to the right. In effect the two eyes will be viewing through different amounts of surface astigmatism. Most of the second generation progressives overcome the problems outlined above by being available in right and left blanks. The design has become asymmetrical instead of symmetrical.

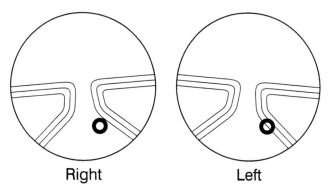

**Figure 22.7** A symmetrical design (viewed from the front) with both lenses inset towards the nasal, achieved by swinging the lens some 10 degrees. The black circles represent the area of the lens a patient would view through if they gazed the reading area to the left. (From A. J. Jarratt by permission.)

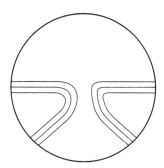

**Figure 22.8** A simple representation of an assymetrical design progressive. (From A. J. Jarratt by permission.)

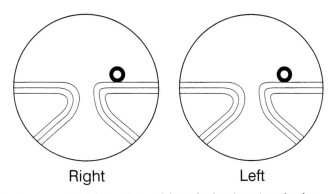

**Figure 22.9** An assymetrical design (viewed from the front) pre-inset by the manufacturer, allowing similar viewing (conditions) for both eyes. The black circles represent the area of the lens a patient would view through if they gazed to the left. (From A. J. Jarratt by permission.)

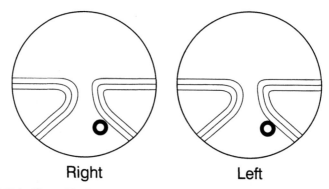

Right          Left

**Figure 22.10** As Figure 22.9 but representing vision through the reading area. (From A. J. Jarratt by permission.)

*Figure 22.8* represents an asymmetrical design where insetting of the reading area is achieved and at the same time the surface astigmatism in the distance portion is kept as level as possible, so as not to intrude too far into the line of peripheral vision. The design in the intermediate and reading areas has been 'balanced' to allow similar viewing conditions for both eyes (*Figure 22.9* and *Figure 22.10*).

## Hard and soft designs

The terms 'hard' and 'soft' are often used as a basis for discussion when referring to progressive lenses. Due to the nature of their design, they will always have areas of surface astigmatism. Designers can, however, affect the placement of this unwanted 'distortion' and so affect the width of the 'corridor' and that of the reading. *Figure 22.11* shows a hard design.

The first generation of progressives were based on the 'hard' principal. The lens has a front spherical distance portion with the areas of surface astigmatism confined to the lower nasal and peripheral areas. This

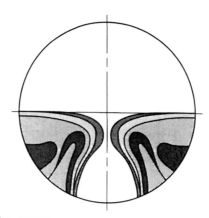

**Figure 22.11** Hard design concept.

concept gives good distortion free distance vision combined with a relatively large reading area. The downside is that the intermediate 'corridor' is rather narrow and the rate of power change rather rapid. Many wearers find the use of such lenses tiring. Adaption to such designs can take longer, but often result in the wearer simply 'giving up' and claiming they are non-tolerant to such a lens.

The width of the intermediate 'corridor' is of prime importance to most patients. Many tasks are undertaken at distances greater than 'reading'. In an effort to reduce non-tolerances the lens designers went back to their drawing boards and attempted to improve upon the progressive concept. The result was second generation 'soft' designs.

The soft designs were based on the principle that the greater area that one can distribute the surface astigmatism over, the wider the intermediate 'corridor' becomes. By moving some of the surface astigmatism up into the distance portion and into the edges of the reading area, a wider intermediate can be formed (*Figure 22.12*).

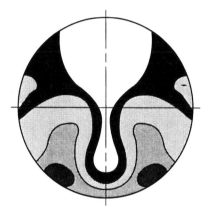

**Figure 22.12** Soft design concept.

However, this does mean that the useful areas of both the distance and the reading are slightly more restricted than in the hard design.

Due to technical advances in progressive lens design we now have lenses that cannot strictly be classified as either hard or soft, but somewhere in between. The word 'firm' has been used to describe such lenses.

## Multifocals versus progressives

*Figure 22.13* demonstrates the fundamental differences experienced when looking through a conventional D-shaped segment and a typical progressive lens.

The magnification of the three broad lines is equal for both lens types but as can be seen, magnification through the progressive is gradual rather than abrupt. However, it can clearly be seen that straight lines, both vertical and horizontal, become 'distorted' around the intermediate and reading areas of the progressive. With time patients learn to avoid

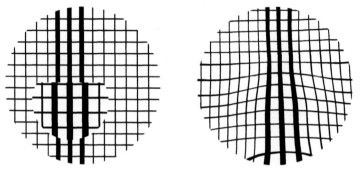

**Figure 22.13** Fundamental differences experienced when looking through a conventional D-shaped segment and a typical progressive lens.

these areas by moving their eyes from top to bottom of their lenses, and moving their head to the left and right to avoid looking through the peripheral areas. Quite often you hear the exclamation, 'Point your nose and adjust your chin'. Patients have to learn to point their nose at what they want to view and then adjust their heads vertically until they obtain clear vision. Then everything from distance through to intermediate and reading will be in focus. Progressive lens wearers get the best from their lenses by moving their head in the direction of gaze rather than trying to view through the lens edges by just moving their eyes.

## Prism thinning

In Chapter 20 reference was made to prism thinning in E-style lenses. The same principal is also used in progressives. Prism thinning, sometimes referred to as cosmetic thinning, has been commonly used since the 1970s.

In order to achieve the reading addition, the front surface radius must progressively shorten in the lower part of the lens. In order to obtain a reasonable blank size in the lower part of the lens, the centre thickness must be made large enough to cope with the progressively shortening radius in the lower regions of the lens. This has the effect of making the lens appear too thick in the distance area, but if it were surfaced down to reduce this centre thickness the overall blank size in the lower part of the lens would be reduced and probably would not allow the lens to be glazed into the chosen frame.

The conventional solution has been to apply a base down prism during surfacing, as a prism with its base down has its thinnest part at the top, making the distance portion thinner and therefore cosmetically more acceptable.

In order that binocular vision is not compromised, the prism must obviously be equally applied to both lenses. The traditional 'across the board' approach of always supplying prism base down equal to two-thirds of the add power is fundamentally flawed. For example, a minus powered progressive fitted at an average height of 4–5 mm above horizontal centre line would actually be worse if prism thinning base down were added. In this instance base up prism thinning would be advantageous.

As referred to in Chapter 20, Norville Optical have developed a system called Intelligent Prism Thinning where factors such as Rx, fitting cross height and frame depth are taken into consideration. After complicated calculations the computer is able to calculate the amount and direction of prism thinning necessary to provide, as near as possible, a substance match at the top and bottom of the lens shape. As the prism has to be equal for both eyes a 'rounding' factor has to be incorporated within the calculation program to ensure that even when the specifications for each lens is different, the prism required is the same. It has to be said that in many instances, Intelligent Prism Thinning means no prism thinning! That is to say, the computer calculates that the best possible substance match between top and bottom can best be achieved by not incorporating additional prism.

Other methods by which the manufacturer attempts to produce thinner progressive lenses includes elliptical shaped blanks. This reduces the effective diameter in the vertical meridian making the overall finished substance of plus lenses thinner than those produced from standard round blanks.

Pre-decentring round blanks is another method by which manufacturers seek to achieve thinner lenses. The physical diameter of the lens is smaller than the effective optical diameter.

## Vocational designs

Another development has been the gradual introduction of progressive lenses specifically designed for differing ranges or tasks. They are designed primarily for close work, having a wider reading area than conventional progressives. They also provide the patient with comfortable intermediate vision. They are not intended for distance vision in the normally accepted sense.

Some manufacturers have a 'family' of progressives, sometimes consisting of three distinct designs. For example, one 'family' of lenses might include a lens for the emerging presbyope, for someone who has never had to wear a reading correction before. There is the lens for the established presbyope who has either worn multifocals or progressives before and, finally, the vocational version for use at intermediate and reading distance. The manufacturers realised that some tasks cannot be satisfied from just one design. For example, a draughtsman may find it very tiring when trying to use a conventional progressive all day, for a task that predominantly involves close work. The manufacturers get around this using the 'family' concept which allows easy transition from one lens type to another. The draughtsman example used above represents a typical situation. Driving to work and at home the conventional progressive is quite adequate, but once in the drawing office, the spectacles are changed for the vocational version.

## Present and future

There are now a multitude of different progressives on the market, from an almost equal multitude of manufacturers. There is one irremovable drawback common to all types of progressive power lenses. This is that the increase in spherical power is inevitably accompanied by an unwanted astigmatic effect. It is not evenly distributed over the whole lens area, and the broad pattern in which it is distributed varies from one type of lens to another. Nevertheless, in some region or regions of the lens, the unwanted astigmatism is bound to reach a maximum value – approximately the same as the maximum increase in the spherical power.

It is the lens designer's dream to create a progressive with no areas of distortion, which unfortunately is just not possible. All they can do is to reduce these distortions to a minimum. Designs will continue to be optimised so that all prescriptions in the range achieve a reasonable performance, but real improvement over existing designs is becoming increasingly difficult to achieve, as there are not the degrees of freedom available to the lens designer for radical change.

In the long term, it is possible that completely different concepts may be used, and of those technologies available, two of the most obvious are liquid crystal lenses and gradient index lens materials. The first of these consists of a lens material with an electronically variable refractive index, whereas gradient index materials have a fixed index gradient over a finite distance in the material. Other options could be diffractive optics or deformable lenses. Whilst some of the above show great theoretical advantages over existing spectacle lenses, none as yet has shown the right combination of optical performance, cosmetic appearance and mechanical stability required to make a commercially successful product. Considering that the 200th anniversary has passed of Benjamin Franklin's bifocal (see Chapter 23) then perhaps there is an assured future for progressive lenses.

So what of the present? First and second generation lenses have been replaced with third and fourth generation. Manufacturers have realised that having one single design of progressives for all stages of presbyopia cannot give all patients the best possible solution to their visual needs. In the lower reading additions the emerging presbyope requires a smooth, gentle power increase. As patients age and their reading addition increases, reduction of aberrations resulting from the greater power changes becomes an important priority. Now is the era of the multi-design concept, where the lens is available in some 12 different designs to cater for the needs of patients at various stages of presbyopia (the design changing as the addition increases).

So what of the future? Several manufacturers have taken the frontiers of progressive technology even further by developing a lens where both the progressive and cylindrical surface are on the back. They claim that by forming the progressive surface on the back it has the effect of enlarging the field of view. Surface astigmatism being equal, the closer the progressive surface is to the eye, the wider the field of view (*Figure 22.14*).

Manufacturers of conventional front surface progressive lenses keep on hand a large stock of semi-finished lens blanks for each base and addition power. The progressive design is already formed on the front surface. The manufacturer selects a blank and surfaces the back surface to the spherical power or cylindrical power demanded by the customer's prescription. In contrast, design work on these lenses begins after the customer's prescription is received. As both progressive and cylindrical

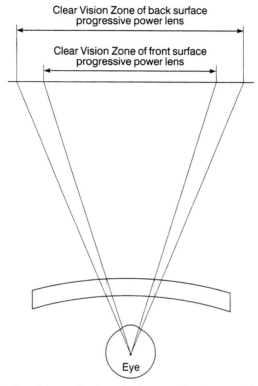

Clear Vision Zone of back surface
progressive power lens

Clear Vision Zone of front surface
progressive power lens

Eye

**Figure 22.14** Ilustration of how a 'back surface' progressive increases the patient's field of vision.

surfaces occupy the same side of the lens, the back surface is entirely customised and optimised to the patients individual requirements. Very sophisticated equipment and techniques are required to obtain a lens of this construction. Is this a template for the future of progressives?

Finally, one has seen an increase in the number of 'short corridor' progressives designed to cater for the present fashion of small shallow eyeshapes. A 'conventional' progressive fitted to this style of frame could result in much of the reading area being 'chopped' off. These modified 'short corridor' progressives attempt to address this problem.

## Common factors

All progressives have certain factors common to one another. When received from the semi-finished manufacturers they come with a series of paint markings to enable the prescription house to position and fabricate the lens. Unlike the traditional multifocals with segments where one at least has some form of reference point such as the segment itself, progressives without paint lines look like ordinary single vision. For this reason, many progressives are treated with a process whereby once the

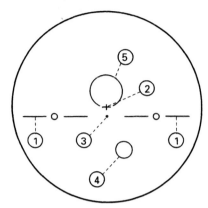

**Figure 22.15** Typical markings seen on a progressive lens prior to surfacing. (1) The 180 degree line that normally has to be kept horizontal. (2) The fitting cross which is normally located central to the patient's pupil when glazed into a frame. (3) The prism checking point for checking prismatic values. (4) The centre of the reading area and normally inset 2.5 mm in relation to the fitting cross. (5) The circle indicating where distance power and axis should be checked.

paint lines, indicating the key areas of the lens, have been removed, they can still be seen when viewed under an ultra-violet light source. *Figure 22.15* is typical of the markings seen on a progressive lens prior to surfacing.

In addition to the markings shown in *Figure 22.15*, all progressives have some form of engraved circles, logos or some other markings, permanently etched into the lens surface, but so designed as not to be visible to the patient or cause an interruption to the line of vision. (Very occasionally, a wearer may notice them but this is extremely rare.) These engravings are very important, for they are the only way that all the original key areas of lens can be identified once the paint lines have been removed. From these engravings all other points on the lens can be re-defined. As they are virtually invisible some skill is required to locate them. It helps if a strong light source is used, preferably against a black background or if the lens has been suitably treated, by positioning under an ultra-violet light source.

The engravings can be circles, squares, triangles, dots or even company logos, but what they all have in common is that they are all placed 34 mm apart, no matter which progressive is being used. They lie in the same plane as the 180 degree line shown in *Figure 22.15*. Underneath these will be found the engraved reading addition on the temporal side, and manufacturer's identification (if any) under the nasal side (*Figure 22.16*).

Some manufacturers place their logo under the addition or elsewhere on the lens leaving the nasal side for other engraved information such as base curve and refractive index of material. Many of these engravings may be abbreviated. For example, a 2.75 addition may only have the first two digits engraved. Similarly a base curve of 5.25 may just be expressed as '5'. Refractive index of 1.70 will be shown as '7'.

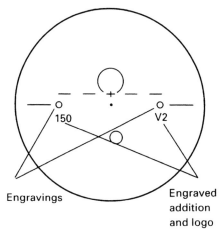

**Figure 22.16** Position of engravings on a progressive lens. (Courtesy of Essilor, Bristol, England.)

Once the engravings have been located, exactly half-way between them is the prism checking point as shown in *Figure 22.15*. This is common to all progressives. The fitting cross as shown in *Figure 22.15* is normally situated directly above the prism checking point, but this is where any uniformity disappears. The vertical distance of the fitting cross above the prism checking point can be either 2, 4 or 6 mm depending upon the manufacturer. Some manufacturer's lenses have the prism checking point and the fitting cross occupying the same position. For this reason it is essential that the manufacturer's technical literature is consulted to ascertain this information. There are even some designs where the fitting cross does not lie directly above the prism checking point, although these are rare (i.e. above but outset from prism checking point).

Correct dispensing and final positioning of progressives is essential for the patient to achieve optimum vision, so extreme care is required by both the profession and the industry.

## Focimeter checking of progressives

Unlike other lenses where once they are positioned correctly in the focimeter, all items are checked such as power, axis, centres and prisms, progressives require a slightly different approach. To begin with there are 'restricted areas' where checking must be performed, to avoid the blended area of the lenses that could cause inaccurate readings (*Figure 22.17*). Restricted areas labelled in *Figure 22.17* are explained as follows:

1 The area for checking distance Rx and axis, usually situated just above the fitting cross. When checking here, ignore any prismatic effects which may be seen.

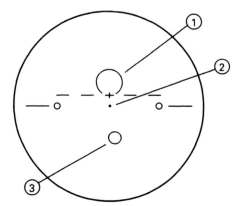

**Figure 22.17** Restricted areas where checking must be performed, to avoid the blended area of the lenses that could cause inaccurate readings. (1) Area for checking distance Rx and axis. (2) Prism checking point. (3) Centre of near vision area.

2 Prism checking point. Situated midway between engravings. This is the optical centre of the lens. It is here that any prescribed prism is checked for accuracy or where the verification of any prism thinning can be confirmed. Ignore power and axis readings at this point.
3 Centre of near vision area. Reading addition is checked here. Remember, as addition is normally incorporated into the front surface, it should be checked front vertex (see Chapter 15).

Some vocational lenses will require different methods of checking. In these instances always refer to the manufacturer's literature.

# Chapter 23
## Franklin (split) and 'bonded' lenses

In the concluding chapter on lenses for the correction of presbyopia, the clock needs to be put back to 1784, an important date in the evolution of optics. It is widely accepted that the first bifocal was described in this year by Benjamin Franklin, an American statesman, philosopher and scientist. He was finding it inconvenient to keep swopping between his separate reading and distance spectacles and therefore came upon the idea of splitting them and using the top part of his distance and the bottom part of his reading in one pair of spectacles. Quite naturally, it was referred to as a Franklin bifocal (*Figure 23.1*), although it must be said that in a letter dated 21st August 1784, he refers to being 'happy in the invention of double spectacles'. It is interesting that he does not claim to have invented bifocals, but that he is satisfied with the outcome.

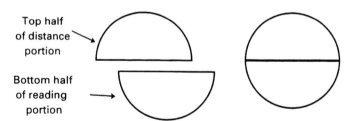

Top half
of distance
portion

Bottom half
of reading
portion

**Figure 23.1** Components of a Franklin.

Requests for Franklin bifocals are still received today, albeit rarely. They are particularly useful where, for example, a prismatic element may be required in the distance or reading only, or indeed different prismatic amounts in distance and reading. Another use, although rare, is where a patient has a different cylinder or axis requirement in the reading to that of the distance. They can also be used if an unusually high or low segment position is required that is not obtainable from a particular type of bifocal, or even simply because the frame is too large for a conventional lens.

In many respects the lens may be considered as a 'perfect bifocal'. Total control over distance and reading centres is obtained, something not always possible with more conventional lenses.

The method of manufacture involves making four lenses (assuming a pair is required): two distance, two reading. A skilled glazer will then split or edge the lenses to half circles. The contact edges must be flat to form a good fit. The edging to the eyeshape is performed in the conventional manner. Either the pressure of the rims will hold the lenses securely together, or some form of epoxy resin will be used to bond the two contact surfaces. Both resin and glass lenses are suitable for making up as Franklin bifocals or, as they are sometimes referred to, split bifocals. By nature of their design, rimless and supra mounts are not suitable for glazing with this lens type. Minus lenses are best suited to the Franklin concept due to their minimal centre substance. Plus lenses tend not to look as neat but this is purely a cosmetic disadvantage (*Figure 23.2*). The concept and advantages of the Franklin are often forgotten but they are often the way of overcoming a particular problem.

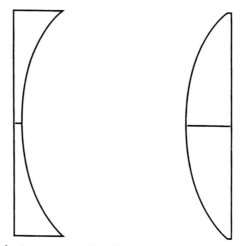

**Figure 23.2** Plus and minus powered Franklin.

The split concept is not limited to bifocals. Trifocals can be fabricated using the same principle. Rather than trying to hold three separate portions (distance, intermediate, reading) together it is more common to make use of an existing E-style bifocal! Distance single vision lenses are made as per normal. A pair of E-style bifocals are made, representing the intermediate and reading powers (*Figure 23.3*). They are then put together to form a trifocal. By way of explanation assume the requirement is to produce the following Rx:

+2.00 DS +1.00 DC × 90
2.00 addition (50% inter)
Franklin split with $2^\Delta$ base in intermediate and reading only

A single vision lens is supplied to the Rx +2.00 DS +1.00 DC × 90, with no prism incorporated. A semi-finished E-style bifocal with a +1.00 addition

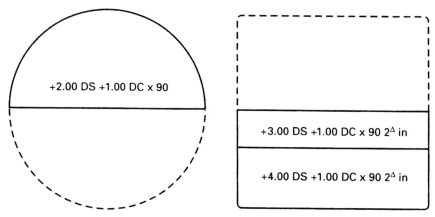

+2.00 DS +1.00 DC x 90

+3.00 DS +1.00 DC x 90 $2^{\Delta}$ in

+4.00 DS +1.00 DC x 90 $2^{\Delta}$ in

**Figure 23.3** Construction of a Franklin trifocal.

is selected. The distance section is worked to +3.00 DS +1.00 DC × 90 (representing a 50% intermediate, i.e. if the reading addition is +2.00 D then 50% of this must be 1.00 D, that is to say the intermediate portion is to be 1.00 D stronger than the distance). The addition of the E-style bifocal blank selected must be +1.00 D, for if this is taken in context, it will give a power in the reading of +4.00 DS +1.00 DC × 90 which represents a +2.00 D addition in comparison to the distance power specified. The prescribed prism is only worked on the E-style lens.

A variation on the Franklin idea is also available on glass lenses. Instead of joining lenses edge to edge it consists of a 'surface to surface' bond. It tends to be used on minus prescriptions. For example, the Rx:

    –10.00 DS
    +2.00 addition

It is known that this can be made in the conventional Franklin by making a –10.00 lens, a –8.00 D lens (reading) and cutting them in such a way as to place them edge to edge. There is always a need for more plus power for reading. In the case of a myope the only way they can receive more plus power is to have less minus, hence the result of –8.00 D for the reading power.

The 'other' method shown diagrammatically below (*Figure 23.4*) entails supplying a –8.00 D lens but not cut in half as would be done for a Franklin. To this lens is bonded a –2.00 D lens that has been cut in half. The advantage of this system is that only two lenses (assuming a pair are required) have to be reduced to half size, and being a lower power the task is easier. When completed, they feel and look like normal E-styles. The disadvantage is that this form does rely on the skill of the surfacer to create two perfect contact surfaces, as of course the back of one lens has to be the same but opposite to that of the front of the other. This is why traditionally this style of lens is made in flat form.

Another option available, and normally confined to glass, is somewhat similar to that described above and is referred to as cemented or bonded

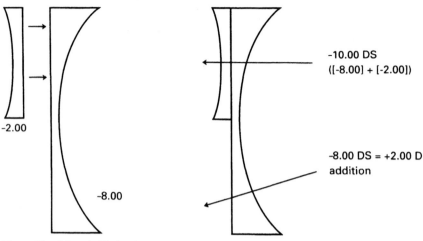

**Figure 23.4** A bonded bifocal.

bifocals. They were introduced in the 1880s and were bonded by a substance referred to as Canada balsam, a process that has survived until the present day with the exception being that a permanent epoxy resin is now used as a final bonding agent whilst the Canada balsam is used by the indusfry to facilitate the manufacture of the small segment components. Any size or shape segment is possible by this method. Even the position is not subject to the normal constraints. The skills of the surfacer are yet again brought into play in the manufacture of these segments as they are so small and wafer thin, yet still need accurate contact curves.

In practice the segment has to be made on what is termed a support lens, as it is too small and thin to produce in the conventional way. Two lenses are selected, one having the contact curve on the inside, the other lens having the opposite curvature on the front (*Figure 23.5*). The support

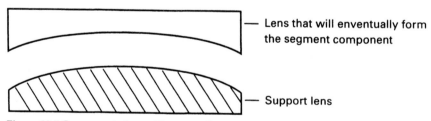

**Figure 23.5** Components for making a small segment.

lens is placed on a hotplate and heated. When the Canada balsam comes into contact with the hot lens it melts and this is spread over the surface. The other lens is then offered to it, and pressed down to remove any air bubbles. The two-lens combination is then left to cool. It is then surfaced as for a normal lens (*Figure 23.6*). The lens combination will then be reheated to soften the balsam and the segment removed (*Figure 23.7*).

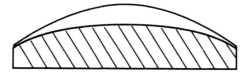

**Figure 23.6** Result when components shown in *Figure 23.5* have been bonded and surfaced.

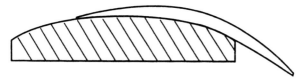

**Figure 23.7** Segment is removed from support lens.

The skill of the glazer is now called upon to lightly run the segment around an edging wheel to remove any very small chips that may have formed on the edges. If needs be, the segment can be shaped, if anything other than a round one is required. It then only remains to position the lens in the correct position on the main distance lens and bond using an epoxy resin that is normally cured to hardness by an ultra-violet light source. They can be applied to either the back or the front of the main lens, depending upon the prescription. Whichever side is decided upon, any cylindrical component would normally be on the opposite side to the segment, thus allowing spherical contact curves.

# igh powered and lenticular lenses

## Some general considerations

Indispensable though they are, lenses of high power have several inherent drawbacks from a wearer's point of view. Of necessity they are thicker than the usual run of lenses, which tends to make them conspicuous if not unsightly. The extra thickness also increases the weight. In addition, they may alter the appearance of the wearer's eyes, making them appear unnaturally larger or smaller. On looking at a medium to high powered minus lens on the wearer's face, a series of concentric images of part of the edge is sometimes noticeable. These are known as power rings or myopic rings. They are formed by repeated reflections and appear to be situated inside the lens, the successive bands becoming fainter from the margin inwards. Although not visible to the wearer, they tend to draw attention, accentuating their thick-edged lenses. The use of anti-reflection coating (see Chapter 26) will improve the appearance somewhat.

One method of reducing the weight and thickness of high powered lenses is to make in lenticular form, where only a central portion, termed the *aperture*, is worked to prescription, the surrounding portion or margin merely acting as a carrier. This expedient, involving as it does a reduction in the field of view, is not always acceptable to the wearer. Lenses not made in this fashion are termed full aperture. Another more acceptable way in which high powers can be made is to use higher index materials, which facilitates the manufacture of thinner lenses.

## High index materials

Firstly, it may help to define what is high index. British Standard 7394 Part 2 advises that 'normal' index should be considered as between 1.48 and 1.53. Any material between 1.54 and 1.63 is considered as 'mid' index, with 1.64 and 1.73 being considered as 'high' index. Any material 1.74 and above is considered as 'very high' index.

Delving more deeply it must be remembered that when the refractive index of a material is referred to, it is implicitly stating a wavelength at which the measurement was taken. It has been common practice to use different wavelengths for measuring the mean refractive index in different parts of the world. In the USA the sodium D-line is used, whereas in the UK it is the helium d-line. France and Germany use the Mercury e-line *Table 24.1* illustrates at what wavelength the various spectral lines are fixed.

**Table 24.1** Spectral lines/wavelengths

| Line | Symbol wavelength (nm) |
|------|------------------------|
| Blue cadmium F' | 479.99 |
| Blue hydrogen F | 486.13 |
| Green mercury e | 546.07 |
| Yellow helium d | 587.56 |
| Yellow sodium D | 589.30 |
| Red cadmium C | 643.85 |
| Red hydrogen C | 656.27 |

By way of explanation, light is but one part of the electro-magnetic spectrum (*Figure 24.1*). The whole range of the spectrum can be imagined as forming one long spectrum of radiations with long wavelengths at one end to very short wavelengths at the other.

The portion of the complete spectrum to which the eye is sensitive, that is the visible spectrum, lies between wavelengths $10^{-4}$ and $10^{-5}$ cm, and forms only a minute fraction of the complete spectrum (*Figure 24.2*). Because the wavelengths are so small they are expressed in terms of nanometres (nm); 1 nm is equal to $10^{-9}$ m (or $10^{-7}$ cm). Therefore, the visible spectrum lies between 380 and 780 nm.

At each end of the visible spectrum there are areas of radiation that cannot be detected by the visual mechanism. From 750 to 500 00 nm there is infra-red (heat). From 10 to 380 nm there is ultra-violet (UV). UV produces chemical and biological activity in living tissue.

Depending upon the wavelength used, the refractive index will vary; this effectively means that one piece of material could have three or more refractive indices. Thus white crown glass usually quoted as 'standard' lens material, has a refractive index of 1.523 for the helium d-line (587.56 nm) and 1.525 for the mercury e-line (546.07 nm). As the index of the material increases, the difference increases, thus a typical 1.700 glass material measured on the d-line, changes to 1.706 on the e-line. The differences are not that great and are not that significant except perhaps in the area of advertising claims where one manufacturer states that their material is of a higher index than any other on the market in that category, but in reality it is just measured at a different wavelength! Hopefully this confusion will be eliminated in the future with the adoption of a single wavelength – the mercury e-line.

Higher refractive index lenses are used to reduce the thickness (and sometimes the weight) compared with 'normal' index lenses. The

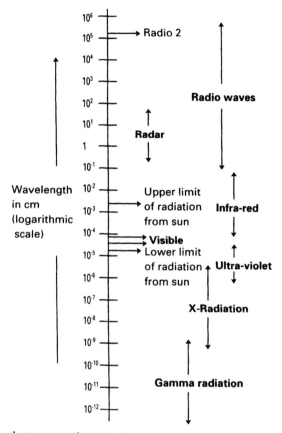

**Figure 24.1** The electro-magnetic spectrum.

thickness is reduced because for a higher refractive index lens material a given curvature will give more power than a normal index. Put in another way, the high index material will deviate light more than a normal material therefore lenses will be flatter and thinner.

An approximate method of assessing the saving in thickness can be determined from what is termed the CVF (curve variation factor). This is normally calculated relative to a 'standard' or 'normal' material.

$$\text{CVF} = (1.523^* - 1)/(n - 1)$$
*for comparison to resin substitute 1.498

Therefore, applying above to 1.700 glass one arrives at an answer of 0.75; consequently a lens made from this material would be very approximately three-quarters of the thickness of an ordinary crown glass lens, or put another way, 25% thinner than crown glass.

If the formula is applied to a 1.600 material, an answer of 0.87 is obtained so a reduction of 13% in the thickness may be expected, and so on.

The earlier high index glasses used for spectacle lenses had a number of drawbacks. They were softer than crown glass, apt to become tarnished, and produced noticeable colour fringes. Moreover, although appreciably thinner than their crown glass counterparts, the lenses were actually heavier because of the greater density of the high index glass. This was due to the dense barium or flint used in their manufacture.

In 1973 a revolutionary new high index material was introduced by Schott (USA) in which they replaced the heavier elements with titanium oxide enabling, for the first time, thinner higher index lenses without an increase in weight.

As a general statement, higher index materials have a greater density than standard materials, which should at first consideration make them heavier, but because the volume of a higher index lens is less than a standard counterpart (due to refractive index and the reduction in curvature) the weight is either the same, or maybe, less.

Before being carried away in the euphoria of higher index lenses, it is necessary to balance the thickness saving and possible weight savings against some of the disadvantages. The ideal lens (which does not exist) would have a constant refractive index at all parts of the visible spectrum (see *Figure 24.2*), but in all practical materials the refractive index varies with wavelength, and unfortunately the variability tends to increase with higher index materials. The effect causes a lens to break up white light into its constituent colours, the colours of the spectrum. The ability of a

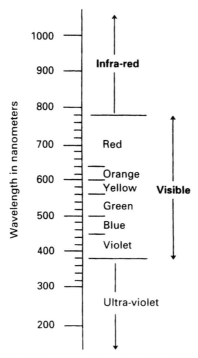

**Figure 24.2** A portion of the electro-magnetic spectrum illustrating ultra-violet, visible and infra-red.

lens to have this effect on light is referred to as its dispersive power. It is usual to express the reciprocal of the dispersive power, its constringence, v-value or Abbe number, the latter being taken from the name of a German physicist, Dr E.K. Abbe (1840–1905), who worked for the Carl Zeiss Jena Company. He was a famous contributor to ophthalmic science, and often accredited with the invention of the focimeter as well as innovative improvements to other measuring devices.

Constringence indicates the degree of chromatic aberration which the wearer would experience under conditions of high contrast. The effect of this is to cause the patient to see colour fringes around the images they view. Typical problems would be viewing black type on white paper through the lower half of the lens, where, in the case of minus lenses, the wearer may see blue fringes beneath the type and red/yellow above. More worrying is the reduction in visual acuity towards the edge of the lenses, often referred to as *off axis blur*, that causes the wearer to notice a decline in quality of vision compared with that through the centre of the lens.

Constringence is the reciprocal of the dispersive power of the material and indicates the degree of chromatic aberration. The lower the Abbe or v-value, the greater the chromatic aberration. Crown glass and normal resin have an Abbe number of around 58. By comparison, some 1.80 glass have a value of 25.4, much lower and therefore whilst being thinner are more likely to cause constringence problems. The above comments must be matched against the unarguable fact that the majority of those prescribed higher index lenses get on well with them and would not go back to 'standard' materials.

The Abbe number may be determined from the following formula:

$$V_e = \frac{n_e - 1}{n_{F'} - n_{C'}}$$

where

$V_e$ = Abbe number for the mercury e-line
$n_{C'}$ = refractive index of the medium at the wavelength of the cadmium C'-line (643.85 nm)
$n_e$ = refractive index of the medium at the wavelength of the mercury e-line (546.07 nm)
$n_{F'}$ = the refractive index of the medium at the wavelength of the cadmium F'-line (479.99 nm)

Alternatively the following formula may be used if basing calculation on the Helium d-line:

$$V_d = \frac{n_d - 1}{n_F - n_C}$$

where

$V_d$ = Abbe number for the helium d-line
$n_C$ = refractive index of the medium at the wavelength of the hydrogen C-line (656.27 nm)

$n_d$ = refractive index of the medium at the wavelength of the
helium d-line (587.56 nm)

$n_F$ = refractive index of the medium at the wavelength of the
hydrogen F-line (486.13 nm)

One other factor to be taken into account is the fact that higher index lenses tend to be more reflective. Listed below are several indices along with percentage reflections that can be expected from each surface (*Table 24.2*). Thus it can be seen that, for example, a crown glass lens of refractive index 1.523 will reflect 8.6% (4.3 × 2) of the available light and therefore could be considered as transmitting to the patient 91.4%. Alternatively, a 1.80 lens would reflect 16.3% of the available light and therefore only transmit 83.7% to the patient. It reflects twice as much as that of the crown lens. this is very apparent cosmetically, the patient being more aware of surface reflections. Fortunately, modern multi-layer anti-reflection coating (see Chapter 26) can reduce residual reflections to around 1–3%.

**Table 24.2** Indices/reflections

| Refractive index | Percentage reflection at each surface |
|---|---|
| 1.498 | 3.97 |
| 1.523 | 4.30 |
| 1.560 | 4.79 |
| 1.600 | 5.33 |
| 1.700 | 6.72 |
| 1.800 | 8.16 |

There is no doubt that the higher index resin market is developing at a rapid rate and it is sure to continue. Prior to 1970 the two principal resin materials were Igard and CR39. This changed when PPG, the original suppliers of CR39, developed a 1.56 resin monomer. This was followed by a 1.60 version from the Japanese chemical company, Toray Industries. Most higher index resin products on the market today are sourced from these companies. Technology has reached new heights with resin materials now available in 1.70 refractive index.

Not intending to be drawn into comparing one manufacturer's product with another, suffice to say there are a multitude of mid or high index products available in both glass and resin, all marketed under various trade names. All allow higher powered lenses to be produced in a more cosmetically acceptable form, or medium powered lenses to be glazed to larger, more fashionable frames than would have otherwise been advisable. *Table 24.3* shows a chart calculated to demonstrate the difference in edge substance for selected powers made in different indices materials. All are calculated on a 65 mm diameter. With the exception of

1.498 index, all substances have been calculated on a 1.2 centre and therefore assume glass. It is generally accepted that 1.498 resin cannot be produced to less than 2 mm centre substance – so this must be taken into account. Some higher index resins can be as thin as 1.0 mm at the centre but for simplicity, have not been shown in the chart.

It is widely agreed that myopes obtain the greater advantages given by higher index materials. They can easily appreciate the reduction in edge substance. That is not to say that hypermetropes do not gain an advantage, it is just that the centre thickness of a plus lens is not quite so tangible as the edge thickness of a minus. *Table 24.4* gives some indication of the savings possible by using higher index materials for plus lenses. All diameters are 65 mm.

**Table 24.3** Substance comparison for minus powers in different indices

| Power | Refractive index | Edge substance |
|-------|------------------|----------------|
| −4.00 | 1.498 | 6.9 |
| −4.00 | 1.523 | 5.8 |
| −4.00 | 1.600 | 5.1 |
| −4.00 | 1.700 | 4.4 |
| −4.00 | 1.800 | 4.0 |
| −8.00 | 1.498 | 11.9 |
| −8.00 | 1.523 | 10.5 |
| −8.00 | 1.600 | 9.0 |
| −8.00 | 1.700 | 7.7 |
| −8.00 | 1.800 | 6.8 |
| −10.00 | 1.498 | 14.1 |
| −10.00 | 1.523 | 12.5 |
| −10.00 | 1.600 | 10.8 |
| −10.00 | 1.700 | 9.2 |
| −10.00 | 1.800 | 8.1 |

**Table 24.4** Substance comparison for plus powers in different indices

| Power | Refractive index | Centre substance |
|-------|------------------|------------------|
| +4.00 | 1.498 | 5.1 |
| +4.00 | 1.523 | 4.8 |
| +4.00 | 1.600 | 4.2 |
| +4.00 | 1.700 | 3.6 |
| +4.00 | 1.800 | 3.2 |
| +8.00 | 1.498 | 9.5 |
| +8.00 | 1.523 | 9.0 |
| +8.00 | 1.600 | 7.8 |
| +8.00 | 1.700 | 6.7 |
| +8.00 | 1.800 | 5.8 |
| +10.00 | 1.498 | 11.5 |
| +10.00 | 1.523 | 10.9 |
| +10.00 | 1.600 | 9.4 |
| +10.00 | 1.700 | 8.1 |
| +10.00 | 1.800 | 7.1 |

## Minus lenticulars

Reducing the edge substance of a minus lens can also be achieved by using some form of lenticular. There are those lenticulars that are created by the surfacing department which tend to have a symmetrical geometry and those created by the glazing department which in many instances do not have the same limitations as those imposed on surfaced lenticulars.

Starting with those types of lenticulars that are created by the skills of the surfacer: the following text applies equally to resin lenses as it does glass. Unlike plus lenticulars that are sometimes purchased by the prescription house in semi-finished form, minus lenticulars are created from 'normal' blanks. The lens in its uncut form undergoes an additional surfacing operation to remove material from its thick marginal zone. The effect is to form a polished margin, the curvature and internal diameter of which can be varied at will. The lens in full aperture form would appear perhaps as *Figure 24.3*.

By surfacing a convex curve on the concave surface of the lens, a lenticular margin can be formed, thereby reducing the edge substance (*Figure 24.4*). The lens is considered as having been 'flattened on plus' or it is said to have a *plus margin*.

Another method is to supply with a plano margin, or 'flattened on flat' as it is sometimes referred to (*Figure 24.5*). This form does not enjoy such a thin edge but unlike that shown in *Figure 24.4* there is no magnification due to convex curve on the margin.

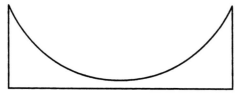

**Figure 24.3** Full aperture minus powered lens.

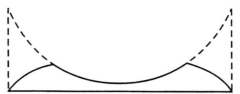

**Figure 24.4** A minus powered lenticular with a plus margin.

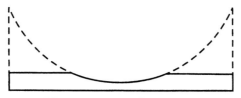

**Figure 24.5** A minus powered lenticular with a plano margin.

The types of lenticular that can be created by a glazer are either what is termed 'hand flattened' or 'profile'. Taking the hand flattened category first: the lens is made in the conventional way by the surfacing department as indeed is the initial glazing. A subsequent operation performed by hand, with the aid of an edging stone or wheel, involves what can be best described as a very heavy safety chamfer (*Figure 24.6*). The result is a lens with a much thinner edge. Normally the margin would be subjected to buffing and polishing. Both glass and resin lend themselves to this method of manufacture.

The other method, profile, is usually just performed on resin lenses. It is referred to as a *step type* lenticular. From the front it will look very much

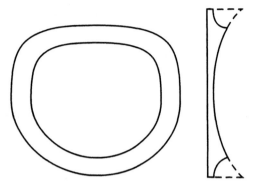

**Figure 24.6** Front and side view of a hand flattened lenticular.

like the diagram to the left in *Figure 24.6*, but from the side it will look as depicted in *Figure 24.7*. It is achieved by edging the lens in the normal manner with a conventional suitable bevel at the edge. It is then placed on another edger with a flat wheel, but offset so that only the back part of the lens will be further edged down, creating the step appearance.

To obtain the same effect in glass material it is normal to bond separate components together. If a –15.00 DS +3.00 DC prescription is to be produced, a 'carrier' lens in flat form would be produced in the power plano +3.00 DC, the cylinder being incorporated on the front surface. Another lens of power –15.00 DS, in flat form, would also be made. This would subsequently be flat edged to the same shape as the frame but several millimetres smaller. This edged, spherical flat lens would then be bonded to the 'carrier'. This would then be edged in the conventional manner resulting in the effect shown in *Figure 24.8*.

Whilst in theory any of the methods described under this section on minus lenticulars can be applied to multifocals as well as single vision, the margin can interfere with any vision through the lower part of the lens and therefore if a segment were in this region, its use may be limited.

**Figure 24.7** Profile, step type lenticular.    **Figure 24.8** Profile, step type lenticular created by bonding components together.

One possible solution for the myopic presbyope could be that shown in *Figure 24.9*. Although a rarity, there are still skilled surfacers who can produce such an item. It can be best visualised as a flat plano carrier into which two different spherical curves have been depressed. The steeper curve for the distance correction is opened out to a slightly larger aperture than the shallower curve for the reading portion, the centres for the two apertures being 8–10 mm apart. Each portion has its independent optical centre, coinciding with the geometrical centre of the respective circle. As shown in the diagram, the two portions meet at a slightly upcurve dividing line. Its curvature varies with the prescription and the diameters and separation of the two apertures. All other factors being equal, an increased reading addition makes it dip closer towards the near optical centre. Any prescribed cylinder is worked on the front surface. In general, its effect will be to cause a slight displacement of the near optical centre from the geometrical centres of the aperture.

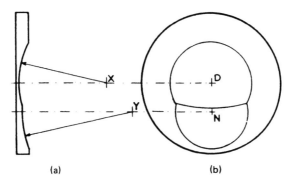

**Figure 24.9** Flattened lenticular; bifocal form: (a) cross-section of lens – X and Y are the centres of curvature of the distance and reading portions respectively; (b) front view of lens – D and N are the distance and reading optical centres respectively.

In concluding this section on minus lenticulars there is also a form generally referred to as blended lenticulars (single vision only). They are available under various trade names in both resin and glass. The edge of the lentic circle has been 'blended' so that it no longer appears as a distinct circle, and is therefore perceived by many as being an improvement on the traditional lenticular design. They are normally supplied to the prescription house in semi-finished form, the back surface (the one containing the blended area) being the finished side, the prescription house having to surface the front to complete the lens (*Figure 24.10*).

## Plus lenticulars

As the need on minus lenses is to reduce the edge substance, on plus it is to reduce the centre substance; this too can be achieved by some form of lenticular. Unlike minus lenticulars which start their life as 'ordinary'

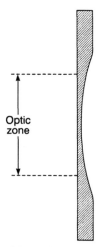

**Figure 24.10** Blended minus powered lenticular.

lenses and rely on the skills of the surfacer or glazer to convert them into lenticulars, resin plus powered lenticulars are supplied to the prescription house in semi-finished form, moulded from one piece of resin. They can be either single vision or bifocals (*Figure 24.11*) and are available in a range of 'bowl', segment size and shapes (the bowl being the term given to the diameter of the central lenticular area). Some even incorporate an aspheric surface (see Chapter 25). Unlike resin lenses where the bowl and segment, if applicable, are created by moulding, glass plus powered lenticulars again rely on the skills of the surfacer.

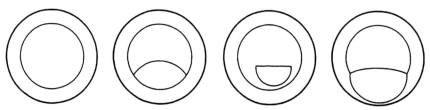

**Figure 24.11** A selection of plus powered lenticular lenses in both single vision and bifocal.

A carrier lens is made, usually in flat form, any cylinder being on the back surface. This allows the bonding of an appropriate bowl to the front. The making of the bowl is somewhat similar to the procedure described in Chapter 23 for making bonded segments. Two lenses that have been cemented together with Canada balsam, plano surface to plano surface, are processed as if they were one lens (*Figure 24.12*). The bowl or *button* as it is sometimes referred to, is removed from the support lens, lightly run around an edging wheel to remove any small chips and is then ready for permanently bonding to the carrier lens.

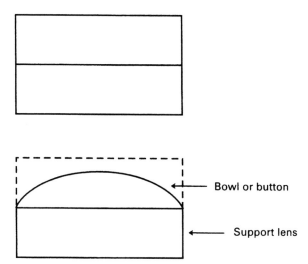

**Figure 24.12** Components to achieve a lenticular 'button'.

Lenticular bifocals can, if necessary, be fabricated by substituting a bifocal lens for the carrier. If a cylinder needs to be incorporated some form of fused bifocal would be used to allow the cylinder surface to be on the back, thus permitting a plano surface to be on the front, providing a contact surface for the lenticular button.

In the concluding section on minus lenticulars mention was made of a form of lens referred to as being 'blended'. A similar type of plus lenticular is also available in resin. Again the manufacturer of the semi-finished blank has developed a blended zone as an alternative to the lenticular button (*Figure 24.13*).

Both single vision and bifocals are available and are normally combined with an aspheric front surface (see Chapter 25).

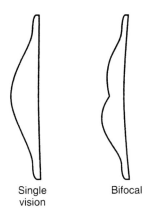

Single
vision

Bifocal

**Figure 24.13** Blended lenses.

# Aspheric lenses

The literal meaning of *aspherical*, derived from Greek, is simply not spherical, e.g. cylindrical. In optics, however, the meaning has been reserved for non-spherical surfaces having the same profile in all meridians. Although at first consideration progressive lenses may not seem to be connected with aspherics, it is unquestionably the technology behind the production of progressive surfaces that has led to the increase in the manufacture of aspherics.

Quite often, a progressive surface is referred to as being aspheric, for it is not spherical as it has to change curvature across the surface to produce the additional power required in the intermediate and reading areas, but as previously stated the term aspheric is reserved for an optical surface which has rotational symmetry about its optical axis. The simplest aspherical surfaces are the conicoids, produced by rotating a conic section about its axis of symmetry. In *Figure 25.1*, for example, the conic section is an ellipse and the rotation of the portion PAQ about the axis XX would produce an ellipsoidal surface of diameter PQ.

There is a much larger family of aspherical surfaces with a more complicated geometry, but the following statements are true of nearly all the convex aspherical surfaces used for spectacle lenses:

1 At the vertex A of the surface, a small portion of the surface is indistinguishable from that of a sphere with its centre at $C_o$. The radius

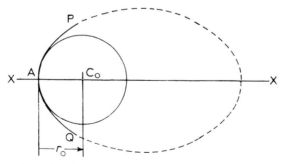

**Figure 25.1** An aspherical surface.

$r_o$ of this sphere is termed the vertex radius of the aspherical surface and is used to calculate its paraxial power.

2 The profile of the surface becomes progressively flatter on plus lenses at increasing distances from its vertex. Minus lenses become progressively steeper. For a given vertex radius, it is the nature and rate of this flattening/steepening that distinguishes one aspherical surface from another.

Why aspherics? Unfortunately strong, non-aspheric lenses leave much to be desired. The wearer notices a great deal of distortion, one effect of which is to make straight lines appear to curve as the head is turned (*Figure 25.2*). Another defect is that the sharpness of vision deteriorates quickly towards the margin of the lens. The result is that the wearer experiences what is termed 'tunnel vision'. This is because light rays which pass through the periphery of a convex lens are brought to a shorter focus than those that pass through the centre. The images formed by a high plus lens will always lack definition in the peripheral area. Expressing the problem in more technical terms, the terminologies *oblique astigmatism* and *curvature error* are used.

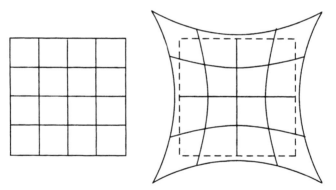

**Figure 25.2** The pin cushion type of distortion which occurs when a grid pattern is viewed through a convex lens.

Oblique astigmatism is considered to be the most serious defect in spectacle lens design. British Standard glossary of terms refers to it as 'an aberation peculiar to pencils of rays obliquely refracted (or reflected) and giving rise to separate tangential and sagittal line foci instead of a single image point'. Oblique astigmatism can be eliminated over a wide range of powers by 'bending' the lens into what is termed optical 'best form'; however, this results in bulbous lenses, which are very often cosmetically unacceptable.

Whilst oblique astigmatism can be considered as a cylindrical blurring, curvature error can be looked on as spherical blurring. It is expressed in such a way as to give the average power at a certain angle away from the optical centre, expressed in dioptres, in comparison with the power at the optical centre.

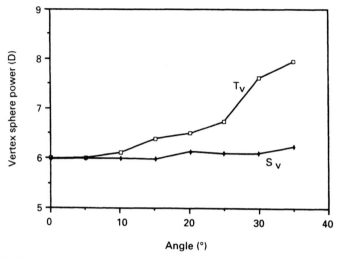

**Figure 25.3** Oblique astigmatism from tangential ($T_v$) and sagittal ($S_V$) errors for a +6.00 DS resin flat lens.

*Figure 25.3* shows diagrammatically the oblique astigmatism through the effect of the tangential and the sagittal errors for a +6.00 DS resin lens made in flat form, for many years, the normal form in which lenses were produced. At the optical centre the power is +6.00 DS, and this continues as the eye is rotated 5 degrees but beyond this, tangential ($T_v$) and sagittal ($S_v$) errors are encountered. Oblique astigmatism is calculated by drawing a vertical line between the two points $T_v$ and $S_v$ as shown in *Figure 25.4*. This is normally performed at an angle of 30 degrees away from the optical centre, a good average. The distance between $T_v$ and $S_v$

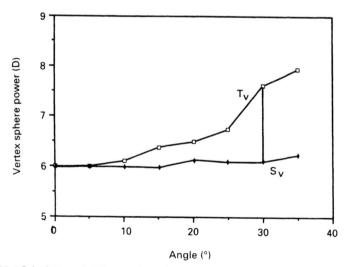

**Figure 25.4** Calculation of oblique astigmatism.

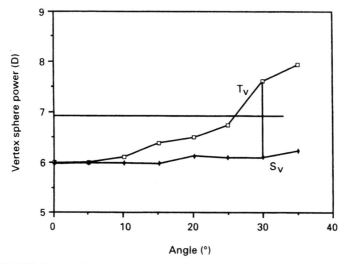

**Figure 25.5** Calculation of curvature error.

measured in dioptres (see vertical scale) is 1.50 dioptres and therefore the lens exhibits 1.50 D of oblique astigmatism.

If the line between $T_v$ and $S_v$ is equally bi-sected and the result noted on the vertical scale, it is possible to calculate the curvature error (*Figure 25.5*). In this instance it touches the vertical scale at +6.87 D and therefore in comparison the power of the lens at the optical centre (+6.00 DS), the lens is shown to exhibit +0.87 D of curvature error.

If the same power lens is made in best form the oblique astigmatism can be reduced to zero (*Figure 25.6*) but pays the price by being very bulbous (–5.25 D inside curve), and subsequently not very flattering in

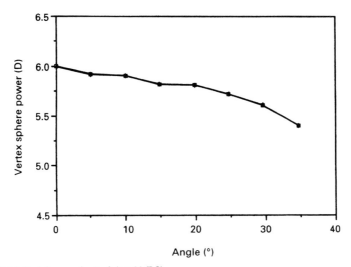

**Figure 25.6** Best form spherical (+6.00 DS).

appearance. Curvature error, incidentally, has also been reduced to −0.40 D, by making the lens in best form. The reader may have noticed that the scale of the vertical line may change in the diagrams used. This is solely to present the graphs in a uniform size.

Now compare the same power lens made up in current manufacturers' stock meniscus form (*Figure 25.7*). Flattening the inside curve to −3.00 D, the bulbousness of the best form has now gone but +0.70 D of oblique astigmatism has been induced. The curvature error is now only +0.15 D.

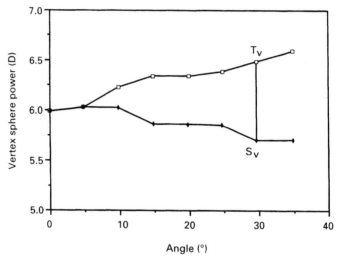

**Figure 25.7** Stock meniscus (+6.00 DS).

So what is the answer? Ideally what is required is a lens that is least bulbous in appearance but does not pay the price in increased oblique astigmatism. It is known that the flat lens gives the least bulbous appearance whilst best form the least oblique astigmatism. The answer is one of the many aspheric design lenses available on the market today. Designs and principles differ greatly. Some eliminate oblique astigmatism, some curvature error, others do not eliminate either of these but reduce both to minimal amounts. *Figure 25.8* depicts a Zeiss Hypal lens in resin material. Oblique astigmatism has been reduced to −0.12 D, with a curvature error of −0.44 D. Alternatively, the lens depicted in *Figure 25.9* has +0.45 D of oblique astigmatism but only −0.03 D of curvature error.

It must be left to others to conclude which of the aberrations is of the greater concern to the wearer, that is to say is it preferable to eliminate oblique astigmatism or curvature error? The ideal lens would have no oblique astigmatism and no curvature error! (The graphs depicted in Figures 25.3–25.9 are the results of practical experiments performed on actual lenses and therefore results may differ slightly to that of theoretical experiments).

A few words at this point about cataracts. In an operation for cataract, the crystalline lens which has become gradually more opaque is removed

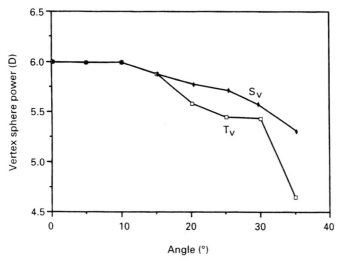

**Figure 25.8** Zeiss Hypal (resin, +6.00 DS).

from the eye. As a result, normal vision is usually restored but a high powered plus lens is needed, due to the absence of the crystalline lens, to bring the retinal image into focus. A patient is referred to as *aphakic* once the crystalline lens has been removed from the eye, and high-powered plus lenses are often referred to as aphakic lenses.

Very common today, due to the improved surgical techniques is for the patient to be fitted with an intra-ocular lens, often referred to as an implant. This consists of a small, man-made 'crystalline' lens being surgically positioned with great precision within the eye to replace the natural lens that has been removed.

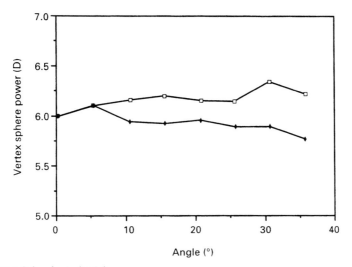

**Figure 25.9** Solaspheric (resin).

So why do aspheric lenses improve the vision for those patients who need high plus powered prescriptions? The non-spherical front surface of an aspheric lens becomes flatter or less convex towards the edge. If a lens measure is placed on a conventional spherical front surface the reading will be consistant regardless of where it is placed. If one repeats the exercise on an aspheric lens, one will immediately see the change of curvature across the surface. Thus, an aspheric surface is spherical on centre but becomes more toroidal as one moves away from the central optical axis. This has the effect of neutralising the aberrations.

One of the earliest designs of aspheric was patented as long ago as 1909 by Von Rohr for Carl Zeiss. In optical terms the design was excellent, but in order to achieve this optical performance it had a rear aspherical surface of some −18.41 D. From a cosmetic point of view the lens was disastrous as it was so bulbous in appearance and was only available in a diameter of 34 mm! Later, Zeiss went on to design a flatter aspheric design which they marketed under the name of Katral. Of course, these lenses were made of glass and were very expensive to produce. It was not until the development of satisfactory optical plastic that aspheric spectacle lenses were produced on a larger scale.

The 1970s saw the introduction of a lens developed by Dr Robert C. Welsh of Miami who called it the *Welsh Four Drop*. This was a departure from previous designs in two respects. First, the asphericity of the front surface was greater, which combined with the shallow rear curve used, gave the lens a considerably flatter appearance. Secondly, the aspherical curve used was not a true aspheric, but a series of blending spherical curves. The concept behind the lens was to have a central clear zone of vision surrounded by an area of rapidly decreasing power where the visual acuity would be less but there would be very much reduced distortion. The use of a flatter aspheric also made a large blank diameter possible compared with previous full aperture aspherics. Because the power dropped by 4 dioptres from centre to edge (i.e. a +12.00 DS lens would be +12.00 DS in the centre gradually reducing to +8.00 DS at the edge) there was a reduced prismatic effect at the edge, and hence a wider field of view than was normally obtainable with a lens in the non-aspheric power range. Several lens types marketed under various trade names are available based on this concept. They have been improved by moving away from the rigid 4 dioptre 'drop' from centre to edge. Instead they have a varying power drop for each blank, the higher bases having more 'drops' than the lower ones.

Whilst variable sphericity lenses give an increase in the visual field it is at the expense of peripheral definition and therefore some lens designers have opted for an alternative to the 'drop' principle. The resulting lenses are often referred to as *blended* or *seamless* lenticulars and are available from several suppliers. They are optically similar to the aspheric lenticular, except that instead of having a sharp dividing line between the powered zone and the carrier lens, the junction is blended so that no dividing line is visible and no 'jump' at the edge of the lenticular aperture takes place (*Figure 25.10*). Compared with the 'drop' type lens they exhibit a wider central field of good acuity, but a more rapid power drop at the lens periphery. The benefit of this is that a larger blank size is obtainable without excessive centre thickness.

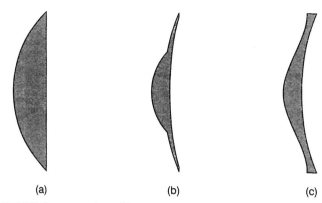

|     |     |     |
| --- | --- | --- |
| (a) | (b) | (c) |

**Figure 25.10** (a) Full aperture lens; (b) lenticular; (c) blended or seamless.

In concluding this section on the traditional use of aspherics, it may help the reader to present a series of comparisons based on the options available.

*Figure 25.11* represents a high powered spherical lens. Note the distortion.

*Figure 25.12* represents a lenticular lens. Note how no distortion is visible but the vision is limited to the lentic aperture and restricts field of view.

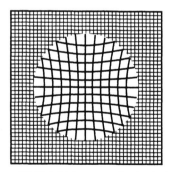

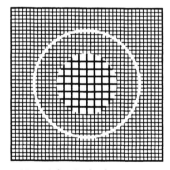

**Figure 25.11** A high powered spherical lens.

**Figure 25.12** A lenticular lens.

*Figure 25.13* represents an aspheric lens of the blended or seamless nature. Notice no distortion in the central area along with peripheral awareness at the edge. Also note the larger diameter of the lens.

*Figure 25.14* represents an aspheric of the 'drop' type.

What of other uses for aspherics? Whereas years ago, one only utilised aspherics for high powered plus lenses, they have now gained in popularity for low powers in both plus and minus. They work on the principle that the thinnest possible lens is one made in flat form. However, as explained earlier the optics of a flat lens are not as good as

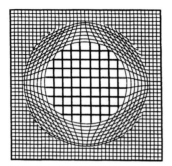

**Figure 25.13** An aspheric blended or seamless lens.

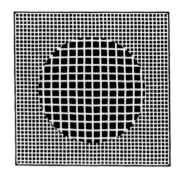

**Figure 25.14** An aspheric drop lens.

those of a curved one. The use of aspherical curvatures on low powers means that one can combine the cosmetic advantages of the 'flattish' appearance but with the optical performance of more curved lenses. Aspherics are therefore thinner and hence lighter than conventional lenses. Some manufacturers are also producing their product in high index materials to make them even thinner.

Seiko have taken aspheric technology to a higher level by developing a lens that has an aspheric surface on both the front and back. Conventional aspheric lenses have their aspheric design incorporated into the front surface. By making the back surface also aspheric, Seiko have produced a lens that reduces unwanted astigmatism even further thereby improving the optical performance of the lens. A conventional aspheric front surface lens works well in meniscus form, however where there is a cylinder involved the design can only be optimum for control of lens aberrations in one of the two principal meridians. If only the front surface is made aspherical, with a conventional toroidal curve on the rear, then the cylindrical power will not be constant for all angles of gaze, as a result of lens aberrations. But if the toroidal surface is also made aspherical, then each principal curvature on the astigmatic surface can be optimised to give a constant cylindrical power for all angles of gaze.

Low power plus aspherics work by effectively introducing negative surface astigmatism to reduce the aberrations at the lens periphery, but at the same time are flattish in form. *Figure 25.15* illustrates very well the comparison between conventional and aspheric lens types. Low powered minus aspherics, on the other hand, increase convexity at the edge which reduces the edge thickness.

The demands of good optical quality and improved cosmetic appearance somewhat contradict each other, and therefore it is down to the lens designers to find a suitable compromise between all of the elements. One element applicable to all types of aspherics is that the design of a lens will only be correct for one combination of base curve and power, thus a different base curve or asphericity should be used for every 0.25 D prescription step. In practice this does not happen because the cost involved would be prohibitive. For this reason a range of base curves are made available along with clear instructions from the manufacturers as to

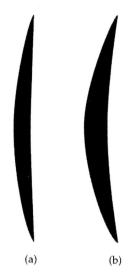

(a)                    (b)

**Figure 25.15** Comparison between (a) aspheric and (b) conventional lenses.

what power should be put on what base. It is absolutely essential that the prescription house does not in any way diminish the features of the lens design by putting powers on the wrong bases. It is quite possible to supply a wide range of prescriptions from one base, but unless the correct curve is used the lens may well not perform correctly.

From this chapter it has hopefully been demonstrated that, put in simplistic terms, there are two 'basic' design concepts, the *drop* and the *blended*. Opticians have the difficult task of deciding whether the patient would prefer the good central visual acuity and low edge distortion of the 'drop' type lens or prefer a wider field of good acuity and more edge distortion as found in the blended designs. The latter is also available in larger blank sizes and therefore sometimes this is the deciding factor.

From the prescription house's point of view, no matter which type the optician selects it is essential that surfacing instruction requirements are accurately arrived at to provide the thinnest and most suitable lens for the patient. In the modern world of optics today with its computers and electronic shape tracing, this should not be difficult to achieve. In conclusion it should be noted that due to the aspheric elements of the lens it is not possible to work prism for decentration as this would cause the optical centre to move away from the centre of the lens thus diminishing the purpose of supplying in aspheric form.

Bifocals are also available in aspheric form, any round segment having a tendency towards oval shape rather than a true round, due to the non-spherical construction of the front surface.

# Chapter 26

# Anti-reflection, tinted and protective lenses

## The electro-magnetic spectrum

The electro-magnetic spectrum is a vast gamut of radiations which include X-rays, ultra-violet rays, visible light, infra-red (heat) rays, radio waves and so on. Although these various radiations seem totally different in their nature and effects, the most fundamental distinction between them is simply their wavelengths. In ophthalmic optics one is concerned with a relatively narrow band of the electro-magnetic spectrum. The wavelengths in this region are extremely short and are expressed in nanometres (nm). This unit of length is one thousand millionth part of a metre or one millionth part of a millimetre (see *Figure 24.1*).

The visible spectrum, embracing those radiations which we perceive as light, is represented in *Figure 26.1*. It extends from about 380–780 nm. Various wavebands within this region are associated with different colour sensations. For example, wavelengths between the approximate limits of 570–590 nm give rise to the sensation of yellow.

In passing it should be mentioned that there are certain wavelengths at which dark lines occur in the solar spectrum. They are named Fraunhofer lines, after their discoverer, and some of them are denoted by single letters. Thus, the wavelengths 587.6 and 546.1 nm mentioned in Chapter 8 and 24 are often referred to as the d-line and e-line respectively, while wavelength 589.3 nm is the mean of the two D-lines at 589.0 and 589.6 nm.

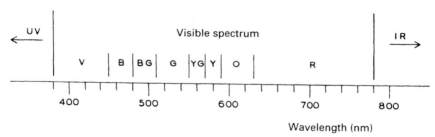

**Figure 26.1** Wavelength and corresponding colour sensation: V, violet; B, blue; BG, blue–green; G, green; YG, yellow–green; Y, yellow; O, orange; R, red; UV, ultra-violet; IR, infra-red.

The radiations emitted by most sources of light and heat, whether natural or artificial, not only include all the wavelengths of the visible spectrum but also extend into the neighbouring regions – the ultra-violet and infra-red. Although not perceived as light, these radiations are capable of doing serious damage to the eyes, if of sufficient intensity.

## The cause of reflections

There are four definable sources of reflection that can cause annoyance to spectacle lens wearers (*Figure 26.2*):

1 *Frontal reflections*, where some of the light incident on the front surface is reflected back towards an observer. This can be disconcerting for the observer, as the wearer's eyes are difficult to observe. Communication between humans relies not just on spoken or written word but by facial expressions, much of which are centred around the eyes reactions. Inability to see the eyes of a person you are talking to, can be rather 'off-putting' as one cannot deduce whether what is being said is actually

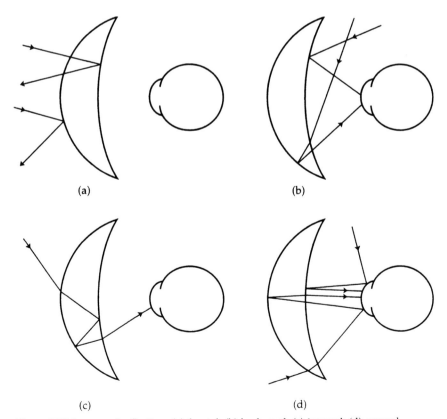

Figure 26.2 Sources of reflection: (a) frontal; (b) backward; (c) internal; (d) corneal.

being understood. These reflections are also annoying from purely a cosmetic point of view as they detract from the overall appearance.

2 *Backward reflections*, where some of the light behind the patient is reflected from the back surface of the lens into his or her eye. This can be particularly annoying at times when reduced lighting conditions are encountered such as at dusk or in driving at night.

3 *Internal reflections*, caused by light being reflected between the two lens surfaces. The amount of reflection caused in this manner will vary depending upon the power and position of the lens in front of the eye.

4 *Corneal reflections*, caused by light being reflected from the surface of the cornea and then interacting with the lens surfaces.

Whilst frontal reflections would appear only to be a cosmetic problem they do reduce the amount of light transmitted through to the eye. Backward, internal and corneal reflections all cause ghost imaging that in turn can lead to reduced visual acuity due to blurring and reduced contrast, which overall reduce the effectiveness of the prescription lens, and thereby reduce its efficiency.

## Reflection at normal incidence

When light travelling in a medium of refractive index $n_1$ is incident on the polished surface of another medium of index $n_2$, the greater part is refracted and passed into the second medium, but a small fraction is reflected. The ratio of the reflected flux to the incident flux is termed the reflectance. If the incidence is exactly normal, the reflectance expressed as a percentage ($P$) can be found from the formula

$$P = 100 \left( \frac{n_1 - n_2}{n_1 + n_2} \right)^2 \text{ per cent}$$

The value of $P$ clearly remains the same if $n_1$ and $n_2$ are interchanged, that is to say, if the light path is reversed.

If one medium is air, the other being a lens material of refractive index $n$, this expression reduces to

$$P = 100 \left( \frac{n - 1}{n + 1} \right)^2 \text{ per cent}$$

*Table 26.1* shows the value of $P$ for the most common lens materials. These figures refer to the d-line wavelength for which the mean refractive index ($n_d$) of the material is measured, and apply to each surface. The total reflectance of a lens is therefore double the figures shown in the right hand column. (Because of multiple internal reflections, the total reflection is not exactly double this value.) Since the refractive index varies with wavelength, the surface reflectance varies accordingly. It is highest at the blue end of the spectrum.

**Table 26.1** Indices/reflections

| Lens material | Mean refractive index $(n_d)$ | Surface reflectance (%) |
|---|---|---|
| CR39 | 1.498 | 4.00 |
| Crown glass | 1.523 | 4.30 |
| Various high index materials | 1.700 | 6.72 |
| | 1.806 | 8.25 |

# Anti-reflection (AR) coatings

Mathematical analysis shows that surface reflectance can be reduced by coating the lens with a film of some material having a lower refractive index than that of the lens. Although there are now two reflections, one at the exposed surface of the film and another at the lens surface, their combined effect produces less reflection than the uncoated surface. In fact, reflections could be almost eliminated by meeting two conditions: (1) that the refractive index of the coating is the square root of that of the lens material and (2) that the thickness of the coating, multiplied by its refractive index, is exactly one-quarter of a wavelength of light – or any odd number of quarter wavelengths. Unfortunately this is not always obtainable. The choice of coating material for resin is very limited. There are several reasons for this including difficulties of adhesion, stress differences and because some are too brittle that they crack when applied to 'flexible' resin lenses. There is also a problem of finding a low enough refractive index material for coating resin. A way around this problem is to apply a coating of a higher refractive index and then apply a 'normal' refractive index layer, possibly silicon oxide, on top of this. For this reason whilst it is possible to have a single layer AR on glass, resin will normally have a minimum of two layers applied to each surface.

Crown glass with a refractive index of 1.523 would need a material with an index of 1.234. The most suitable material available for glass is magnesium fluoride which has a refractive index of around 1.38, so whilst it is not so well suited for crown glass its performance is better on higher index materials. Also, the two necessary conditions can be met for only one wavelength. For these and other reasons, single-layer on glass or double-layer on resin coatings cannot reduce the reflectance by much more than one-half. Single- and double-layer coatings are designed to give their maximum effect in the middle and brightest region of the visible spectrum. The reflectance gradually increases towards both the violet and red ends of the spectrum. As a result, the coated surface presents the characteristic purplish appearance which is usually described as a *bloom*.

The limitation of single-layer AR coating can be overcome by *multi-layer* coatings which are now capable of almost extinguishing surface reflections from one end of the visible spectrum to the other. Most requests for some form of anti-reflection coating will therefore be of the multi variety.

Caution should be taken when comparing claims by various manufacturers with regard to the performance of their coatings. It may prove
useful at this stage to examine a reflectance graph (*Figure 26.3*). The
percentage reflection is shown on the vertical scale to the left. Part of the
electro-magnetic spectrum (the visible element) is shown on the scale at the
bottom. Using the two scales one can determine the percentage reflectance
at any wavelength by noting the position on the graph.

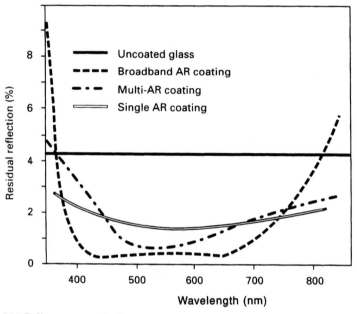

**Figure 26.3** Different types of AR coatings compared to one another.

A variation on the multi coating has been developed and is referred to
generally as *broadband*. It can be deduced from the graph that both
broadband and multi-AR have a very similar performance at 550 nm;
however, the broadband reduces reflections across many more wavelengths, unlike the multi that steeply curves away to the right and the left
of the 550 nm position.

Anti-reflection coatings work because by interposing a transparent
layer (the coating we call AR) we cause two reflections, the first from the
surface layer itself and the second from the lens surface. If the thickness
of the layer is made a quarter of a wavelength thick, the two reflected rays
will be out of phase with one another by half a wavelength. This is
because the ray reflected from the lens surface has to travel through the
layer and then back again. Being out of phase with one another they
effectively cancel or eliminate each other, thus destroying the reflection.

By building up layers of alternate high and low refractive index
materials in pairs on each surface of the lens, it is possible to reduce
reflections over a broader visible spectrum. Typically the thicker pairs

cancel the central spectral range and the thin pairs the blue and red regions at the edges of the visible spectrum.

With spectacle lenses both the curvature and the angle that light hits and reflects off the lens is significant in how effective the coating is. It is very difficult to achieve a totally uniform AR across the whole lens surface. It soon becomes apparent that coating technology is very complex, requiring powerful computers making many calculations.

## Application of AR coatings

Application takes place in a chamber from which the air has been evacuated to a very low pressure, thus providing a vacuum (*Figure 26.4*). The better the vacuum, the further the coating material will travel before it collides with another molecule. Coating machines normally operate at a pressure of 0.000001 millibar (atmospheric pressure is 1000 millibar).

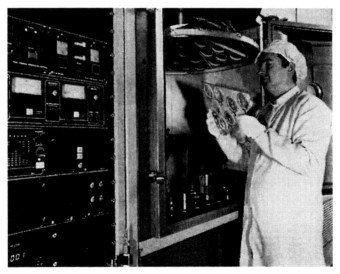

**Figure 26.4** Vacuum chamber lens preparation.

The system then relies on chemicals being deposited upon the lens surface under some form of heat, the chemical vaporising into a gaseous state. The lens surfaces are charged electrically with respect to the remainder of the chamber and therefore there is attraction between them and the chemical.

Original machines were of the 'Bell-Jar' design where the 'Bell' housing would be brought down over the area containing the lenses and a vacuum created. These machines are still in use today, mainly for vacuum tinting of glass lenses and for the application of single AR.

To achieve the uniformity of coating for multi-layer/broadband AR extreme accuracy and consistency of coating thickness is required. In simplistic terms, the farther the lenses are from the coating source (crucible), the better the coating application. For this reason, larger machines, referred to as 'Box' coaters have been developed. They are capable of holding many more lenses than the original 'Bell' type machines, but being so large they require massive vacuum pumping systems incorporated.

Earlier machines relied upon passing electrical current through the crucible to evaporate the coating material which was fine for glass (as it withstands the high temperatures) but not so good for resin, which would simply melt!

Techniques had to be developed to overcome this, hence electronic beam guns fire a charged beam at the chemicals, achieving evaporation at much lower temperatures to those previously used. This, coupled with the use of sophisticated microprocessor controls of pressure, temperature and evaporation rate, combined with other technological advances with regard to adhesion of the AR to the lens surface, has allowed the application of very durable coatings to most lens types.

The end result is lenses that have an enhanced cosmetic appeal, fewer ghost images, improved contrast and therefore improved optical performance. Preparation is, however, as important as the end result, and without proper preparation the quality and adhesion of the AR is adversely affected.

Prior to being placed in the vacuum chamber, lenses will have been cleaned using high tech ultrasonic cleaning systems, in ultra-clean, humidity controlled 'clean rooms'. As resin retains moisture, the lenses will be subjected to several hours in special ovens to de-hydrate them prior to the vacuum coating process.

With a price tag well over £1 million for such 'Box' coaters it is no wonder that it is only the largest prescription houses that can justify (or even afford) such technology.

The system described above relies on evaporating chemicals by the use of heat onto the lens surface. An alternative method in both cost and size is also available. Its referred to as a 'splutter' coating, the technology of which is less expensive and the machine size much smaller than the previously described 'Box' coaters.

The system employs an electro-magnetic field to create a plasma which 'splutters' the coating materials, such as zirconium, titanium and silicon onto the lens surface in a uniform manner. The system allows the lenses to be much closer to the source of the coating material, hence the saving in size.

Although the alternative system described above is readily available, it must be said that the majority of AR coating will be entrusted to the larger specialist prescription houses using the 'Box' coating systems.

## Tinted lenses in general

Tinted lenses or filters as they are sometimes referred to, are used to protect the eyes from glare or harmful radiations, their mode of action being to intercept a proportion of the light or radiant energy that would otherwise enter the eyes.

The prescribing of a suitable tint to meet an individual need requires careful consideration where one must be guided by three of its physical properties: (1) its transmission in various important regions of the spectrum (e.g. in the ultra-violet and infra-red), (2) the overall depth of tint (the current technical term for which is luminous transmittance, formerly known as integrated visible transmission) and (3) its colour. An adequate understanding of these properties requires some knowledge of the optics of reflection, absorption and transmission.

## Regulations

Under recent CEN regulations it is necessary to classify tint densities by a filter category number based on the transmission characteristics of the lens as defined by BS EN 1836 (1997). There are five categories under the 'Sunglare Filters' classification (*Table 26.2*).

The end wearer should be informed as to which category the tinted lenses come under and the usage/restrictions that apply.

**Table 26.2** 'Sunglare Filters' classification

| Transmittance range (%) | Description | Usage | Restrictions | Filter category |
|---|---|---|---|---|
| 81–100 | clear or very light tint | comfort/indoors/ cosmetic | none | 0 |
| 44–80 | light tint | low sunlight | not suitable for night driving | 1 |
| 19–43 | medium tint | medium sunlight | not suitable for night driving | 2 |
| 9–18 | dark tint | bright sunlight | not suitable for night driving; some may not be suitable for any driving | 3 |
| 4–8 | very dark tint | very bright sunlight | not be suitable for any driving | 4 |

## Methods of lens tinting

Lenses made from white crown glass and standard optical resin transmit some 90–92% of visible light, the loss being almost entirely due to the two surface reflections. Higher index materials in both glass and resin reflect even more light. A spectacle lens is said to be tinted if the transmission is deliberately decreased by any means, either over the whole of the visible spectrum and its neighbouring regions, or merely a part of it.

Spectacle lenses may be tinted in three different ways. First, the material itself may have been tinted during the course of its manufacture. Such tints are referred to as *solid* or *integral*. Next, the tint may be produced by a deposited *surface coating* designed not to extinguish but to intensify reflection. The transmission is modified in the desired manner by reflection instead of absorption. The third process, applied to resin lenses, is *dyeing* by immersion in a coloured liquid which permeates into the surface.

*Integral tints*

For many centuries this was the only method by which a glass lens could be tinted. Various oxides were added to the batch materials to give the lenses a specific colour. It should be said that the colour of the lens is somewhat immaterial, the important factor being what wavelength the tint absorbs. Cerium added to the batch mix would give rise to pinkish tints whilst cobalt or iron oxides would give rise to green tinted lenses. Light passing through a homogeneous material suffers a continuous loss by absorption. The loss can best be visualised by imaging the lens or filter to be made up of a number of very thin layers, each of which absorbs a constant proportion (and therefore transmits a constant proportion) of the radiant energy emerging from the previous layer. This proportion is not necessarily the same for all wavelengths. By adding the various metallic oxides or other compounds to the glass constituents, the absorption can be deliberately increased in almost any desired way, both within and beyond the visible spectrum. If the absorption is uniform within the visible spectrum, the tint imparted to the material will be grey or neutral. Selective absorption gives rise to a definitive hue, however pale. Thus, a relatively higher absorption in the red region of the spectrum would tend to produce a greenish tint.

The effect of thickness on the percentage of light transmitted can be illustrated by the following example. Suppose that, for a given wavelength, a certain material absorbs about 40% per millimetre of thickness, that is, it transmits 60%. The second millimetre transmits 60% of this 60, that is 36%, while the third millimetre transmits 60% of 36, which is 21.6%, and so on.

By way of another example, the effect of reflections off the front and back surfaces of the lens need also to be taken into consideration. Suppose it is assumed that 4% of incident light is lost by reflection at each surface and that a known tint absorbs 25% light for every 2 mm of thickness. Further suppose that a lens is to be made from this material and that the finished thickness will be 6 mm. How do we determine the transmission at the thickest part (optical centre) of the lens? The solution is shown below:

Reflection loss at front surface 4%, therefore 96% transmittance.

Total 6 mm $\begin{cases}$ first 2 mm absorbs 25% so transmits 75%, therefore $96 \times 75 = 72\%$ <br> next 2 mm absorbs 25% so transmits 75%, therefore $72 \times 75 = 54\%$ <br> next 2 mm absorbs 25% so transmits 75%, therefore $54 \times 75 = 40.5\%$ $\end{cases}$

and finally          Reflection loss at back surface 4%, therefore 96% transmittance therefore $40.5 \times 96 = 38.88\%$

The finished lens (6 mm thick) will have a transmission value of 38.88% LTF.

Since white crown glass available today absorbs less than 0.1% per millimetre throughout the visible spectrum, it remains free from discernible colour even at considerable thicknesses. Integral glass tints held the field for centuries and include many internationally famous trade names such as Crookes and Rayban. Only a brief description will be given here. Crookes glass was traditionally made in four shades. The palest, shade Alpha, had a faint pink coloration if viewed edgewise but the next in order of density, A2, was of a pale blue tint. The darker shades, B and B2, were both described as neutral in colour. All four shades, particularly the darkest, were strongly absorbent in the ultra-violet region, which was one of their merits. A peculiarity of shades Alpha and A2 was a sharp reduction of transmission in the yellow band of the visible spectrum. This, incidentally, made them effectively darker in sodium street lighting.

Pinkish tints also tended to have absorptive properties in the ultra-violet region, but they were mainly prescribed to attenuate the light in a pleasing way. A wide range of olive–green and blue–green glasses were available, each in several shades. In general, these glasses showed a marked transmission peak in the green region of the spectrum, with good absorption in the ultra-violet and even more in the infra-red, especially up to about 1500 nm. Brown tints had the merit of not greatly disturbing the natural appearance of colours, even in the darker shades. The best known of these glasses is probably the Zeiss Umbral.

Due to the problems of manufacturers having to produce all their products in all the different bases and additions (if applicable) in all the various tints, and the prescription houses having the problem of stocking these, it is no wonder that integral, or as they are more commonly known, solid tints, have all but disappeared from the optical scene. Add to this the problem caused by a combination of high power and solid tint, whereby there is a change in density across the lens due to the change in thickness from centre to edge, and the fact that unless both prescriptions are identical, there could be a tint match problem between right and left, it is no wonder that with a few exceptions, solid tints are becoming increasingly difficult to obtain, more so in any form of multifocal or progressive. There is still a small market in specialist tints such as those worn for laser and X-ray protection, etc., but for normal prescription wear they are now a rarity.

Although uncommon, some resin materials can be manufactured in a solid tinted form. Special ultra-violet and blue light absorbing lenses, as indeed some polycarbonates, are made from solid tinted material.

### Surface coating/tinting

Glass lenses can be tinted in a similar manner to that already described for AR coatings. In a vacuum chamber chemicals are deposited onto normally the back surface to form a thin film of tint (AR coatings are applied to both surfaces). The wearer benefits because the depth of tint is uniform over the whole lens area, whatever the power and thickness of the lens. The prescription house benefits because it is spared the necessity for specially working lenses in coloured materials and keeping stocks of the necessary blanks. Solid tints work by absorbing wavelengths whereas surface coated lenses, often referred to as vacuum coated lenses, work by reflecting back specific wavelengths.

Another objection to solid tints is that because they absorb light energy, this expresses itself in the form of heat which might irradiate the eye. By use of a vacuum tint this does not occur as the energy is reflected away, thus eliminating the possibility of irradiation.

By positioning of special plates above the crucibles containing the tinting chemical it is possible to impart a graduated vacuum tint onto the lens surface. The process also lends itself to the application of silver or chromium to create mirrored lenses that allow the wearer to see out but the observer cannot see in. To ensure exact colour match on any pair it is essential that both lenses are placed in the vacuum chamber together; it is therefore not advisable to supply half pairs where vacuum coating is involved.

### Dye tinting

Compared to vacuum coating, the dye tinting of resin lenses could best be described as an 'art' rather than a scientific process. Much depends on the skills of the tinting operative to produce a tint of the correct colour and density. BS 7394 Part 2 (1994) states that with the exception of solid/integral tints, the transmission value of a tint should be within 8% of that requested. In addition, there should be no more that 3% difference in transmission between a pair of lenses.

Resin lenses can be tinted by immersion in a tank or container of dye. The tank or container is normally housed in a unit that allows heat to be transferred to the dye. In simplistic terms the longer the lenses remain in the dye, the more they will absorb, thus making them darker. The dye penetrates the lens material and becomes part of the substrata. It cannot be rubbed off – it has become part of the lens itself. From dyes of the three primary colours, red, yellow and blue it is possible to make all the other colours that one would require. Green, for example, is a mixture of blue and yellow. Brown is a mixture of red and blue with perhaps a little yellow.

The dyes can be purchased in either powder or liquid form which are then mixed with either deionised water or water that has been previously boiled to remove any chlorine. Once the dye has been mixed it is brought up to a temperature of between 92 and 96°C (195–205°F). As lenses are normally tinted in pairs, unlike vacuum coating where as many as 50 or more lenses may be in the chamber at any one time, individual requirements for specials can be easily catered for. Interesting tint combinations can be created, the only limitation in many respects being one's imagination. Graduated and double graduated effects are reasonably easy to achieve with the aid of a pulley mechanism which gradually lifts the lenses out of the tint tank, thus imparting more tint on one part of the lens than the other.

A word of caution. One is not able to predict how a pair of lenses will react when immersed into a tint bath. Even though both may be of the same material and indeed from the same manufacturer, the 'take up' rate between the right and the left may be different. This can be due to a number of factors. It could even be that one lens has been in storage longer than the other and thereby reacts differently from the newer one when immersed into the tint bath.

To try to reduce problems to a minimum always try to ensure that if a pair of lenses are to be tinted, that they both come from the same manufacturer, for although many companies make resin lenses each manufacturer's product is unique and not necessarily of exactly the same 'recipe' as another; they may cure the lenses differently or for a different length of time. This has an effect on how a pair of lenses will react when introduced to a tint.

Higher index resin materials exhibit different characteristics that sometimes prevent them from being tinted to the darker shades or indeed having graduated tints applied. Guidelines on these limitations are normally given by both the manufacturers and the prescription house. Some resin materials such as polycarbonate are not tintable in the accepted sense but in this instance it is the hardcoat (more about this later in the chapter) that accepts the tint rather than the lens itself. This again presents tint limitations.

As the majority of lenses supplied to patients today are of a resin material, dye tinting is by far the most convenient and popular method. It is not uncommon for tinted lenses to be combined with AR coatings or indeed hardcoating or an ultra-violet protector (more about this later in the chapter). Because dye tints are absorbed into both surfaces equally, they are not affected by the power of the lens and will therefore have an even tint regardless of prescription.

In order to obtain a good quality tint certain factors have to be taken into consideration and good housekeeping practiced. For example, before tinting the lenses should be cleaned to remove any grease or even focimeter ink marks. This can be achieved by using an alcohol solution such as methylated spirits. An ultrasonic unit may also be employed. There are also preparation fluids that can be purchased. These further clean the lenses and prepare the surfaces to receive the tint, by slightly altering the surface chemistry of the lens.

Many consider it good tinting practice to slightly overtint lenses and then briefly place in bleach or decolourant for a few seconds in order to remove the tint from close to the surface. This reduces the tendency for tints to fade with time and by many it is considered essential if lenses are to be AR coated for this entails the lenses being put through a very strict cleaning regime that can lighten the tint if the above procedures are not followed.

There are two other important factors to consider. Every time a lens is tinted the dye solution becomes very slightly weaker as, of course, the dye has transferred from the solution to the lens substrate, therefore diluting and weakening the solution. Over a prolonged period the operative will note that it takes longer to produce a certain density tint. Evaporation caused by heating the fluid somewhat counteracts the dilution problem but tint strength should be monitored with either more tint being added or the complete solution changed.

The second important factor to consider is oxidisation which takes place once the dye solution is exposed to the atmosphere. This gradual change tends to give the tint a slight 'reddish' tinge. If a unit is processing a large number of tints, the effect of oxidisation will probably not be noticed as the tint will have become diluted and probably changed before this can take place.

As dye materials and solvent chemicals from the tinting process can be released into the drainage system it is important that care be exercised. For example many manufacturers now supply bio-degradable dyes that at the same time are non-toxic. Good manufacturing techniques can also reduce or eliminate the need for other chemicals such as alcohol, acetone, etc.

## Transmission data

In some cases, tinted lenses are prescribed just to give relief to patients unusually sensitive to light. In other cases, the intention is to provide eye protection in condition of exposure to harmful radiations in the ultra-violet and/or infra-red regions of the spectrum. The colour of a tint, however produced, gives very little indication of its transmission in these regions. Before a prescriber can judge the usefulness of any particular tint, he needs to be given certain data. It is the responsibility of the manufacturer or supplier to provide this information.

The percentage of radiant energy transmitted by a lens at any given wavelength is termed the transmittance. This may be expressed either as a decimal fraction or, more usually, as a percentage; for example, either as 0.65 or as 65%. Losses by surface reflection are included in this figure. If the transmittance is plotted as a graph over a range of wavelengths, the result is a transmission curve (*Figure 26.5*). The vertical scale indicates the percent transmittance and the base scale represents part of the electro-magnetic spectrum expressed in nanometres. The transmission curve is

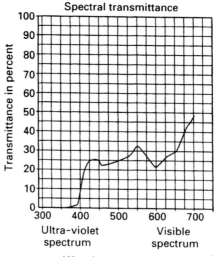

**Figure 26.5** A transmission graph.

plotted across the graph. By using the chart it is very easy to determine the transmittance at any particular wavelength. For example at 550 nm we can determine that the transmittance is in the region of 32%. One simply moves up the 550 nm line until the transmission curve crosses it, then refer to the scale to the left.

There is a dilemma that the reader needs to appreciate when a tint and an AR are combined. Suppose a grey tint having a 75% transmission (LTF) has been requested combined with a broadband AR. The prescription house has the facility to tint the lenses and when checked on a transmission meter they display 75%. If the lenses are then AR coated this will reduce reflection by about 8% (or increase transmission by 8%) so the tint now has an effective transmission of 83%!

The problem gets more complicated if the effect of reflections is taken into account at the tinting stage. Accepting the average reduction in reflections on a lens are 8%, then should the tint when placed in the transmission meter now read 67% LTF (75–8)? Whilst this is the incorrect LTF, the application of AR will increase the transmittance by approximately 8% and therefore the lens will have an LTF of 75% (67 + 8).

The situation is further complicated in that it is generally accepted that due to additional processing in ultrasonic units prior to application of AR, resin tints do tend to lighten a little and therefore many of those performing the tinting process, compensate by making the tint a little darker. It was mentioned earlier in the chapter that procedures can be adopted to minimise the lightening effect by using bleach or decolourant to remove any surplus dye from the lens surfaces.

## Photochromic lenses

Photochromism, the phenomenon by which absorption of electromagnetic energy causes reversible change in colour of a material has been known to scientists since 1800 and hundreds of natural organic chemical compounds possess this ability. Two ingenious research chemists, Dr W. H. Armistead and S. D. Stookey, at Corning Incorporated (formerly Corning Glass Works), in the USA developed and harnessed this phenomenon in 1964 to produce a lens which changed colour to suit the lighting conditions. That is to say it changed to a dark colour when exposed to sunlight but lightened again when indoors or in areas of lower illumination.

A photochromic glass lens contains billions of microscopic silver halide crystals (about 5 nm in diameter). When exposed to direct sunlight these microcrystals disassociate into free silver particles which then cluster together to form silver colloides. These colloides absorb ultra-violet light, thus darkening the lens. When the activating illumination is removed, the silver colloides split apart into free silver particles which regroup with the trapped halides and re-form into silver halide microcrystals. As this happens the lens clears. Being trapped within the glass the microcrystals are available for lightening and darkening the lens indefinitely.

There were drawbacks with the early lenses in as much that they were rather slow to react, especially clearing. In time Pilkington Special Glass also became involved in research and development of photochromics. Both Corning and Pilkington developed what is termed second generation photochromics that have a faster reacting time, hence the original first generation were eventually phased out. There are even third generation photochromics on the market now with even faster darkening and lightening times.

The choice of photochromic lenses today is bewildering and it is not the purpose of this chapter to attempt to list them, but rather to describe them in general terms. There are certain characteristics applicable to all photochromics that are worth developing, to understand how and why they work and the differences between them.

All are somewhat temperature dependant. Assuming the same degree of illumination, they will be darker when its colder and lighter when its warmer. This is slightly ironic as of course they are looked upon as a sunglass lens to be used in warm conditions. Because they react more in colder climates, there are some photochromics where the manufacturer issues a warning stating that if the centre substance is to be greater than 3 mm, they should not be worn in freezing or cold conditions as the lens would darken to virtually zero transmission!

Lens thickness has an effect on the density of the tint. The silver halides run evenly through the lens, and therefore the thicker the lens, the more of them there is to absorb the light, hence the tint would be darker. Care must be exercised when looking at transmission graphs or curves put out by the various photochromic manufacturers. They are all normally based on a 2 mm thick sample at a specific stated temperature. Any variance in these values will effect the transmission characteristics.

Linked to transmission charts or curves we have the consideration as to whether a lens is classed as a *narrow swing* or *wide swing*. All photochromics available would generally fall into one of these categories. A narrow swing would be a lens that normally changes from a light to a medium dark comfort tint, e.g. 90–50% LTF, on the other hand a wide swing would change from light to a dark tint, perhaps 87–22% LTF. The latter tends to be the most popular as of course they go very light and very dark and therefore the patient does not need to keep changing spectacles as the intensity of the light changes through the day. Although unusual, but available nevertheless, there are some lenses that start dark and go even darker. Because of their restricted swing they would fall into the narrow swing category.

With regard to fused multifocals, there were some initial difficulties due to the fact that the photochromic properties were affected by the heat used in the fusing process. However, these have now been overcome.

As photochromic lenses tend to improve with age, the more light/dark cycles that they go through the better they perform. It is not uncommon for patients supplied with a new pair of photochromics to complain they do not react as well as their old pair. They are forgetting that their old pair was probably supplied two years previous and have gone through many light/dark cycles. Their new spectacles need a short running in period to achieve full reaction. Because of the above it is recommended that lenses are always replaced in pairs to ensure best possible tint match.

Like solid tints there will be a variation between densities if there is a marked difference between the prescriptions for the right and left lens as indeed there will be a variation from centre to edge on high powers.

Glass photochromics come in two basic colours, grey or brown. Technically it is possible to obtain others, but demand has to be sufficient to justify running the mix of that particular colour. It has been attempted in the past but it seems to have settled down to a choice normally between grey or brown. Developments have also allowed a limited availability of higher index photochromics.

So what of resin photochromics? Photochromic resin lenses utilise a significantly different photochromic technology to that used for glass. Achieving a high performance resin photochromic has not been an easy task and involves numerous chemical balancing acts. Many early attempts were based on a principle similar to that used for dyeing resin lenses. They had very limited success and were not generally accepted by the profession, industry or, indeed, the general public.

The turning point came in 1987 when the research and development division of PPG Industries embarked upon research and experimentation into producing an organic photochromic system for resin lenses. The effort resulted in the first commercially successful resin photochromic ophthalmic lens, followed by test marketing of the first generation of Transition lenses. The promising results of the test markets led to the formation of Transitions Optical Inc. in 1990.

Transition Optical supplies to the lens manufacturers a special monomer called CR 307 from which they mould their lenses. The manufacturers then send the lenses to Transitions Optical who subject them to their unique imbibing process.

With this technique it is possible to provide a uniform distribution of millions of photosensitive molecules within the front surface to depths of several microns. They become an integral part of the lens and not a coating that can wear or rub off. The process of imbibing can be best illustrated by imaging a piece of standard laboratory filter paper saturated with the photochromic compounds and then allowed to air dry. The result is a paper with a compound evenly dispersed throughout. By placing the paper on the lens surface and heating both lens and paper the compound will transfer and imbibe into the lens surface. Penetrations depth of the compound is in the region of 100–150 µm. The advantage of this system is that no matter what the prescription, the tint density is uniform.

Over a period of approximately two years, resin photochromics will unfortunately degrade due to their exposure to ultra-violet radiation, unlike glass where the reaction is locked in permanently, for the life of the lens.

As with glass, resin photochromics are temperature dependent and will get darker at colder temperatures than hotter ones. As most climates with high temperatures also have very intense ultra-violet levels, this will partially counter the temperature dependence.

Advances in photochromic technology has meant that second and third generation resin photochromics have been developed. It has also been possible to combine the technology with higher index materials, including polycarbonate.

A word of warning. As the photochromic elements are incorporated into the front surface, lenses are not suitable for facetting (i.e. some rimless mounts). Whilst the main part of the lens would retain its photochromic reaction, the facetted edges would not, leading to an area of 'no-colour' surrounding the lens, which many patients would not find acceptable.

With care, most resin photochromics can be AR coated; however, it must be remembered that this application will affect the transmission of the lens in two ways. Firstly, AR coating reduces the amount of ultra-violet reaching the lens and as ultra-violet is an important element in photochromic activation this will affect the overall performance. Secondly, the affect of an AR is to reduce reflections thereby increasing transmittance, therefore AR-coated lenses will not be considered as dark as uncoated.

The latest development in resin photochromics has been by Corning, the originators of glass photochromics. Over five years in development, and picking up some 25 patents along the way, their new material is called SunSensors. It has several advantages over its rivals. The photochromic elements are contained within the material and do not have to be imparted at a later date. This means that production is quicker and more efficient. Being within the lens the photochromic reaction is far less prone to fatigue and will therefore give any lens a longer lifespan. Even though within the lens, only the outer surfaces react so there is no marked colour difference between centre and edge on higher power prescriptions.

The material is available in 1.555 index as standard and will therefore allow thinner lenses to be produced. It is also remarkably light having a specific gravity of only 1.168.

Available in grey or brown it retains its 'colour' throughout the change from light to dark back to light again. Some previous designs exhibited shifts from the true grey or the brown during this process.

SunSensors are truly the nearest equivalent to glass photochromics in relation to their transmission values. A common complaint from patients in the past is that resin photochromics did not react as well as their glass. As discussed all photochromics be they glass or resin, are temperature dependent. Corning patient literature warns that under conditions of extreme cold, the light transmission could fall below the minimum 8% required for driving – a unique claim for resin photochromics!

In the clear state the material has a transmittance of approximately 85% darkening to approximately 17% for the grey version and 20% for the brown. Working closely with Signet Armorlite Inc. a range of single vision bifocal and progressive lenses are available in this new material.

In conclusion, all photochromics, both glass and resin are excellent ultra-violet absorbers. (More about ultra-violet later in this chapter.)

## Bonded equitint lenses

Early in the chapter it was mentioned that any solid integral tint made in high plus or minus prescriptions would exhibit a marked difference between the density of that tint from centre to edge. Plus lenses will be dark at the centre going lighter towards the edge; minus lenses will be darker at the edge, lightening towards the centre. There is also the problem of tint matching when there is significant difference in power between the two lenses.

One possible solution is to bond a sliver of tinted material to a clear prescription lens. For example, if our need was to supply a –7.00 DS in photochromic the answer could be to make up the –7.00 DS in white glass (this could be crown or high index) and bond to it using an epoxy resin described in Chapter 23, a thin layer of photochromic material (*Figure 26.6*).

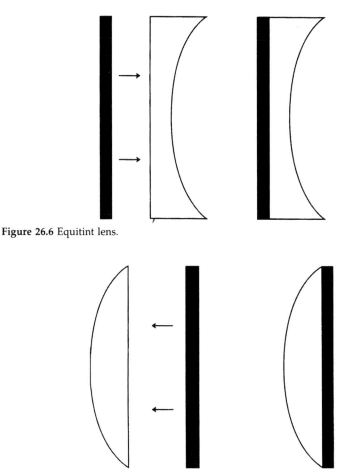

**Figure 26.6** Equitint lens.

**Figure 26.7** Equitint lens.

The above would also apply to a solid non-photochromic tint. Plus powers can also be catered for by the bonding technique as shown in *Figure 26.7*. This, however, is not recommended for photochromic lenses due to the photochromic layer having to be placed on the back surface. This has the result of the white lens filtering out some of the light that causes the photochromic lens to change colour and therefore it does not darken as much.

The bonding technique is also very useful for supplying tinted lenses that would otherwise be out of range. It means that the prescription can be fabricated in white glass, for which a greater variety of substances and diameters is available, and the tint sliver can then be bonded. With some slight adaptions the bonding technique can be used for multifocals as well as single vision. Whilst it is possible under certain circumstances to bond resin to resin or indeed resin to glass, by far the majority of requests are for glass to glass.

## Hardcoating

With growth in usage of resin lenses it soon became apparent that whilst patients enjoyed the lightness of resin they objected to the way that it scratched more readily than traditional glass. The advent of higher index resins, which generally tend to be softer than ordinary CR39 accelerated the search for a solution. It is difficult to quantify the ability of a hardcoat to resist scratching and this is, and has been, the subject of much debate. The main problem is that there are so many different types of scratches. Hardcoats are normally very good at preventing the numerous small scratches which occur during normal everyday wear, but they cannot prevent deep scratches due to accident or major abuse. Nothing, not even diamond is scratchproof!

Generally it is accepted that the harder a material, the more brittle it is. To prevent hardcoats from cracking, they must be very thin relative to the lens thickness. They are normally between 0.5 and 10 μm thick. (Typically this is 10–20 times thicker than an AR coating.)

Hardcoats can be applied to a lens either in the form of a lacquer or by vacuum deposit. The former by either a 'dip' or 'spin' method, which technically is less expensive and normally allows tinting, the latter uses more expensive vacuum technology (similar to AR coating) which produces a thinner layer (normally silica) that is harder than lacquer, but due to its thinner nature does not appear to offer as much protection. Any tinting has to be preformed before application.

Lacquer technology is continually developing. At one time those hardcoating lacquers that allowed tinting where often less scratch resistant than those that did not. Today there is very little difference between tintable and non-tintable hardcoats with regard their ability to resist scratching.

What are the optical effects of hardcoating? Providing the coating material has the same refractive index as that of the lens it is being applied to – none, assuming it has been applied properly. Once applied, the hardcoat is difficult to discern with the possible exception of 'teardrop' in the area of any segment. The main effect of a mismatch between indices of lens and coating material is to change the surface reflections slightly. However as most hardcoating materials have an index very similar to that of the lens material the effect is not significant. With the application of an AR, it becomes even less significant as the hardcoat is relatively thick compared to the AR and so the lens index becomes somewhat irrelevant.

There can be a problem if the hardcoat layer is not exactly equal thickness across the lens surface. Interference pattern similar to 'oil on water' can be the result, therefore spoiling the cosmetic effect.

There are several methods by which a scratch resistance (not scratchproof) coating can be applied to a resin lens.

There is what is termed the *spin method*, where the lenses are mounted individually on a rotating spindle and a small amount of polymer is placed on the lens surface which is then spun at high speed, the centrifugal force of the spinning lens taking the polymer to the edge, creating a scratch resistant coating. On any straight top multifocal the segment does tend to create an obstruction to the smooth flow of the polymer across the lens surface so it is not uncommon to see very small ripples (or teardrops as they are sometimes called) in the area around the segment. An inexperienced eye would find difficulty in detecting these. After spinning, the coating would be inspected before proceeding to repeat the procedure for the other side of the lens. Once the operator is satisfied with the result the coating will be cured on to the lens by ultra-violet or thermal curing methods. If at the inspection stage some defect is discovered, then providing the polymer has not been cured, it can be removed and the lens retreated.

Another method for imparting a hardcoat on a resin lens is by a process known as *dipping*. With this method several lenses are mounted in a rack and immersed into a polymer solution (*Figure 26.8*) and then lifted back out. Any residue is allowed to run off. There is still the problem caused by the liquid being interrupted by the shaped segments but careful placing of the lens in the rack enables the 'teardrop' to be kept to a minimum. The

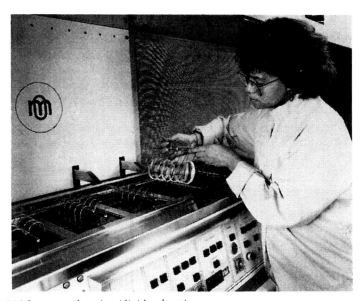

Figure 26.8 Lenses undergoing 'dip' hardcoating.

polymer used is similar to that used for spin coating although the solids-to-solvent ratio and the viscosity are changed to suit the different production techniques. The dipping method lends itself to volume production. Room temperature and humidity are important to prevent deterioration of the polymer, and therefore climate controls and clean room regimes are important to ensure quality of the coating process. Ultrasonic cleaning and stain-free drying systems are also an essential ingredient.

Through improved technology a hardcoat chemical can also be applied to resin lenses by means of *vacuum coating*, similar to that already described for AR coating. It is generally accepted that this is not so resistant to scratching as the spin/dip methods. The cost of this technology and the time a lens has to spend in the vacuum chamber means that it is probably the least used method of hardcoating.

Yet another method whereby a scratch resistance coating can be imparted on to a resin lens is that known as *in-mould* scratch resistant coating. This is performed by the semi-finished lens manufacturer who, during the initial casting, incorporates a scratch resistant coating to the front surface. In principle this is a good way to make a hardcoating since it will be inherently well bonded to the lens surface. The drawbacks are that it is only possible to coat the front surface and therefore after surfacing it will be necessary to apply a spin hardcoating to the back. There are those who say there is no need to coat the back as inevitably it is the front surface that takes the greatest wear and tear. It is best to check with your prescription house as to their policy regarding this.

An additional consideration of in-mould hardcoats is the compatibility with other manufacturers AR coating processes or indeed, their hard-coating if they have a policy of coating the back. Many prescription houses would prefer to have a 'bare' lens, allowing them to have total control over any coating processes.

In-mould hardcoats are not suitable for dip hardcoating as this method applies polymer to both sides of the lens at the same time and would therefore cause problems to the side already coated!

A word of caution, straight top segments that have been hardcoated can cause problems when checking on a lensmeter. If the distance optical centre is within approximately 3 mm of the segment top, the lensmeter can sometimes detect lacquer run-off along the top of the segment ridge, which can lead to an incorrect power reading. To avoid this, move lens vertically so one is checking power at approximately 5 mm above the segment top.

In conclusion, it should be noted that with the exception of the vacuum method of applying a hardcoat all other methods are normally applied to the lens in its uncut form.


## Water resistant coatings

Also referred to as hydrophobic coating. Applying this type of coating can overcome to a great extent the major drawback for users of multi-layer AR coatings. It is a paradox that the better and more effective the AR, the greater chance that it will show smudges and marks. It is not a case of the lens becoming more dirty because it has been AR treated; the

AR will just exhibit the smudges and marks more clearly. Because of this, water resistant coatings were developed. They work on a similar principle to that of wax polishing the paintwork of a car. It creates a low surface wetting angle which allows the water to run off rather than wetting and drying on the painted surface. When applied to a lens it causes the water and grease to form smaller droplets which in turn have a smaller area of contact with the lens surface, meaning that they cannot adhere so firmly and therefore can be removed easier. In simplistic terms the coating makes the surface more slippery, thus leading to less adhesion of the droplets.

It is performed after any AR coating has been applied by either dipping in a 'solution' of chemical or as part of the vacuum process. The thickness of the hydrophobic layer can be measured in numbers of molecules and is therefore even thinner than the AR coating layer it is applied to.

## Ultraviolet (UV) inhibitors

Despite the sun being some 93 million miles away from earth, with its temperature of 27 million degrees Fahrenheit, its intense light floods us with waves of UV.

It is an established fact that exposure to UV radiation can cause cancer of the skin. The probability is that it can also cause opacity of the crystalline lens. The levels of UV need not be high because the effect on the lens is cumulative over a period of years. This is significant for three reasons: (1) People are living longer and the incidence of cataracts does increase dramatically with age, hence more people are likely to suffer from them. (2) The ozone layer has been depleted and it has been estimated a decrease in ozone of only 2.5% could cause an increase of 10% in the incidence of skin cancer. It is logical to assume that a similar increase in cataracts would result. (3) Increasing leisure time means that more people are spending more time in outdoor pursuits and holidays, often in areas of high UV luminance, for example skiing and watersports where reflection increases already high levels of UV by about 85 and 10%, respectively.

We are becoming increasingly exposed to UV light and it is a matter of simple prudence to help ourselves by wearing protective filters. Just as skin can be sunburned with too much sun, so can the eye. In its milder form this can lead to symptoms some time after the actual exposure. The eyes feel red and sandy and there may be some swelling and even some temporary loss of vision. In its more severe form some of the corneal epithelial cells may be damaged, causing quite intense pain and taking weeks or months fully to recover. The retina can also be put at risk because longer wave UV light can reach the retina, causing blanching and lesions.

*Figure 26.9* is a pictorial representation of the source of UV and how different elements absorb it. The UV section of the electro-magnetic spectrum covers a wavelength region from 100 nm, where it merges with X-rays, to 380 nm, where it merges with visible light. For convenience, UV radiation is subdivided into three elements, UVC, UVB and UVA:

*UVC.* Wavelengths below 280 nm are effectively filtered out by the ozone layer surrounding the earth. The amount of absorption varies and is

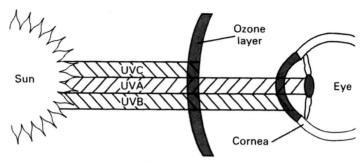

**Figure 26.9** Components of UV light.

reduced near to the equator and at high altitudes due to the reduced atmospheric thickness.

*UVB.* Wavelengths between 280 and 315 nm are responsible for sunburn and snow blindness. The amount of UV affecting a person is substantially increased by reflection from surfaces such as snow, sand, concrete and water.

*UVA.* Possibly the most dangerous area between 315 and 380 nm causing chronic damage to the eye, especially low dose exposure over a long period of time.

It is necessary to protect ocular tissues as much as possible from the effects of UV. The cornea absorbs UV radiation below 300 nm, the lower portion of UVB. It is susceptible to UV-related problems such as pterygia and pingueculae, snow blindness and photokeratitis.

The crystalline lens absorbs UV radiation below 380 nm (UVA). Continuous exposure of the lens to near UV (300–380 nm) may result in cumulative photochemical damage. With ageing, the lens absorbs more UVA, generating more pigments. The nucleus or core of the lens becomes more yellow so that with further exposure and ageing, cataracts develop. Patients who have cataracts removed, therefore, lose a significant intraocular filter. Lenses suitably treated are essential to offset this loss in postoperative cataract patients.

It is possible to impart into a resin lens, in a similar way to that already described for tinting, a UV inhibitor. Resin is naturally more UV absorbing than Crown glass, that is to say it absorbs up to approximately 350 nm in comparison to glass at approximately 300 nm. However, resin can be subsequently treated to bring this figure up to about 400 nm where the eye begins to encounter the less harmful visible light. The UV inhibitor is normally contained in a similar tank or pot to that used for tinting of resin. However, immersion times are longer to ensure adequate protection is given and the lenses emerge with normally a very slight yellowish hue to them. The UV inhibitor is not classed as a tint but it does give some slight residue colour to the lens. If the cut off point is brought close to 400 nm then the lens will still retain a 'white' appearance, but as soon as absorption moves above 400 nm, the lenses begin to show some yellowness.

If required, a tint and UV inhibitor can be incorporated into a lens. In this instance the UV treatment would normally be done first followed by the tinting. If it were done the other way around it is possible that the tint might contaminate the UV due to the increased immersion time required for UV treatment. It is advisable that any dark tint should be combined with a UV treatment. The pupil of the eye will increase in size in response to a dark tint and could therefore receive an excessive amount of UV radiation.

BS 7394 Part 2 (1994) clearly defines what constitutes a UV absorber (*Table 26.3*). The reader is urged to obtain a copy for fuller reference purposes.

**Table 26.3** Classification by UV absorption

| Classification term | Minimum percentage absorption[a] at any wavelength within the range: | |
| --- | --- | --- |
| | UV-B[b] | UV-A[c] |
| UV-B absorber | 99 | 50 |
| UV absorber | 99 | 95 |

[a]Centred at distance design reference point of the lens.
[b]UV-B extends between wavelengths 280 and 315 nm.
[c]UV-A extends between wavelengths 315 and 380 nm.

*Figure 26.10* illustrates the difference between an untreated CR39 lens and one that has had a UV inhibitor applied.

Notice how the plot of the untreated lens begins to turn upwards at around 350 nm. In comparison, the treated lens causes the plot to turn just before 400 nm indicating the lens is absorbing ultra-violet radiation up to this point.

Some manufacturers will go even further and provide protection beyond 400 nm into the blue element of the spectrum as it is believed that

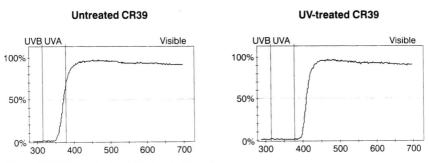

**Figure 26.10** Untreated and UV-treated CR39.

this too can cause discomfort. These lenses tend to have a definite colour incorporated. One such example is a variation on the glass photochromic theme which produces lenses that could best be described as 'spectral control'. They have been 'engineered' to filter specific wavelengths of light to enhance visibility and block those wavelengths that are harmful to the eye.

A name synonymous with 'spectral control' is Serengeti. By subjecting the lenses to a process referred to as hydrogen firing it is possible to engineer the molecular structure of the photochromic glass thereby introducing layers of silver. The silver becomes an integral part of the lens and produces a permanent barrier to ultra-violet radiation.

The lenses also help to relieve what is often termed 'blue blur' which is caused by short blue light wavelengths focusing in front of the retina instead of the back where other wavelengths focus. This natural phenomenon reduces the sharpness of an image causing eyestrain and fatigue. 'Spectral control' lenses, such as Serengeti, block some of the blue light. They should not block all blue light because this would distort the colours seen through the lenses. Blue light as well as enough green, yellow and red light, are necessary to keep colour perception balanced and natural looking. As a result, the lenses provide and improve contrast which in turn enhances the wearer's vision.

As a general statement, high index materials in both glass or resin normally provide greater UV protection than their more standard counterparts. The application of a UV inhibitor can normally be performed on either edged or uncut lenses.

## Polarised lenses

There are some naturally occurring polarisers in nature. Calcite has natural properties. In 1808 Etienne Louis Malus, a French military engineer and researcher, was looking across a garden through calcite and found that in the image he saw the brilliant glare from the sun had been extinguished! This 'experiment' can be considered as the first use of a polariser for the elimination of glare.

Edwin Land, the founder of the Polaroid Corporation developed the first commercially viable synthetic polariser in the early 1930s. His original intent was to use it to block glare from oncoming car headlights. By 1935 American Optical made available the first sunwear polarisers. When ophthalmic polarisers started to appear there were problems with both the quality and stability of the lenses – they tended to delaminate very easily (split apart).

Technological advances mean that today's resin polarised lenses do not suffer delamination or colour match problems. They are now available in a wide range of lens types and normally two colours, grey and brown. Several different densities of these two colours may be offered, the lighter ones allowing over-tinting with the opportunity to change the colour for cosmetic reasons.

At the heart of any polarised lens is the polarised filter. The filter is created by having iodine crystals randomly imbedded into a translucent film base, almost like cellophane. The film is then stretched in one direction causing the random crystals to become aligned in parallel rows. This causes a situation similar to that of light passing through a venetian blind, it only allows light through in a single direction. For example, only light waves orientated in the same direction as the vertical 'slats' in the polarised 'vertical blind' get through.

The film is then cut into spherical shapes and formed into specific curves.

Under clean room conditions the film, the moulds and the liquid monomer are brought together, the positioning of the film, close to the front mould is critical. The entire assembly is then cured, with the film becoming an integral part of the lens.

It used to be the case that minus powered polarised lenses were much thicker at the centre than a standard resin lens to avoid going through the polarised lamination. Because today's technology allows the polarised film to be positioned so close to the front surface, this is no longer an issue, the lenses being able to be processed as if made from conventional material.

It may be appropriate at this time to dispel the myth concerning 'Can we have a clear polariser?' As described above it is the colour blocking properties of the aligned crystals themselves which allows polarised lenses to block out the light in certain directions, so if the aligned crystals were perfectly clear all light would pass through, much as a perfectly clear venetian blind would not work to block out light coming through a window!

Polarised lenses are promoted as a means of reducing glare. But what is glare? It can be defined as an 'optical phenomenon in which reflections create polarised light on flat surfaces'. Poor visual accommodation in the human eye results in extreme discomfort and aggravated eyestrain. Simply, it becomes very hard to see. Ordinary tinted lenses may 'soften' the effect of glare, but they can only do that by reducing the total amount of light allowed to enter the eye. Taken to an extreme, the only way ordinary tinted lenses can protect the wearer from glare is by making the tint so dark you cannot even see through it!

Glare can be found everywhere. Reflections off cars, bodies of water, snow, sand or even haze, where polarised light bounces off particles in the air. Whatever the season, whether summer or winter, early mornings or late afternoons, glare can be present.

As people get older it appears they are more sensitive to glare and possibly slower to recover from the effects of it. After eye surgery, such as a cataract operation, patients appear to become more sensitive to glare. It is generally accepted that contact lens wearers are more sensitive to glare and preliminary findings are suggesting that those that have undergone vision corrective surgery, are also affected.

To better understand how polarisers work, imagine, or better still, obtain two polarising filters, turned at 90 degrees to each other, the first blocks all but vertical light waves, the second blocks all but horizontal light waves. Result – darkness – no light gets through.

Glass polarised lenses are also available and are often combined with photochromic elements.

## Conclusion

In concluding the first part of this chapter on AR, tinting and associated treatments it must be said that compatibility of all these different processes can give rise to problems. Each individual treatment is fine in its own right, but prescription houses have to develop systems that allow one or more of these coatings to be combined. For example it is not unusual to receive a request for a CR39 lens to be UV treated, tinted, hardcoated, AR coated and water resistant treated. Procedures have to be developed to allow this, taking into account such considerations as to what order the various coatings are applied, whether the lenses are in uncut or edged form and the technical problems of combining the various coatings together. Will the adhesion be affected? Will the UV inhibitor still be effective? All these questions have to be satisfied before a prescription house can market these products and their various combinations.

## Protection against impact

So far, this chapter has dealt with how eyes can be protected against certain radiation by some form of tint or treatment being utilised. But what about physical protection against some form of impact? Not only is some form of protection required due to certain occupational hazards, not forgetting certain professions such as police and armed forces, but with increased leisure time people are participating in sport or other activities that could put their sight at risk. Others at risk include children, who by their playful nature probably have more knocks and bumps during the day than the average adult. What about those unfortunate people who only have the use of one eye? How important it is that they protect the only good eye they have!

For ease of classification, when one talks in terms of safety lenses, they normally fall into two distinct categories: those for general, everyday or dresswear, and those for industrial use. Safety requirements and standards will vary from country to country. For example, in the USA, patients are not permitted to wear glass lenses of any kind unless they have been treated in some way to make them more impact resistant. No such requirement exists in the UK at the moment.

Although safety requirements may vary around the world, what they do have in common is that the lenses should withstand the impact of specific diameter steel balls dropped from pre-determined heights, the test for dresswear not being so stringent as for industrial. There are also various projectile tests consisting of small calibre steel balls being fired from a gun at a pair of safety spectacles, mounted in a frame and resting upon a dummy head.

What are the options available? For the purposes of this chapter we will concentrate on ophthalmic lenses mounted in spectacle frames. Over-specs or those offering protection against other elements such as gas, dust, chemical, etc. will not be included. It may be as well to consider each material in turn with an explanation of how additional strength can be incorporated.

*Glass.* At one time the most popular material for the manufacture of spectacle lenses, but now in decline. It is ironic really that for a long time the most popular material available for spectacle lenses was renowned as one of the most brittle materials available. They will break, even from quite a low force impact. If a glass lens or sheet of glass for that matter is struck, the side that is hit will be compressed and the opposite surface will be put under tension, causing it to crack or fracture. Minus powered lenses are particularly prone to fracture due to their thinner centre substances, although sometimes the thicker edge provides rigidity thus preventing breakage. Plus lenses, on the other hand, being thicker at the centre, are more likely to withstand impact.

There are two methods by which glass lenses can be toughened. One of them is thermal or heat treatment. The lenses are made in the normal manner except they have to comply with certain minimum centre and edge substance requirements. The edged lenses are then placed in a suitably heated ceramic oven where the temperature of the glass will be raised to something in the region of 600–700°C. The length of time the lenses remain in the oven will depend upon a combination of their size, weight and type of glass, but charts are available to assist the operative. After the designated time has elapsed they are removed and sprayed with cold air. This causes the outer layers to cool more rapidly than the central core putting them into a state of compression, and the inner core into tension. When such a lens receives any form of impact, the side opposite the blow will stay in compression (or is not put under tension) and therefore fracture is less likely. Lenses normally emerge from the toughening process, very fractionally larger. This needs to be taken into account by the glazers as further edging of the lenses after toughening is not possible as it would reduce the compression/tension set up within them. Prescription houses will normally only guarantee a toughened product for 24 months, as any scratching or knocks that the lens may receive effectively reduces its strength little by little.

A 100% check is made on all toughened lenses. This normally consists of dropping a steel ball from a pre-determined height, the diameter and height depending on if the spectacles are being worn for dress or industrial wear. The test is simple; if the lens breaks it has failed! Every time a safety lens receives a knock it loses some of its strength and therefore to minimise this for the test procedure, it is normally performed whilst the lens is still warm. One can identify a heat toughened lens by observing it between two crossed polarised filters. A pattern similar to that shown in *Figure 26.11* will be seen.

A slight variation on above, and only available through Norville Optical is a process referred to as thin toughening. It is a thermal treatment as described above, but controlled, and the lenses cooled in such a manner that they can be of a thinner substance than those used for conventional thermal toughening. The pattern observed through polarised filters is slightly different to that of conventional thermal toughening (*Figure 26.12*). It has more of a mottled appearance.

When considering any form of safety lens it must be borne in mind that no prescription house guarantees that they will not break when receiving an impact. They certainly are less likely to but they still can break. The

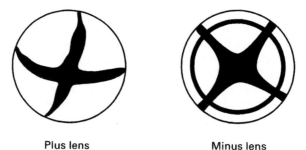

Plus lens                    Minus lens

**Figure 26.11** Toughened lenses observed through crossed polarised filters. (After Jalie, M. *Principles of Ophthalmic Lenses*, ADO, by permission.)

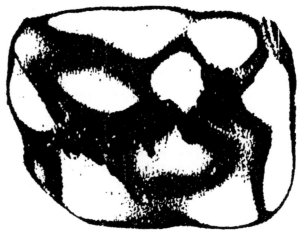

**Figure 26.12** A thin toughened lens observed through crossed polarised filters. (Courtesy of Norville Optical, Gloucester, England.)

guarantee is that if breakage does occur the broken pieces will not be sharp and jagged, which obviously can damage the eye. In the case of glass toughened lenses they will crumble into a mosaic of small pieces of reasonably uniform size, and are unlikely to cause serious ocular injury.

Not all lens materials are suitable for thermal toughening. Photochromics have to be treated in a slightly different manner as the heat of the toughening can affect the photochromic properties. Normally a secondary heat process is performed to restore the correct photochromic activity. High index lenses in general are not suitable for thermal toughening. Certain lens types, namely E-style, prism controlled or any lens fitted to a supra or rimless, are not suitable either.

Another means by which glass lenses can be toughened is by chemical treatment. This particular method has not really gained acceptance in the UK but is used extensively in the USA. The process again involves edged lenses, this time being immersed in a bath of chemicals, normally sodium nitrate, heated to around 450–460°C, for several hours. During this time there is a transfer between the potassium ions in the chemicals and the sodium ions on the surface of the lens material. The potassium ions being larger than the sodium ones, have the result of creating compression layers near the surface of the lens as the ions push together. This has effectively the same result as the thermal treatment; compression/tension is set up within the lens. The compression depth should exceed 75 μm (0.075 mm) to be effective. The resulting strength of the lens is greater than that obtained from the thermal method, with the added advantage that the lenses do not have to be as thick as they would have been had they been thermal treated. Unfortunately, no strain pattern can be observed when viewing through crossed polarised filters.

The chemical method is more costly as different chemical baths are needed for the different index materials. For example, photochromics require a different mix and lower temperatures. All lenses have to go through a pre-heat process before entering the bath, and then a cooling down period must be allowed for. The baths must be constantly checked for purity as they become contaminated with sodium ions. The chemicals used have to be treated with great care as they are quite dangerous. The great advantage of the system is of course the fact that lenses of different shapes and sizes can be treated in batches rather than individually. The process is also suitable for all glass types providing appropriate bath mixtures and temperatures are used.

*Resin.* By its very nature, resin is much safer to wear before the eye. Specific requests for safety lenses in resin need no additional treatment other than perhaps leaving the lens slightly thicker than normal for additional robustness.

*Polycarbonate.* The strongest material from which a lens can be made. A brief outline of its characteristics have already been given in Chapter 2.

# Chapter 27

# Lens surfacing/manufacturing

## General considerations

A prescription house will always prefer to start with a semi-finished lens blank. The mass producers make these available in a reasonably comprehensive range of curves and are thus able to achieve production runs at a unit cost not normally possible in one-off systems.

The majority of semi-finished blanks have the outside (convex) surface finished. It is left to the laboratory to surface the concave side as required by the individual prescription. Indeed, in many parts of the world prescription houses carry a set of tools for working concave surfaces only. Some countries, however, including the UK, still have a demand for solid bifocals with segments on the concave side and must therefore carry a set of plus working tools as well. These laboratories have the advantage of being able, when necessary, to start from unworked material, surfacing both sides and producing lenses with curvatures not possible from stock semi-finished blanks.

When surfacing the second side of a lens to prescription, the aim is not only to produce a good surface but also to achieve the standard of optical accuracy required for the finished lens. This includes the prescribed lens and prism powers, but in the case of multifocals the optical centre position and orientation of the cylinder axis (when applicable) must both be correct in relation to the segment.

## Surfacing instructions

In the surfacing shop, jobs are normally accompanied by a ticket or docket containing the necessary instructions. These comprise, depending on the prescription, some or all of the following particulars:

1 The surface curve to be worked, or, in the case of toroidal surfaces, the curve in each of the two principal meridians. The *curve* refers to the spectacle tool numbering according to the refractive index adopted for this purpose. Some prescription houses may substitute radii of curvature rather than actual curve.
2 The cylinder axis or base curve meridian.

3 The centre thickness of the lens, or for some plus lenses, the minimum edge thickness required.

4 The prismatic effect to be worked. If both vertical and horizontal prisms are prescribed, they must be replaced by the single resultant prism.

5 The prism base setting. In some laboratories it is the practice to use the 360 degree protractor for this purpose.

6 The prism thickness difference.

7 Nominal and actual curves of the semi-finished lens.

8 Lens diameter.

9 Trepan or crib instructions. This is the name given to the process whereby the blank being used is reduced to a diameter more compatible with the size of the frame that it is to be eventually glazed into. For example, a lens may only be available in a 70 mm diameter, but a frame may only be a 46 eyesize. Why surface a full blank when most of it will be edged away? The blank would therefore probably be trepaned down to 60 or 65 mm depending on the decentration requirements. The lens would now be easier to surface and in the case of plus prescriptions, allow a thinner centre substance to be obtained without chipping.

Calculation of optimum centre thicknesses for plus lenses of even moderate power can become extremely complicated. A combination, for example, of an asymmetrical lens shape, a strong cylinder at an oblique axis, decentration, and prescribed prism, would present quite a challenge even with the assistance of calculation tables. Playing for safety may result in a lens unacceptably thick, while errors may lead to rejects.

Many computer programs have been written to take care of all the calculations, complex or otherwise, that are needed to print out complete surfacing tickets or dockets. Calculation of curves and substance have already been discussed in Chapters 8 and 10.

## Blank selection

The next stage is to select a semi-finished or 'rough' blank to which specific curves are to be imparted as dictated by the surfacing instruction docket. The processes of achieving surfacing instructions and blank selection can be reversed, i.e. some prescription houses will select the blank first and calculate the surfacing instructions around them, whilst others will allow the computer to choose the appropriate blanks and make their selection on this.

Consideration on blank selection should be to use the smallest possible blank that will allow the prescription to be achieved accurately. Some computer lens design programs will automatically calculate this. If not, then this has to be assessed taking such factors as lens shape, decentration, segment or fitting cross requirements into account. It is also important to ensure that the blank selected is of sufficient substance to achieve the instructions on the docket.

The task of blank selection can be a skill in itself due to the quantity and variety of lenses that have to be held in a comprehensive prescription house.

## Marking for surfacing

Can also be referred to as *stampout* or *markup*. It is evident that the lens must be correctly located for the different surfacing stages. This can be achieved by marking a series of lines on the lens to indicate the correct alignment of the cylinder axis (especially when a multifocal or progressive is involved), prism (with apex and base clearly marked), calibrating points for checking substances, and R or L to indicate right or left, and normally some form of reference to avoid any possible mix-ups. Marking can be performed freehand using a paint brush and either water based or oil based paint, and a protractor. Alternatively, one can use various fine marking-pens or china pencils. More likely, however, is for the use of some form of marking up machine available from several manufacturers. The lens is placed on an illuminated scale/grid and positioned as per requirements dictated by the surfacing instruction docket. The marking head or rubber is then brought down onto the lens, having previously been inked to apply one or more marking lines. It is important to ensure that the marking device is very sturdy and does not deviate from its intended position in the course of operation.

The markings required on the lens vary according to the blocking system employed. Some systems only require a centre dot to be applied, the axis and prism settings being made on the blocker itself.

## Blocking

To hold the lens firmly and accurately for surfacing, a metal button is used to which the lens is blocked (*Figure 27.1*). For a great many years, pitch was the medium used. In ophthalmic work it has largely been superseded by low melting point alloys. Various kinds are used with

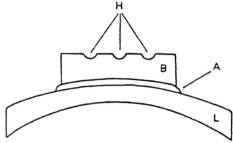

**Figure 27.1** Lens blocked for surfacing: H, driving pin location holes; B, button; A, alloy or wax; L, lens.

melting points ranging from about 47 to 85°C. The lower melting point alloys are generally more stable but are also much more expensive. It was a logical development to cast the button in alloy and block the lens to it in the same operation. Care must also be exercised in the choice of alloys used for resin lenses, for if they melt at too high a temperature this may cause damage to the lenses.

In an effort to find a more environmentally friendly and less expensive alternative to alloy, various wax blocking systems have been developed. Being more temperature sensitive, wax blocking systems work better in an air-conditioned environment. If the ambient temperature is too high, it is possible that the lenses will move on the block causing inaccuracies to occur during the surfacing process.

The blocking machine consists of a reservoir for the alloy or wax, with a heater and one or more casting moulds, a means of controlling the flow and an ejector to remove the blocked-on lens. To ensure adhesion of the alloy or wax to the lens, a coating of lacquer is normally applied before blocking, either by brush or by spraying. An alternative, especially for resin lenses, takes the form of a plastics film supplied in rolls and coated on one side with an adhesive. By means of a vacuum operated applicator the film is affixed to the lens and trimmed to size. Not only does this film give a good surface to take the alloy or wax but at the cleaning stage it has merely to be peeled off. Further cleaning is minimal.

Care needs to be exercised during blocking to ensure that the lens is seated on the blocker in such a way as to ensure that at no stage is it tilted, for this would cause unwanted prism to be incorporated. Certain lens types, namely large segments, E-style and progressives, have to be handled and positioned carefully to avoid leakage of the alloy from around the lens or incorrect pressure which allows the lens to tilt, thereby imparting unwanted prism.

On occasions where prism is required to be incorporated into the lens, some blockers have adjustments that angle it to achieve desired prismatic results. Others will have special rings, appropriately angled. Where very large amounts of prism are required it is not unusual to block with as much prism as possible with the remaining amount being obtained by a prism ring on the generator (see section on generating below).

It will soon become apparent that like so many other tasks in optics, every stage of manufacture is so very dependent on the previous stage. In this instance the blocking can only be as accurate as the marking-up lines that have been placed on the lens by the previous operator.

To avoid warpage or waviness in resin lenses it is essential to ensure that the blocking machines are checked on a regular basis to ensure they are not operating too hot.

# Trepanning/cribbing

This process has already been detailed in Chapter 2 and at the beginning of this chapter. It should be noted that some of today's modern generators (see below) have the capacity to trepan/crib during the generating cycle thereby removing the need for a separate operation.

## Generating

This is the name given to the process whereby the correct curvature(s) are cut into the lens surface and it is reduced to within a few tenths of a millimetre of its final centre substance. That is to say a small allowance is made for the subsequent smoothing and polishing operations that will in themselves remove some very small amounts of material. How much an allowance is made will depend upon whether the lenses are resin, high index resin, standard glass, high index glass or photochromic, etc.

It is essential, more so with resin lenses, that the material is kept as cool as possible whilst it is being worked. Generators, as they are called (*Figure 27.2*), are normally equipped with coolant systems that remove the debris to a filtering point as well as keeping the material cool.

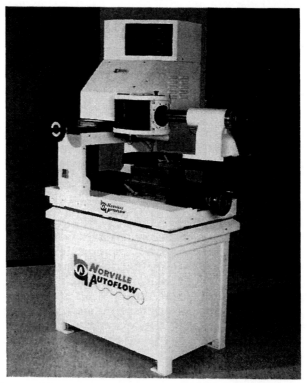

**Figure 27.2** A manual lens generator. (Picture courtesy of Norville Optical, Gloucester, England.)

Various types of cutting wheels (*Figure 27.3*) are available to be fitted to generators. Most are diamond impregnated or electroplated wheels. Some will employ carbide discs screwed into what is termed a crown. These wheels or discs are available in different diameters, the smaller ones being used to facilitate the cutting of high curves. The type and size of wheel used will depend on the material and powers being processed.

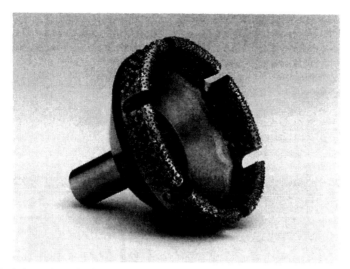

**Figure 27.3** A cutting wheel.

A recent development has been the introduction of what is termed *dry cutting*. Instead of a water or coolant being used to remove the debris, a strong vacuum source is connected to the generator. It is important when using this system that the integrity of the vacuum is checked on a regular basis and the resulting powder disposed of safely. Dry cut is only suitable for resin lenses.

Before diamond impregnated generators were available a process known as roughing would be employed. This consisted of rubbing the lens against a tool of the required radius of curvature using a coarse abrasive to wear the unwanted material away. This process is still used today on extremely high curves that are out of the range of the generators. In this instance the nearest curve possible would be cut into the lens, the final curve being roughed in by hand as described.

At one time two types of generator were available, those that cut sphere curves and those that cut toroidal surfaces (base curve and cross curve). Spherical generators have all but disappeared, the toric generator simply cutting a base curve the same as the cross curve to produce a sphere. In fact the proof of a good toric generator is how good a sphere it cuts!

Designs of generators vary tremendously. On some the radii of curvature is set up by calibrated wheels whilst on others the data is input via keyboard. Some have dual spindles to allow the operator to load and input data for one lens whilst the generator is cutting another.

As one has seen dramatic advancement in motor car refinements, so too have generators become highly sophisticated technological pieces of equipment, capable of being set to a wide variety of parameters, some even with self-analysis systems to advise what has gone wrong in the case of a breakdown. Dials and slides have been replaced with display screens and keyboards.

Latest development include single point cutting tools combined with revolutionary multi-axis turning technology. This type of generator works on a principle similar to that of a lathe. The precise control and synchronisation of each axis via sophisticated computer programme, results in a lens with extremely accurate curves and a surface finish superior to a conventional ground or milled surface. In most cases this will eliminate the need for first fining (see Smoothing section).

The single point tool is normally of polycrystalline construction and is only suitable for resin/organic materials. See *Figure 27.4.*

Another innovative concept is the ability of these generators to not only cut the correct curve(s) onto the lenses but to produce the smoothing/polishing tools as well. Accuracy can be greatly increased because if

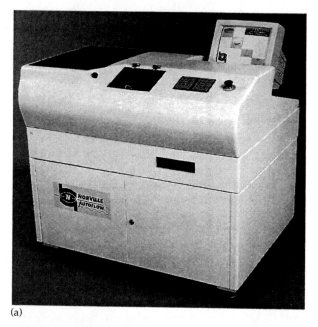

(a)

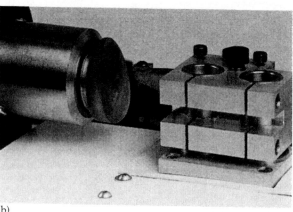

(b)

**Figure 27.4** (a) A multi-axis generator. (b) Single point cutting tool as used on this generator. (Pictures courtesy of Norville Optical, Gloucester, England.)

required lens and tool curves can be cut to the nearest 0.01 of a dioptre rather than rounding to the nearest 0.06 or 0.12.

The use of robotics is also expanding with lenses being placed in trepaners/cribbers and generators automatically, and removed in a similar way and passed along to the next operation.

The surface quality of some generators is so good that the need to smooth is eliminated, the lenses going straight to polishing process (resin only)!

## Smoothing

Generated surfaces can vary both in the surface finish and accuracy. Smoothing or fining is used to produce a suitable finish that will readily take a polish, and to obtain the true curve(s) required.

For glass lenses a one step smooth system is operated unless, as mentioned earlier, it is necessary to smooth in a curve due to generator limitations, in which case a double or even triple smooth may be required. Resin lenses can be smoothed or fined in a one or two step process depending on the type of curvatures involved and the type of machinery being used.

Before the lens can be mounted into the smoothing or fining machines a suitable tool or lap has to be selected. These are normally made in aluminium (although they can be made in a type of plastics). The principle behind smoothing or fining is that the lens is allowed to rub against the tool or lap of the same radius of curvature of that required to obtain the prescription. Some form of abrasive is introduced between the lens surface and the tool or lap face. This causes material to be removed by abrasion, produced by a repeated or continuous relative motion of the lens and tool. The tool or laps can be essentially of two types, *mushroom* or *minus laps* (*Figure 27.5*) or *saucer* or *plus laps* (*Figure 27.6*). The saucer variety are rarely used due to the fact that most lenses today are surfaced on the concave side.

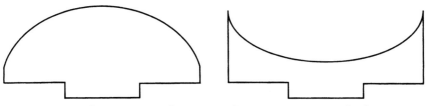

**Figure 27.5** A mushroom or minus lap.          **Figure 27.6** A saucer or plus lap.

Whereas years ago tools would have been made from cast iron and the lens smoothed by direct contact with the tool, because of the fact that they rapidly became worn and had to be constantly retrued it is now standard practice to use some form of smoothing pad applied to the tool surface. As this effectively changes the radius of the tool and therefore the final curvature, a compensation has to be made when initially making the tool. This allowance is referred to as the 'pad compensation'. Mushroom or

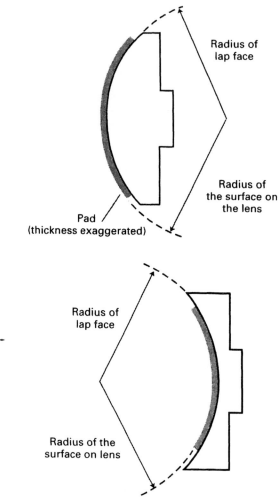

**Figure 27.7** The effect of a pad when applied to a lap. (Courtesy of Worshipful Company of Spectacle Makers.)

minus laps must have their radius shortened by the thickness of the pad whereas hollow or plus tools must have their radius increased by the thickness of the pad (*Figure 27.7*).

Another consideration is that the radius necessary to produce a specific curve on glass will be different to that required for resin. For example, the radius of a 9.50 D curve on glass would be

$$r = \frac{1000\,(n-1)}{F}$$

$$r = \frac{1000\,(1.523-1)}{9.5}$$

$$r = \frac{523}{9.50}$$

$$r = 55.05\,\text{mm}$$

To obtain the same curvature on standard CR39 would require

$$r = \frac{1000\,(n-1)}{F}$$

$$r = \frac{1000\,(1.498-1)}{9.5}$$

$$r = \frac{498}{9.50}$$

$$r = 52.42\,\text{mm}$$

The shorter radius would effectively cause the tool to be more greatly curved. Because of the above it is normal practice for those prescription houses that surface both glass and resin to have separate racks of tools for each material. For indices other than standard, the procedure is either to have tools cut for that index or convert the curvatures/radii to one of the standard materials. For example a 10.00 curve on a 1.701 material would have a radius of 70.1 mm

$$r = \frac{1000\,(n-1)}{F}$$

$$r = \frac{1000\,(1.701-1)}{10}$$

$$r = \frac{701}{10}$$

$$r = 70.1\,\text{mm}$$

If we apply

$$F = \frac{1000\,(n-1)}{r}$$

we obtain 7.46 (assuming crown glass tooling). Therefore, to produce a 10.00 curve on a material of 1.701 we would either use a 10.00 tool cut for that index or a 7.50 (nearest to 7.46) cut for standard glass material.

Having selected the tool, we now have to apply a pad to facilitate the smoothing process. Pads can either be impregnated with an abrasive which means that they can be used with just water running through the machine, or they can be of the type that need what is described as a coarse abrasive mixed with water to create a smoothing slurry. Pads used for glass tend to be of the latter variety whereas pads used for resin tend to be of the former.

The pads normally have an adhesive backing to hold them on the tool although there are some available that adhere simply by pressure and friction. Most pads are only used once and then disposed of, a new pad being used for each new lens.

A wide variety of sizes and grades of pads are available. Most are circular in shape with cutouts to allow them to lie smoothly on the more higher curve tools, and to help facilitate the flow of any liquid compounds. Their grades are generally specified either by the grit size of the impregnating abrasive or the average micron size of the particles. One of the roughest grades is a 400 grit pad, little used today. More common are the 600 grit or 15 micron type.

Having selected the tool and the pad attached they, along with the lens, are mounted into the smoothing machine. Two types are available, either those designed for spheres or those designed for torics. On spherical lenses it is advantageous to have both tool and lens rotating, with one oscillating over the other. The tool is rotated but there is no separate drive on the lens. Nevertheless, as it is moved across the tool as indicated, the revolution of the tool imparts some rotational movement to the lens despite the pressure of the driving pin.

A much more complicated mechanism is needed for smoothing and polishing toroidal surfaces. Whatever the system employed it must meet the following requirements:

1 The cylinder axis or base curve meridian of the lens must remain parallel to that of the tool during the whole of its travel. Some means of constraint is therefore essential.
2 The relative motion of tool and lens must ensure that the abrasive action is evenly distributed over the whole lens area.
3 The actual path of the lens over the tool must not be too quickly or simply repetitive or there will be a tendency to produce a wavy pattern on the surface.
4 The mechanical arrangement for imparting the separate motions of lens and tool must be free from bias or misalignment, tending to produce curvature errors.

Today's toric smoothers can quite easily be used for spheres as well. The machines allow for pressures, strokes and times to be varied depending on the type of material being smoothed, the smoothing agent or pad, the diameter and the curvature.

## Polishing

Essentially a similar operation to that of smoothing inasmuch that similar machines and the same tools are used. However, a different type of pad is employed along with an abrasive slurry which is now so fine it may be considered as a polish. Also polishing times, pressure and strokes of the machines may have to be altered.

The quality of the resulting polished surface depends very much on the smoothing operation previously performed. It is important that the polishing slurry is kept clean and uncontaminated to avoid scratches, sleeks and other quality problems. For resin lenses in particular, it is important to ensure that the slurry does not become too warm so most polishing machines have some form of chiller attached to ensure correct temperatures are maintained, although some manufacturers have developed polishes that they claim do not need chilling thereby removing the necessity of chilling units. Humidity of the general area in which polishing is performed is also important. If it is allowed to reach 90%, polishing becomes difficult.

The pads used for polishing have what can only be described as a 'velveteen' feel to them. Polishing is normally a one step process and the pad is disposed of after each lens is complete. The polishing slurry should be regularly filtered with a mesh to take out any foreign bodies such as any bits of pad that may have contaminated it. Depending upon throughput, the polish will last between 3 and 5 days before it has to be changed, although some topping-up may be performed in the interim. If scratches become a problem, the polish will most certainly have to be changed.

A recent development has been chiller/coolant units that serve several polishing machines. Manufacturers claim that polish need only be changed once a year, with just the occasional 'top-up'.

## Deblocking and cleaning

The lens must now be separated from its holder. *Knocking off* is the method used in some laboratories. It consists of giving the block a sharp tap. *Crimping* is another method which can be used if the whole block is cast. The block is squeezed to deform it slightly, after which it can be pulled away from the lens surface. An alternative method for alloy blocking is melting off. The lens and block are dipped into water which is held at a slightly higher temperature than the alloy's melting point. Rinsing the lens and block before deblocking is advisable. If the polishing compound is allowed to dry, its removal becomes much more difficult in the final cleaning of the lens. Moreover, any that is left on the block will be carried away with the alloy in the melting-off process, thus fouling it.

All traces of any varnish, tape and paint used must now be removed from the lens. Ultrasonic baths can be used at various stages of cleaning. In this late stage of manufacture, any damage to the surface which occurs is particularly unwelcome. The necessity for wiping the lens – possibly the most likely source of scratches – is reduced to a minimum by vapour drying systems.

From a health and safety point of view, it is advisable to wear protective gloves when handling alloy blocks and smoothing and polishing materials.

## Alternative methods of lens manufacture

Alternative methods for producing a lens have been developed. The first attempt was the concept of the mini-lab system based on a scaled down version of the surfacing laboratory described earlier in this chapter. As it is a miniaturised version of a full scale laboratory, the only limitation is governed by what semi-finished lenses are chosen to stock and the number of smoothing/polishing tools. Developed for the glazing house that wanted to offer just that 'little extra' and the 'in-store lab' that wanted to offer a 'one hour service', the mini lab is very versatile. It is not limited to one supplier for components and virtually any type of lens material can be surfaced (although in practice this tends to be a standard resin) and any make of branded lens can be surfaced. The resulting lens quality should be the same as that produced by a larger surfacing laboratory.

Lens casting is another alternative to the 'traditional' method of surfacing. It is not as versatile as the mini-lab system previously described. Much depends on the number and type of moulds held in stock. The principle is very similar to that used by the major lens casting manufacturers except instead of using CR39 that has to be heat cured for some considerable time and is also subject to shrinkage problems, an ultra-violet cured material is substituted that also happens to be less prone to shrinkage.

The quality of lenses made by the casting system relies very much on the cleanliness of the environment and the amount of attention given by the operator to mould cleaning.

Another important limitation of this system is the non-availability of special substance plus lenses. If for example it was required to cast a lens for a small frame, the lens produced would be the same substance as that required to glaze a medium to large frame. The process is governed by the mould availability. If one was surfacing a lens by conventional or mini-lab systems, adjustments/compensations could be made to allow a thinner lens for the smaller eyesize.

An advantage of the lens casting system is that some have a facility for applying a hardcoating liquid over the front mould before introducing the casting chemical, thus producing a lens with an in-mould front hardcoat.

A variation of the lens casting system is a process referred to as a surface casting. As indicated earlier, one of the major problems in casting CR39 is the shrinkage factor (up to 14%). For low powered lenses the shrinkage is insignificant compared to that of high powers. The difference in shrinkage around the edge compared to that in the central area can be considerable. The resulting stress can cause the lens to be rejected and at worse, even cause the moulds to fracture. In addition, whilst in the process of solidifying, CR39 exotherms, i.e. gives off heat. This limits the speed at which thick lens can be cast.

To overcome these difficulties, the surface casting system uses an existing single vision lens, with the correct distance prescription and then allows a very thin bifocal or progressive sliver to be cast onto the front. Usually CR39 can be used as the shrinkage factor is virtually eliminated because the sliver is so thin. The system does, however, rely on single vision lenses with very accurately formed front surfaces because any difference between the front and the mould curves will result in power errors.

Finally as an alternative to surfacing or casting there is a system perhaps best described as wafer laminating. It involves gluing/bonding a front wafer which incorporates the bifocal/progressive element onto a rear wafer which has the distance prescription. An ultra-violet curing adhesive forms the bonding agent. Its probably the quickest of any system, taking less than 10 min, but obviously the range offered depends on the number of components stocked. As with casting, the system does not allow reduced centre substance for small plus powered lenses.

* * * * *

Congratulations on reaching the end of the book (apart from the Appendices). It was never the intention that it covered all aspects of manufacturing optics and there are plenty of good books around that go into much more detail on specific subjects. It is hoped, however, that it has given you an overview of the world of optics and spurred you on to find out more, to read some of the other books, for now you have a good basic understanding – reading those other books will be less of a daunting task because you now speak and have a command of the 'language' of optics.

I said in the preface 'ENJOY'. I hope you have and now you must 'congratulate' yourself on having got this far.

**Strive for even greater achievements.**

**Part Four**

# Appendices

# Vertex power allowances

If the thickness of a lens could be ignored, its back vertex power would be the algebraic sum of its surface powers. In fact, the lens thickness increases the effective power of a convex front surface. To neutralise this increase, a vertex power allowance must usually be made. Either the plus power of the front surface must be reduced or the minus power of the back surface increased.

## Front surface allowance

In mass-produced lenses the allowance is usually on the front surface. In the prescription laboratory, the necessity for making front surface allowances arises mainly when finishing solid bifocals with the segment on the back surface. Suppose, for example, that the prescription in the plus cylinder transposition is

+4.00 DS +2.00 DC

The blank selected would probably have a DP curve of −400 D. If so, the nominal base and cross curves would be +8.00 D and +10.00 D respectively. If the finished lens is to have a centre thickness of 5.5 mm, reference to *Table 1* shows the required vertex power allowances to be 0.22 D and 0.35 D. The actual base curve should therefore be reduced to +7.78 D and the cross curve to +9.65 D.

The table was computed from the formula

$$\text{VPA} = \frac{tF_N^2}{1000\,n + tF_N}$$

where VPA denotes the vertex power allowance, $F_N$ the nominal (uncompensated) front surface power and $t$ the centre thickness in mm.

Alternatively, the value of $F_1$, the actual or compensated front surface power required, can be calculated directly from

$$F_1 = \frac{1000\,F_N}{1000 + (t/n)\,F_N}$$

*Table 1* was computed for a refractive index of 1.523 and *Table 2* for 1.498.

To a reasonable standard of approximation, the tabulated values can be adjusted for a different refractive index $n'$ by multiplying them by $(1.523/n')$.

**Table 1** Front surface vertex power allowances ($n = 1.523$)

| Nominal front surface power | Centre thickness of lens (mm) | | | | | | | | | | | | | | | | | | | | |
|---|---|---|---|---|---|---|---|---|---|---|---|---|---|---|---|---|---|---|---|---|---|
| | 2.0 | 2.5 | 3.0 | 3.5 | 4.0 | 4.5 | 5.0 | 5.5 | 6.0 | 6.5 | 7.0 | 7.5 | 8.0 | 8.5 | 9.0 | 9.5 | 10.0 | 10.5 | 11.0 | 11.5 | 12.0 |
| 2.50 | 0.01 | 0.01 | 0.01 | 0.01 | 0.02 | 0.02 | 0.02 | 0.02 | 0.02 | 0.03 | 0.03 | 0.03 | 0.03 | 0.03 | 0.04 | 0.04 | 0.04 | 0.04 | 0.04 | 0.05 | 0.05 |
| 2.75 | 0.01 | 0.01 | 0.01 | 0.02 | 0.02 | 0.02 | 0.02 | 0.03 | 0.03 | 0.03 | 0.03 | 0.04 | 0.04 | 0.04 | 0.04 | 0.05 | 0.05 | 0.05 | 0.05 | 0.06 | 0.06 |
| 3.00 | 0.01 | 0.01 | 0.02 | 0.02 | 0.02 | 0.03 | 0.03 | 0.03 | 0.04 | 0.04 | 0.04 | 0.04 | 0.05 | 0.05 | 0.05 | 0.06 | 0.06 | 0.06 | 0.06 | 0.07 | 0.07 |
| 3.25 | 0.01 | 0.02 | 0.02 | 0.02 | 0.03 | 0.03 | 0.03 | 0.04 | 0.04 | 0.04 | 0.05 | 0.05 | 0.05 | 0.06 | 0.06 | 0.06 | 0.07 | 0.07 | 0.07 | 0.08 | 0.08 |
| 3.50 | 0.02 | 0.02 | 0.02 | 0.03 | 0.03 | 0.04 | 0.04 | 0.04 | 0.05 | 0.05 | 0.06 | 0.06 | 0.06 | 0.07 | 0.07 | 0.07 | 0.08 | 0.08 | 0.09 | 0.09 | 0.09 |
| 3.75 | 0.02 | 0.02 | 0.03 | 0.03 | 0.04 | 0.04 | 0.05 | 0.05 | 0.05 | 0.06 | 0.06 | 0.07 | 0.07 | 0.08 | 0.08 | 0.09 | 0.09 | 0.09 | 0.10 | 0.10 | 0.11 |
| 4.00 | 0.02 | 0.03 | 0.03 | 0.04 | 0.04 | 0.05 | 0.05 | 0.06 | 0.06 | 0.07 | 0.07 | 0.08 | 0.08 | 0.09 | 0.09 | 0.10 | 0.10 | 0.11 | 0.11 | 0.12 | 0.12 |
| 4.25 | 0.02 | 0.03 | 0.04 | 0.04 | 0.05 | 0.05 | 0.06 | 0.06 | 0.07 | 0.08 | 0.08 | 0.09 | 0.09 | 0.10 | 0.10 | 0.11 | 0.12 | 0.12 | 0.13 | 0.13 | 0.14 |
| 4.50 | 0.03 | 0.03 | 0.04 | 0.05 | 0.05 | 0.06 | 0.07 | 0.07 | 0.08 | 0.08 | 0.09 | 0.10 | 0.10 | 0.11 | 0.12 | 0.12 | 0.13 | 0.14 | 0.14 | 0.15 | 0.15 |
| 4.75 | 0.03 | 0.04 | 0.05 | 0.05 | 0.06 | 0.07 | 0.07 | 0.08 | 0.09 | 0.09 | 0.10 | 0.11 | 0.12 | 0.12 | 0.13 | 0.14 | 0.14 | 0.15 | 0.16 | 0.16 | 0.17 |
| 5.00 | 0.03 | 0.04 | 0.05 | 0.06 | 0.06 | 0.07 | 0.08 | 0.09 | 0.10 | 0.10 | 0.11 | 0.12 | 0.13 | 0.14 | 0.14 | 0.15 | 0.16 | 0.17 | 0.17 | 0.18 | 0.19 |
| 5.25 | 0.04 | 0.04 | 0.05 | 0.06 | 0.07 | 0.08 | 0.09 | 0.10 | 0.11 | 0.12 | 0.12 | 0.13 | 0.14 | 0.15 | 0.16 | 0.17 | 0.17 | 0.18 | 0.19 | 0.20 | 0.21 |
| 5.50 | 0.04 | 0.05 | 0.06 | 0.07 | 0.08 | 0.09 | 0.10 | 0.11 | 0.12 | 0.13 | 0.14 | 0.15 | 0.15 | 0.16 | 0.17 | 0.18 | 0.19 | 0.20 | 0.21 | 0.22 | 0.23 |
| 5.75 | 0.04 | 0.05 | 0.06 | 0.07 | 0.09 | 0.10 | 0.11 | 0.12 | 0.13 | 0.14 | 0.15 | 0.16 | 0.17 | 0.18 | 0.19 | 0.20 | 0.21 | 0.22 | 0.23 | 0.24 | 0.25 |
| 6.00 | 0.05 | 0.06 | 0.07 | 0.08 | 0.09 | 0.10 | 0.12 | 0.13 | 0.14 | 0.15 | 0.16 | 0.17 | 0.18 | 0.19 | 0.21 | 0.22 | 0.23 | 0.24 | 0.25 | 0.26 | 0.27 |
| 6.25 | 0.05 | 0.06 | 0.08 | 0.09 | 0.10 | 0.11 | 0.13 | 0.14 | 0.15 | 0.16 | 0.17 | 0.19 | 0.20 | 0.21 | 0.22 | 0.23 | 0.25 | 0.26 | 0.27 | 0.28 | 0.29 |
| 6.50 | 0.06 | 0.07 | 0.08 | 0.10 | 0.11 | 0.12 | 0.14 | 0.15 | 0.16 | 0.18 | 0.19 | 0.20 | 0.21 | 0.23 | 0.24 | 0.25 | 0.27 | 0.28 | 0.29 | 0.30 | 0.32 |
| 6.75 | 0.06 | 0.07 | 0.09 | 0.10 | 0.12 | 0.13 | 0.15 | 0.16 | 0.17 | 0.19 | 0.20 | 0.22 | 0.23 | 0.25 | 0.26 | 0.27 | 0.29 | 0.30 | 0.31 | 0.33 | 0.34 |
| 7.00 | 0.06 | 0.08 | 0.09 | 0.11 | 0.13 | 0.14 | 0.16 | 0.17 | 0.19 | 0.20 | 0.22 | 0.23 | 0.25 | 0.26 | 0.28 | 0.29 | 0.31 | 0.32 | 0.34 | 0.35 | 0.37 |
| 7.25 | 0.07 | 0.08 | 0.10 | 0.12 | 0.14 | 0.15 | 0.17 | 0.18 | 0.20 | 0.22 | 0.23 | 0.25 | 0.27 | 0.28 | 0.30 | 0.31 | 0.33 | 0.35 | 0.36 | 0.38 | 0.39 |
| 7.50 | 0.07 | 0.09 | 0.11 | 0.13 | 0.14 | 0.16 | 0.18 | 0.20 | 0.22 | 0.23 | 0.25 | 0.27 | 0.28 | 0.30 | 0.32 | 0.34 | 0.35 | 0.37 | 0.39 | 0.40 | 0.42 |
| 7.75 | 0.08 | 0.09 | 0.11 | 0.13 | 0.15 | 0.17 | 0.19 | 0.21 | 0.23 | 0.25 | 0.27 | 0.28 | 0.30 | 0.32 | 0.34 | 0.36 | 0.38 | 0.39 | 0.41 | 0.43 | 0.45 |
| 8.00 | 0.08 | 0.10 | 0.12 | 0.14 | 0.16 | 0.18 | 0.20 | 0.22 | 0.24 | 0.26 | 0.28 | 0.30 | 0.32 | 0.34 | 0.36 | 0.38 | 0.40 | 0.42 | 0.44 | 0.46 | 0.47 |
| 8.25 | 0.08 | 0.10 | 0.12 | 0.14 | 0.17 | 0.19 | 0.21 | 0.23 | 0.26 | 0.28 | 0.30 | 0.32 | 0.34 | 0.36 | 0.38 | 0.40 | 0.42 | 0.44 | 0.46 | 0.48 | 0.50 |
| 8.50 | 0.09 | 0.11 | 0.13 | 0.15 | 0.18 | 0.20 | 0.22 | 0.24 | 0.28 | 0.30 | 0.32 | 0.34 | 0.36 | 0.38 | 0.41 | 0.43 | 0.45 | 0.47 | 0.49 | 0.51 | 0.53 |
| 8.75 | 0.09 | 0.12 | 0.14 | 0.16 | 0.19 | 0.21 | 0.23 | 0.25 | 0.29 | 0.31 | 0.34 | 0.36 | 0.38 | 0.41 | 0.43 | 0.45 | 0.48 | 0.50 | 0.52 | 0.54 | 0.56 |
| 9.00 | 0.10 | 0.12 | 0.15 | 0.17 | 0.20 | 0.22 | 0.24 | 0.27 | 0.31 | 0.33 | 0.36 | 0.38 | 0.41 | 0.43 | 0.45 | 0.48 | 0.50 | 0.53 | 0.55 | 0.57 | 0.60 |
| 9.25 | 0.11 | 0.13 | 0.16 | 0.18 | 0.21 | 0.23 | 0.26 | 0.28 | 0.33 | 0.35 | 0.38 | 0.40 | 0.43 | 0.45 | 0.48 | 0.50 | 0.53 | 0.55 | 0.58 | 0.60 | 0.63 |
| 9.50 | 0.11 | 0.14 | 0.17 | 0.19 | 0.22 | 0.25 | 0.27 | 0.30 | 0.34 | 0.37 | 0.40 | 0.42 | 0.45 | 0.48 | 0.50 | 0.53 | 0.56 | 0.58 | 0.61 | 0.64 | 0.66 |

|  | | | | | | | | | | | | | | | | | | | | | |
|---|---|---|---|---|---|---|---|---|---|---|---|---|---|---|---|---|---|---|---|---|---|
| 9.75 | | 0.15 | 0.18 | 0.21 | 0.24 | 0.27 | 0.30 | 0.33 | 0.36 | 0.39 | 0.42 | 0.45 | 0.48 | 0.50 | 0.53 | 0.56 | 0.59 | 0.61 | 0.64 | 0.67 | 0.70 |
| 10.00 | 0.12 | 0.16 | 0.19 | 0.22 | 0.26 | 0.29 | 0.32 | 0.35 | 0.38 | 0.41 | 0.44 | 0.47 | 0.50 | 0.53 | 0.56 | 0.59 | 0.62 | 0.64 | 0.67 | 0.70 | 0.73 |
| 10.25 | 0.13 | 0.17 | 0.20 | 0.24 | 0.27 | 0.30 | 0.33 | 0.37 | 0.40 | 0.43 | 0.46 | 0.49 | 0.52 | 0.55 | 0.59 | 0.62 | 0.65 | 0.68 | 0.71 | 0.74 | 0.77 |
| 10.50 | 0.14 | 0.18 | 0.21 | 0.25 | 0.28 | 0.32 | 0.35 | 0.38 | 0.42 | 0.45 | 0.48 | 0.52 | 0.55 | 0.58 | 0.61 | 0.65 | 0.68 | 0.71 | 0.74 | 0.77 | 0.80 |
| 10.75 | 0.15 | 0.19 | 0.22 | 0.26 | 0.30 | 0.33 | 0.37 | 0.40 | 0.44 | 0.47 | 0.51 | 0.54 | 0.57 | 0.61 | 0.64 | 0.68 | 0.71 | 0.74 | 0.77 | 0.81 | 0.84 |
| 11.00 | 0.16 | 0.20 | 0.23 | 0.27 | 0.31 | 0.35 | 0.38 | 0.42 | 0.46 | 0.49 | 0.53 | 0.57 | 0.60 | 0.64 | 0.67 | 0.71 | 0.74 | 0.78 | 0.81 | 0.84 | 0.88 |
| 11.25 | 0.16 | 0.20 | 0.24 | 0.28 | 0.32 | 0.36 | 0.40 | 0.44 | 0.48 | 0.52 | 0.55 | 0.59 | 0.63 | 0.66 | 0.70 | 0.74 | 0.77 | 0.81 | 0.85 | 0.88 | 0.92 |
| 11.50 | 0.17 | 0.21 | 0.25 | 0.30 | 0.34 | 0.38 | 0.42 | 0.46 | 0.50 | 0.54 | 0.58 | 0.62 | 0.66 | 0.69 | 0.73 | 0.77 | 0.81 | 0.84 | 0.88 | 0.92 | 0.96 |
| 11.75 | 0.18 | 0.22 | 0.27 | 0.31 | 0.35 | 0.39 | 0.44 | 0.48 | 0.52 | 0.56 | 0.60 | 0.64 | 0.68 | 0.72 | 0.76 | 0.80 | 0.84 | 0.88 | 0.92 | 0.96 | 1.00 |
| 12.00 | 0.19 | 0.23 | 0.28 | 0.32 | 0.37 | 0.41 | 0.45 | 0.50 | 0.54 | 0.58 | 0.63 | 0.67 | 0.71 | 0.75 | 0.79 | 0.84 | 0.88 | 0.92 | 0.96 | 1.00 | 1.04 |
| 12.25 | 0.19 | 0.24 | 0.29 | 0.34 | 0.38 | 0.43 | 0.47 | 0.52 | 0.56 | 0.61 | 0.65 | 0.70 | 0.74 | 0.78 | 0.83 | 0.87 | 0.91 | 0.95 | 1.00 | 1.04 | 1.08 |
| 12.50 | 0.20 | 0.25 | 0.30 | 0.35 | 0.40 | 0.45 | 0.49 | 0.54 | 0.59 | 0.63 | 0.68 | 0.72 | 0.77 | 0.82 | 0.86 | 0.90 | 0.95 | 0.99 | 1.04 | 1.08 | 1.12 |
| 12.75 | 0.21 | 0.26 | 0.31 | 0.36 | 0.41 | 0.46 | 0.51 | 0.56 | 0.61 | 0.66 | 0.71 | 0.75 | 0.80 | 0.85 | 0.89 | 0.94 | 0.98 | 1.03 | 1.08 | 1.12 | 1.16 |
| 13.00 | 0.22 | 0.27 | 0.32 | 0.38 | 0.43 | 0.48 | 0.53 | 0.58 | 0.63 | 0.68 | 0.73 | 0.78 | 0.83 | 0.88 | 0.93 | 0.98 | 1.02 | 1.07 | 1.12 | 1.16 | 1.21 |
| 13.25 | 0.23 | 0.28 | 0.34 | 0.39 | 0.45 | 0.50 | 0.55 | 0.61 | 0.66 | 0.71 | 0.76 | 0.81 | 0.86 | 0.91 | 0.96 | 1.01 | 1.06 | 1.11 | 1.16 | 1.21 | 1.25 |
| 13.50 | 0.24 | 0.29 | 0.35 | 0.41 | 0.46 | 0.52 | 0.57 | 0.63 | 0.68 | 0.74 | 0.79 | 0.84 | 0.89 | 0.95 | 1.00 | 1.05 | 1.10 | 1.15 | 1.20 | 1.25 | 1.30 |
| 13.75 | 0.24 | 0.30 | 0.36 | 0.42 | 0.48 | 0.54 | 0.59 | 0.65 | 0.71 | 0.76 | 0.82 | 0.87 | 0.93 | 0.98 | 1.03 | 1.09 | 1.14 | 1.19 | 1.24 | 1.29 | 1.34 |
| 14.00 | 0.25 | 0.31 | 0.38 | 0.44 | 0.50 | 0.56 | 0.62 | 0.67 | 0.73 | 0.79 | 0.85 | 0.90 | 0.96 | 1.01 | 1.07 | 1.12 | 1.18 | 1.23 | 1.29 | 1.34 | 1.39 |
| 14.25 | 0.26 | 0.33 | 0.39 | 0.45 | 0.51 | 0.58 | 0.64 | 0.70 | 0.76 | 0.82 | 0.88 | 0.93 | 0.99 | 1.05 | 1.11 | 1.16 | 1.22 | 1.27 | 1.33 | 1.38 | 1.44 |
| 14.50 | 0.27 | 0.34 | 0.40 | 0.47 | 0.53 | 0.60 | 0.66 | 0.72 | 0.78 | 0.85 | 0.91 | 0.97 | 1.03 | 1.09 | 1.14 | 1.20 | 1.26 | 1.32 | 1.37 | 1.43 | 1.49 |
| 14.75 | 0.28 | 0.35 | 0.42 | 0.48 | 0.55 | 0.62 | 0.68 | 0.75 | 0.81 | 0.87 | 0.94 | 1.00 | 1.06 | 1.12 | 1.18 | 1.24 | 1.30 | 1.36 | 1.42 | 1.48 | 1.54 |
| 15.00 | 0.29 | 0.36 | 0.43 | 0.50 | 0.57 | 0.64 | 0.70 | 0.77 | 0.84 | 0.90 | 0.97 | 1.03 | 1.10 | 1.16 | 1.22 | 1.28 | 1.34 | 1.41 | 1.47 | 1.53 | 1.59 |
| 15.25 | 0.30 | 0.37 | 0.44 | 0.52 | 0.59 | 0.66 | 0.73 | 0.80 | 0.86 | 0.93 | 1.00 | 1.07 | 1.13 | 1.20 | 1.26 | 1.32 | 1.39 | 1.45 | 1.51 | 1.57 | 1.64 |
| 15.50 | 0.31 | 0.38 | 0.46 | 0.53 | 0.61 | 0.68 | 0.75 | 0.82 | 0.89 | 0.96 | 1.03 | 1.10 | 1.17 | 1.23 | 1.30 | 1.37 | 1.43 | 1.50 | 1.56 | 1.62 | 1.69 |
| 15.75 | 0.32 | 0.40 | 0.47 | 0.55 | 0.63 | 0.70 | 0.77 | 0.85 | 0.92 | 0.99 | 1.06 | 1.13 | 1.20 | 1.27 | 1.34 | 1.41 | 1.48 | 1.54 | 1.61 | 1.67 | 1.74 |
| 16.00 | 0.33 | 0.41 | 0.49 | 0.57 | 0.65 | 0.72 | 0.80 | 0.87 | 0.95 | 1.02 | 1.10 | 1.17 | 1.24 | 1.31 | 1.38 | 1.45 | 1.52 | 1.59 | 1.66 | 1.72 | 1.79 |
| 16.25 | 0.34 | 0.42 | 0.50 | 0.58 | 0.67 | 0.74 | 0.82 | 0.90 | 0.98 | 1.05 | 1.13 | 1.20 | 1.28 | 1.35 | 1.42 | 1.50 | 1.57 | 1.64 | 1.71 | 1.78 | 1.84 |
| 16.50 | 0.35 | 0.44 | 0.52 | 0.60 | 0.69 | 0.77 | 0.85 | 0.93 | 1.01 | 1.09 | 1.16 | 1.24 | 1.32 | 1.39 | 1.47 | 1.54 | 1.61 | 1.69 | 1.76 | 1.83 | 1.90 |
| 16.75 | 0.36 | 0.45 | 0.53 | 0.62 | 0.71 | 0.79 | 0.87 | 0.96 | 1.04 | 1.12 | 1.20 | 1.28 | 1.35 | 1.43 | 1.51 | 1.58 | 1.66 | 1.73 | 1.81 | 1.88 | 1.95 |
| 17.00 | 0.37 | 0.46 | 0.55 | 0.64 | 0.73 | 0.81 | 0.90 | 0.98 | 1.07 | 1.15 | 1.23 | 1.31 | 1.39 | 1.47 | 1.55 | 1.63 | 1.71 | 1.78 | 1.86 | 1.93 | 2.01 |
| 17.25 | 0.38 | 0.47 | 0.57 | 0.66 | 0.75 | 0.84 | 0.92 | 1.01 | 1.10 | 1.18 | 1.27 | 1.35 | 1.43 | 1.51 | 1.60 | 1.68 | 1.76 | 1.83 | 1.91 | 1.99 | 2.06 |
| 17.50 | 0.39 | 0.49 | 0.58 | 0.68 | 0.77 | 0.86 | 0.95 | 1.04 | 1.13 | 1.22 | 1.30 | 1.39 | 1.47 | 1.56 | 1.64 | 1.72 | 1.80 | 1.88 | 1.96 | 2.04 | 2.12 |
| 17.75 | 0.40 | 0.50 | 0.60 | 0.70 | 0.79 | 0.88 | 0.98 | 1.07 | 1.16 | 1.25 | 1.34 | 1.43 | 1.51 | 1.60 | 1.69 | 1.77 | 1.85 | 1.94 | 2.02 | 2.10 | 2.18 |
| 18.00 | 0.42 | 0.52 | 0.62 | 0.72 | 0.81 | 0.91 | 1.00 | 1.10 | 1.19 | 1.28 | 1.38 | 1.47 | 1.55 | 1.64 | 1.73 | 1.82 | 1.90 | 1.99 | 2.07 | 2.15 | 2.24 |
| 18.25 | 0.43 | 0.53 | 0.63 | 0.73 | 0.83 | 0.93 | 1.03 | 1.13 | 1.22 | 1.32 | 1.41 | 1.50 | 1.60 | 1.69 | 1.78 | 1.87 | 1.95 | 2.04 | 2.13 | 2.21 | 2.29 |

*Continued*

**Table 1** *Continued*

| Nominal front surface power | Centre thickness of lens (mm) | | | | | | | | | | | | | | | | | | | | |
|---|---|---|---|---|---|---|---|---|---|---|---|---|---|---|---|---|---|---|---|---|---|
| | 2.0 | 2.5 | 3.0 | 3.5 | 4.0 | 4.5 | 5.0 | 5.5 | 6.0 | 6.5 | 7.0 | 7.5 | 8.0 | 8.5 | 9.0 | 9.5 | 10.0 | 10.5 | 11.0 | 11.5 | 12.0 |
| 18.50 | 0.44 | 0.55 | 0.65 | 0.75 | 0.86 | 0.96 | 1.06 | 1.16 | 1.26 | 1.35 | 1.45 | 1.54 | 1.64 | 1.73 | 1.82 | 1.91 | 2.00 | 2.09 | 2.18 | 2.27 | 2.35 |
| 18.75 | 0.45 | 0.56 | 0.67 | 0.77 | 0.88 | 0.98 | 1.09 | 1.19 | 1.29 | 1.39 | 1.49 | 1.58 | 1.68 | 1.78 | 1.87 | 1.96 | 2.06 | 2.15 | 2.24 | 2.33 | 2.41 |
| 19.00 | 0.46 | 0.57 | 0.69 | 0.79 | 0.90 | 1.01 | 1.12 | 1.22 | 1.32 | 1.43 | 1.53 | 1.63 | 1.72 | 1.82 | 1.92 | 2.01 | 2.11 | 2.20 | 2.29 | 2.38 | 2.47 |
| 19.25 | 0.47 | 0.59 | 0.70 | 0.82 | 0.93 | 1.04 | 1.14 | 1.25 | 1.36 | 1.46 | 1.56 | 1.67 | 1.77 | 1.87 | 1.97 | 2.06 | 2.16 | 2.26 | 2.35 | 2.44 | 2.54 |
| 19.50 | 0.49 | 0.60 | 0.72 | 0.84 | 0.95 | 1.06 | 1.17 | 1.28 | 1.39 | 1.50 | 1.60 | 1.71 | 1.81 | 1.91 | 2.01 | 2.11 | 2.21 | 2.31 | 2.41 | 2.50 | 2.60 |
| 19.75 | 0.50 | 0.62 | 0.74 | 0.86 | 0.97 | 1.09 | 1.20 | 1.31 | 1.43 | 1.54 | 1.64 | 1.75 | 1.86 | 1.96 | 2.06 | 2.17 | 2.27 | 2.37 | 2.47 | 2.56 | 2.66 |
| 20.00 | 0.51 | 0.64 | 0.76 | 0.88 | 1.00 | 1.12 | 1.23 | 1.35 | 1.46 | 1.57 | 1.68 | 1.79 | 1.90 | 2.01 | 2.11 | 2.22 | 2.32 | 2.42 | 2.52 | 2.62 | 2.72 |
| 20.25 | 0.52 | 0.65 | 0.78 | 0.90 | 1.02 | 1.14 | 1.26 | 1.38 | 1.50 | 1.61 | 1.72 | 1.84 | 1.95 | 2.06 | 2.16 | 2.27 | 2.38 | 2.48 | 2.58 | 2.69 | 2.79 |
| 20.50 | 0.54 | 0.67 | 0.80 | 0.92 | 1.05 | 1.17 | 1.29 | 1.41 | 1.53 | 1.65 | 1.77 | 1.88 | 1.99 | 2.10 | 2.22 | 2.32 | 2.43 | 2.54 | 2.64 | 2.75 | 2.85 |
| 20.75 | 0.55 | 0.68 | 0.81 | 0.94 | 1.07 | 1.20 | 1.32 | 1.45 | 1.57 | 1.69 | 1.81 | 1.92 | 2.04 | 2.15 | 2.27 | 2.38 | 2.49 | 2.60 | 2.70 | 2.81 | 2.92 |
| 21.00 | 0.56 | 0.70 | 0.83 | 0.97 | 1.10 | 1.23 | 1.35 | 1.48 | 1.60 | 1.73 | 1.85 | 1.97 | 2.09 | 2.20 | 2.32 | 2.43 | 2.54 | 2.66 | 2.77 | 2.87 | 2.98 |
| 21.25 | 0.58 | 0.72 | 0.85 | 0.99 | 1.12 | 1.26 | 1.39 | 1.51 | 1.64 | 1.77 | 1.89 | 2.01 | 2.13 | 2.25 | 2.37 | 2.49 | 2.60 | 2.72 | 2.83 | 2.94 | 3.05 |
| 21.50 | 0.59 | 0.73 | 0.87 | 1.01 | 1.15 | 1.28 | 1.42 | 1.55 | 1.68 | 1.81 | 1.93 | 2.06 | 2.18 | 2.30 | 2.42 | 2.54 | 2.66 | 2.78 | 2.89 | 3.00 | 3.11 |
| 21.75 | 0.60 | 0.75 | 0.89 | 1.04 | 1.18 | 1.31 | 1.45 | 1.58 | 1.72 | 1.85 | 1.98 | 2.10 | 2.23 | 2.35 | 2.48 | 2.60 | 2.72 | 2.84 | 2.95 | 3.07 | 3.18 |
| 22.00 | 0.62 | 0.77 | 0.91 | 1.06 | 1.20 | 1.34 | 1.48 | 1.62 | 1.75 | 1.89 | 2.02 | 2.15 | 2.28 | 2.41 | 2.53 | 2.65 | 2.78 | 2.90 | 3.02 | 3.13 | 3.25 |
| 22.25 | 0.63 | 0.78 | 0.93 | 1.08 | 1.23 | 1.37 | 1.51 | 1.65 | 1.79 | 1.93 | 2.06 | 2.20 | 2.33 | 2.46 | 2.59 | 2.71 | 2.84 | 2.96 | 3.08 | 3.20 | 3.32 |
| 22.50 | 0.65 | 0.80 | 0.95 | 1.11 | 1.26 | 1.40 | 1.55 | 1.69 | 1.83 | 1.97 | 2.11 | 2.24 | 2.38 | 2.51 | 2.64 | 2.77 | 2.90 | 3.02 | 3.15 | 3.27 | 3.39 |
| 22.75 | 0.66 | 0.82 | 0.98 | 1.13 | 1.28 | 1.43 | 1.58 | 1.73 | 1.87 | 2.01 | 2.15 | 2.29 | 2.43 | 2.56 | 2.70 | 2.83 | 2.96 | 3.08 | 3.21 | 3.34 | 3.46 |
| 23.00 | 0.67 | 0.84 | 1.00 | 1.15 | 1.31 | 1.46 | 1.61 | 1.76 | 1.91 | 2.06 | 2.20 | 2.34 | 2.48 | 2.62 | 2.75 | 2.89 | 3.02 | 3.15 | 3.28 | 3.40 | 3.53 |
| 23.25 | 0.69 | 0.85 | 1.02 | 1.18 | 1.34 | 1.49 | 1.65 | 1.80 | 1.95 | 2.10 | 2.24 | 2.39 | 2.53 | 2.67 | 2.81 | 2.94 | 3.08 | 3.21 | 3.34 | 3.47 | 3.60 |
| 23.50 | 0.70 | 0.87 | 1.04 | 1.20 | 1.37 | 1.53 | 1.68 | 1.84 | 1.99 | 2.14 | 2.29 | 2.44 | 2.58 | 2.72 | 2.87 | 3.00 | 3.14 | 3.28 | 3.41 | 3.54 | 3.67 |
| 23.75 | 0.72 | 0.89 | 1.06 | 1.23 | 1.39 | 1.56 | 1.72 | 1.88 | 2.03 | 2.19 | 2.34 | 2.49 | 2.63 | 2.78 | 2.92 | 3.06 | 3.20 | 3.34 | 3.48 | 3.61 | 3.74 |
| 24.00 | 0.73 | 0.91 | 1.08 | 1.25 | 1.42 | 1.59 | 1.75 | 1.91 | 2.07 | 2.23 | 2.38 | 2.54 | 2.69 | 2.83 | 2.98 | 3.13 | 3.27 | 3.41 | 3.55 | 3.68 | 3.82 |
| 24.25 | 0.75 | 0.93 | 1.11 | 1.28 | 1.45 | 1.62 | 1.79 | 1.95 | 2.11 | 2.27 | 2.43 | 2.59 | 2.74 | 2.89 | 3.04 | 3.19 | 3.33 | 3.47 | 3.61 | 3.75 | 3.89 |
| 24.50 | 0.76 | 0.95 | 1.13 | 1.31 | 1.48 | 1.65 | 1.82 | 1.99 | 2.16 | 2.32 | 2.48 | 2.64 | 2.79 | 2.95 | 3.10 | 3.25 | 3.40 | 3.54 | 3.68 | 3.82 | 3.96 |
| 24.75 | 0.78 | 0.97 | 1.15 | 1.33 | 1.51 | 1.69 | 1.86 | 2.03 | 2.20 | 2.36 | 2.53 | 2.69 | 2.85 | 3.00 | 3.16 | 3.31 | 3.46 | 3.61 | 3.75 | 3.90 | 4.04 |
| 25.00 | 0.79 | 0.99 | 1.17 | 1.36 | 1.54 | 1.72 | 1.90 | 2.07 | 2.24 | 2.41 | 2.58 | 2.74 | 2.90 | 3.06 | 3.22 | 3.37 | 3.53 | 3.68 | 3.82 | 3.97 | 4.11 |

**Table 2** Front surface vertex power allowances ($n = 1.498$)

| Nominal front surface power | Centre thickness of lens (mm) | | | | | | | | | | | | | | | | | | | | |
|---|---|---|---|---|---|---|---|---|---|---|---|---|---|---|---|---|---|---|---|---|---|
| | 2.0 | 2.5 | 3.0 | 3.5 | 4.0 | 4.5 | 5.0 | 5.5 | 6.0 | 6.5 | 7.0 | 7.5 | 8.0 | 8.5 | 9.0 | 9.5 | 10.0 | 10.5 | 11.0 | 11.5 | 12.0 |
| 2.50 | 0.01 | 0.01 | 0.01 | 0.01 | 0.02 | 0.02 | 0.02 | 0.02 | 0.02 | 0.03 | 0.03 | 0.03 | 0.03 | 0.03 | 0.04 | 0.04 | 0.04 | 0.04 | 0.05 | 0.05 | 0.05 |
| 2.75 | 0.01 | 0.01 | 0.02 | 0.02 | 0.02 | 0.02 | 0.03 | 0.03 | 0.03 | 0.03 | 0.03 | 0.04 | 0.04 | 0.04 | 0.04 | 0.05 | 0.05 | 0.05 | 0.05 | 0.06 | 0.06 |
| 3.00 | 0.01 | 0.01 | 0.02 | 0.02 | 0.02 | 0.03 | 0.03 | 0.03 | 0.04 | 0.04 | 0.04 | 0.04 | 0.05 | 0.05 | 0.05 | 0.06 | 0.06 | 0.06 | 0.06 | 0.07 | 0.07 |
| 3.25 | 0.01 | 0.02 | 0.02 | 0.02 | 0.03 | 0.03 | 0.03 | 0.04 | 0.04 | 0.05 | 0.05 | 0.05 | 0.06 | 0.06 | 0.06 | 0.07 | 0.07 | 0.07 | 0.08 | 0.08 | 0.08 |
| 3.50 | 0.02 | 0.02 | 0.02 | 0.03 | 0.03 | 0.04 | 0.04 | 0.04 | 0.05 | 0.05 | 0.06 | 0.06 | 0.06 | 0.07 | 0.07 | 0.08 | 0.08 | 0.08 | 0.09 | 0.09 | 0.10 |
| 3.75 | 0.02 | 0.02 | 0.03 | 0.03 | 0.04 | 0.04 | 0.05 | 0.05 | 0.06 | 0.06 | 0.06 | 0.07 | 0.07 | 0.08 | 0.08 | 0.09 | 0.09 | 0.10 | 0.10 | 0.10 | 0.11 |
| 4.00 | 0.02 | 0.03 | 0.03 | 0.04 | 0.04 | 0.05 | 0.05 | 0.06 | 0.06 | 0.07 | 0.07 | 0.08 | 0.08 | 0.09 | 0.09 | 0.10 | 0.10 | 0.11 | 0.11 | 0.12 | 0.12 |
| 4.25 | 0.02 | 0.03 | 0.04 | 0.04 | 0.05 | 0.05 | 0.06 | 0.07 | 0.07 | 0.08 | 0.08 | 0.09 | 0.09 | 0.10 | 0.11 | 0.11 | 0.12 | 0.12 | 0.13 | 0.13 | 0.14 |
| 4.50 | 0.03 | 0.03 | 0.04 | 0.05 | 0.05 | 0.06 | 0.07 | 0.07 | 0.08 | 0.09 | 0.09 | 0.10 | 0.11 | 0.11 | 0.12 | 0.12 | 0.13 | 0.14 | 0.14 | 0.15 | 0.16 |
| 4.75 | 0.03 | 0.04 | 0.04 | 0.05 | 0.06 | 0.07 | 0.07 | 0.08 | 0.09 | 0.10 | 0.10 | 0.11 | 0.12 | 0.12 | 0.13 | 0.14 | 0.15 | 0.15 | 0.16 | 0.17 | 0.17 |
| 5.00 | 0.03 | 0.04 | 0.05 | 0.06 | 0.07 | 0.07 | 0.08 | 0.09 | 0.10 | 0.10 | 0.11 | 0.12 | 0.13 | 0.14 | 0.15 | 0.15 | 0.16 | 0.17 | 0.18 | 0.18 | 0.19 |
| 5.25 | 0.04 | 0.04 | 0.05 | 0.06 | 0.07 | 0.08 | 0.09 | 0.10 | 0.11 | 0.11 | 0.13 | 0.13 | 0.14 | 0.15 | 0.16 | 0.17 | 0.18 | 0.19 | 0.19 | 0.20 | 0.21 |
| 5.50 | 0.04 | 0.05 | 0.06 | 0.07 | 0.08 | 0.09 | 0.10 | 0.11 | 0.12 | 0.13 | 0.14 | 0.15 | 0.16 | 0.17 | 0.18 | 0.19 | 0.19 | 0.20 | 0.21 | 0.22 | 0.23 |
| 5.75 | 0.04 | 0.05 | 0.06 | 0.07 | 0.09 | 0.10 | 0.11 | 0.12 | 0.13 | 0.14 | 0.15 | 0.16 | 0.17 | 0.18 | 0.19 | 0.20 | 0.21 | 0.22 | 0.23 | 0.24 | 0.25 |
| 6.00 | 0.05 | 0.06 | 0.07 | 0.08 | 0.09 | 0.11 | 0.12 | 0.13 | 0.14 | 0.15 | 0.16 | 0.17 | 0.19 | 0.20 | 0.21 | 0.22 | 0.23 | 0.24 | 0.25 | 0.26 | 0.28 |
| 6.25 | 0.05 | 0.06 | 0.08 | 0.09 | 0.10 | 0.12 | 0.13 | 0.14 | 0.15 | 0.16 | 0.18 | 0.19 | 0.20 | 0.21 | 0.23 | 0.24 | 0.25 | 0.26 | 0.27 | 0.29 | 0.30 |
| 6.50 | 0.06 | 0.07 | 0.08 | 0.10 | 0.11 | 0.12 | 0.14 | 0.15 | 0.16 | 0.18 | 0.19 | 0.20 | 0.22 | 0.23 | 0.24 | 0.26 | 0.27 | 0.28 | 0.30 | 0.31 | 0.32 |
| 6.75 | 0.06 | 0.08 | 0.09 | 0.10 | 0.12 | 0.13 | 0.15 | 0.16 | 0.18 | 0.19 | 0.21 | 0.22 | 0.23 | 0.25 | 0.26 | 0.28 | 0.29 | 0.30 | 0.32 | 0.33 | 0.35 |
| 7.00 | 0.06 | 0.08 | 0.10 | 0.11 | 0.13 | 0.14 | 0.16 | 0.18 | 0.19 | 0.21 | 0.22 | 0.24 | 0.25 | 0.27 | 0.28 | 0.30 | 0.31 | 0.33 | 0.34 | 0.36 | 0.37 |
| 7.25 | 0.07 | 0.09 | 0.10 | 0.12 | 0.14 | 0.15 | 0.17 | 0.19 | 0.20 | 0.22 | 0.24 | 0.25 | 0.27 | 0.29 | 0.30 | 0.32 | 0.33 | 0.35 | 0.37 | 0.38 | 0.40 |
| 7.50 | 0.07 | 0.09 | 0.11 | 0.13 | 0.15 | 0.17 | 0.18 | 0.20 | 0.22 | 0.24 | 0.25 | 0.27 | 0.29 | 0.31 | 0.32 | 0.34 | 0.36 | 0.37 | 0.39 | 0.41 | 0.42 |
| 7.75 | 0.08 | 0.10 | 0.12 | 0.14 | 0.16 | 0.18 | 0.20 | 0.21 | 0.23 | 0.25 | 0.27 | 0.29 | 0.31 | 0.33 | 0.34 | 0.36 | 0.38 | 0.40 | 0.42 | 0.44 | 0.45 |
| 8.00 | 0.08 | 0.11 | 0.13 | 0.15 | 0.17 | 0.19 | 0.21 | 0.23 | 0.25 | 0.27 | 0.29 | 0.31 | 0.33 | 0.35 | 0.37 | 0.39 | 0.41 | 0.42 | 0.44 | 0.46 | 0.48 |
| 8.25 | 0.09 | 0.11 | 0.13 | 0.16 | 0.18 | 0.20 | 0.22 | 0.24 | 0.26 | 0.29 | 0.31 | 0.33 | 0.35 | 0.37 | 0.39 | 0.41 | 0.43 | 0.45 | 0.47 | 0.49 | 0.51 |
| 8.50 | 0.10 | 0.12 | 0.14 | 0.17 | 0.19 | 0.21 | 0.23 | 0.26 | 0.28 | 0.30 | 0.32 | 0.35 | 0.37 | 0.39 | 0.41 | 0.43 | 0.46 | 0.48 | 0.50 | 0.52 | 0.54 |
| 8.75 | 0.10 | 0.13 | 0.15 | 0.18 | 0.20 | 0.22 | 0.25 | 0.27 | 0.30 | 0.32 | 0.34 | 0.37 | 0.39 | 0.41 | 0.44 | 0.46 | 0.48 | 0.51 | 0.53 | 0.55 | 0.57 |

*Continued*

**Table 2** Continued

| Nominal front surface power | Centre thickness of lens (mm) | | | | | | | | | | | | | | | | | | | | |
|---|---|---|---|---|---|---|---|---|---|---|---|---|---|---|---|---|---|---|---|---|---|
| | 2.0 | 2.5 | 3.0 | 3.5 | 4.0 | 4.5 | 5.0 | 5.5 | 6.0 | 6.5 | 7.0 | 7.5 | 8.0 | 8.5 | 9.0 | 9.5 | 10.0 | 10.5 | 11.0 | 11.5 | 12.0 |
| 9.00 | 0.11 | 0.13 | 0.16 | 0.19 | 0.21 | 0.24 | 0.26 | 0.29 | 0.31 | 0.34 | 0.36 | 0.39 | 0.41 | 0.44 | 0.46 | 0.49 | 0.51 | 0.53 | 0.56 | 0.58 | 0.61 |
| 9.25 | 0.11 | 0.14 | 0.17 | 0.20 | 0.22 | 0.25 | 0.28 | 0.30 | 0.33 | 0.36 | 0.38 | 0.41 | 0.44 | 0.46 | 0.49 | 0.51 | 0.54 | 0.56 | 0.59 | 0.61 | 0.64 |
| 9.50 | 0.12 | 0.15 | 0.18 | 0.21 | 0.23 | 0.26 | 0.29 | 0.32 | 0.35 | 0.38 | 0.40 | 0.43 | 0.46 | 0.49 | 0.51 | 0.54 | 0.57 | 0.59 | 0.62 | 0.65 | 0.67 |
| 9.75 | 0.13 | 0.16 | 0.19 | 0.22 | 0.25 | 0.28 | 0.31 | 0.34 | 0.37 | 0.40 | 0.42 | 0.45 | 0.48 | 0.51 | 0.54 | 0.57 | 0.60 | 0.62 | 0.65 | 0.68 | 0.71 |
| 10.00 | 0.13 | 0.16 | 0.20 | 0.23 | 0.26 | 0.29 | 0.32 | 0.35 | 0.38 | 0.42 | 0.45 | 0.48 | 0.51 | 0.54 | 0.57 | 0.60 | 0.63 | 0.65 | 0.68 | 0.71 | 0.74 |
| 10.25 | 0.14 | 0.17 | 0.21 | 0.24 | 0.27 | 0.31 | 0.34 | 0.37 | 0.40 | 0.44 | 0.47 | 0.50 | 0.53 | 0.56 | 0.59 | 0.63 | 0.66 | 0.69 | 0.72 | 0.75 | 0.78 |
| 10.50 | 0.15 | 0.18 | 0.22 | 0.25 | 0.29 | 0.32 | 0.36 | 0.39 | 0.42 | 0.46 | 0.49 | 0.52 | 0.56 | 0.59 | 0.62 | 0.66 | 0.69 | 0.72 | 0.75 | 0.78 | 0.81 |
| 10.75 | 0.15 | 0.19 | 0.23 | 0.26 | 0.30 | 0.34 | 0.37 | 0.41 | 0.44 | 0.48 | 0.51 | 0.55 | 0.58 | 0.62 | 0.65 | 0.69 | 0.72 | 0.75 | 0.79 | 0.82 | 0.85 |
| 11.00 | 0.16 | 0.20 | 0.24 | 0.28 | 0.31 | 0.35 | 0.39 | 0.43 | 0.46 | 0.50 | 0.54 | 0.57 | 0.61 | 0.65 | 0.68 | 0.72 | 0.75 | 0.79 | 0.82 | 0.86 | 0.89 |
| 11.25 | 0.17 | 0.21 | 0.25 | 0.29 | 0.33 | 0.37 | 0.41 | 0.45 | 0.48 | 0.52 | 0.56 | 0.60 | 0.64 | 0.67 | 0.71 | 0.75 | 0.79 | 0.82 | 0.86 | 0.89 | 0.93 |
| 11.50 | 0.17 | 0.22 | 0.26 | 0.30 | 0.34 | 0.38 | 0.42 | 0.47 | 0.51 | 0.55 | 0.59 | 0.63 | 0.67 | 0.70 | 0.74 | 0.78 | 0.82 | 0.86 | 0.90 | 0.93 | 0.97 |
| 11.75 | 0.18 | 0.23 | 0.27 | 0.31 | 0.36 | 0.40 | 0.44 | 0.49 | 0.53 | 0.57 | 0.61 | 0.65 | 0.69 | 0.73 | 0.77 | 0.81 | 0.85 | 0.89 | 0.93 | 0.97 | 1.01 |
| 12.00 | 0.19 | 0.24 | 0.28 | 0.33 | 0.37 | 0.42 | 0.46 | 0.51 | 0.55 | 0.59 | 0.64 | 0.68 | 0.72 | 0.76 | 0.81 | 0.85 | 0.89 | 0.93 | 0.97 | 1.01 | 1.05 |
| 12.25 | 0.20 | 0.25 | 0.29 | 0.34 | 0.39 | 0.43 | 0.48 | 0.53 | 0.57 | 0.62 | 0.66 | 0.71 | 0.75 | 0.80 | 0.84 | 0.88 | 0.93 | 0.97 | 1.01 | 1.05 | 1.09 |
| 12.50 | 0.21 | 0.26 | 0.31 | 0.35 | 0.40 | 0.45 | 0.50 | 0.55 | 0.60 | 0.64 | 0.69 | 0.74 | 0.78 | 0.83 | 0.87 | 0.92 | 0.96 | 1.01 | 1.05 | 1.09 | 1.14 |
| 12.75 | 0.21 | 0.27 | 0.32 | 0.37 | 0.42 | 0.47 | 0.52 | 0.57 | 0.62 | 0.67 | 0.72 | 0.76 | 0.81 | 0.86 | 0.91 | 0.95 | 1.00 | 1.05 | 1.09 | 1.14 | 1.18 |
| 13.00 | 0.22 | 0.28 | 0.33 | 0.38 | 0.44 | 0.49 | 0.54 | 0.59 | 0.64 | 0.69 | 0.74 | 0.79 | 0.84 | 0.89 | 0.94 | 0.99 | 1.04 | 1.09 | 1.13 | 1.18 | 1.23 |
| 13.25 | 0.23 | 0.29 | 0.34 | 0.40 | 0.45 | 0.51 | 0.56 | 0.61 | 0.67 | 0.72 | 0.77 | 0.82 | 0.88 | 0.93 | 0.98 | 1.03 | 1.08 | 1.13 | 1.17 | 1.22 | 1.27 |
| 13.50 | 0.24 | 0.30 | 0.36 | 0.41 | 0.47 | 0.53 | 0.58 | 0.64 | 0.69 | 0.75 | 0.80 | 0.85 | 0.91 | 0.96 | 1.01 | 1.06 | 1.12 | 1.17 | 1.22 | 1.27 | 1.32 |
| 13.75 | 0.25 | 0.31 | 0.37 | 0.43 | 0.49 | 0.55 | 0.60 | 0.66 | 0.72 | 0.77 | 0.83 | 0.89 | 0.94 | 0.99 | 1.05 | 1.10 | 1.16 | 1.21 | 1.26 | 1.31 | 1.36 |
| 14.00 | 0.26 | 0.32 | 0.38 | 0.44 | 0.50 | 0.56 | 0.62 | 0.68 | 0.74 | 0.80 | 0.86 | 0.92 | 0.97 | 1.03 | 1.09 | 1.14 | 1.20 | 1.25 | 1.30 | 1.36 | 1.41 |
| 14.25 | 0.27 | 0.33 | 0.40 | 0.46 | 0.52 | 0.58 | 0.65 | 0.71 | 0.77 | 0.83 | 0.89 | 0.95 | 1.01 | 1.07 | 1.12 | 1.18 | 1.24 | 1.29 | 1.35 | 1.40 | 1.46 |
| 14.50 | 0.28 | 0.34 | 0.41 | 0.47 | 0.54 | 0.61 | 0.67 | 0.73 | 0.80 | 0.86 | 0.92 | 0.98 | 1.04 | 1.10 | 1.16 | 1.22 | 1.28 | 1.34 | 1.39 | 1.45 | 1.51 |
| 14.75 | 0.28 | 0.35 | 0.42 | 0.49 | 0.56 | 0.63 | 0.69 | 0.76 | 0.82 | 0.89 | 0.95 | 1.01 | 1.08 | 1.14 | 1.20 | 1.26 | 1.32 | 1.38 | 1.44 | 1.50 | 1.56 |
| 15.00 | 0.29 | 0.37 | 0.44 | 0.51 | 0.58 | 0.65 | 0.71 | 0.78 | 0.85 | 0.92 | 0.98 | 1.05 | 1.11 | 1.18 | 1.24 | 1.30 | 1.36 | 1.43 | 1.49 | 1.55 | 1.61 |
| 15.25 | 0.30 | 0.38 | 0.45 | 0.52 | 0.60 | 0.67 | 0.74 | 0.81 | 0.88 | 0.95 | 1.01 | 1.08 | 1.15 | 1.21 | 1.28 | 1.34 | 1.41 | 1.47 | 1.54 | 1.60 | 1.66 |
| 15.50 | 0.31 | 0.39 | 0.47 | 0.54 | 0.62 | 0.69 | 0.76 | 0.83 | 0.91 | 0.98 | 1.05 | 1.12 | 1.18 | 1.25 | 1.32 | 1.39 | 1.45 | 1.52 | 1.58 | 1.65 | 1.71 |
| 15.75 | 0.32 | 0.40 | 0.48 | 0.56 | 0.64 | 0.71 | 0.79 | 0.86 | 0.93 | 1.01 | 1.08 | 1.15 | 1.22 | 1.29 | 1.36 | 1.43 | 1.50 | 1.57 | 1.63 | 1.70 | 1.76 |
| 16.00 | 0.33 | 0.42 | 0.50 | 0.58 | 0.66 | 0.73 | 0.81 | 0.89 | 0.96 | 1.04 | 1.11 | 1.19 | 1.26 | 1.33 | 1.40 | 1.47 | 1.54 | 1.61 | 1.68 | 1.75 | 1.82 |

| | | | | | | | | | | | | | | | | | | | | | |
|---|---|---|---|---|---|---|---|---|---|---|---|---|---|---|---|---|---|---|---|---|---|
| 16.25 | 0.34 | 0.43 | 0.51 | 0.59 | 0.68 | 0.76 | 0.84 | 0.91 | 0.99 | 1.07 | 1.15 | 1.22 | 1.30 | 1.37 | 1.44 | 1.52 | 1.59 | 1.66 | 1.73 | 1.80 | 1.87 |
| 16.50 | 0.36 | 0.44 | 0.53 | 0.61 | 0.70 | 0.78 | 0.86 | 0.94 | 1.02 | 1.10 | 1.18 | 1.26 | 1.34 | 1.41 | 1.49 | 1.56 | 1.64 | 1.71 | 1.78 | 1.85 | 1.93 |
| 16.75 | 0.37 | 0.46 | 0.54 | 0.63 | 0.72 | 0.80 | 0.89 | 0.97 | 1.05 | 1.13 | 1.22 | 1.30 | 1.37 | 1.45 | 1.53 | 1.61 | 1.68 | 1.76 | 1.83 | 1.91 | 1.98 |
| 17.00 | 0.38 | 0.47 | 0.56 | 0.65 | 0.74 | 0.83 | 0.91 | 1.00 | 1.08 | 1.17 | 1.25 | 1.33 | 1.41 | 1.50 | 1.57 | 1.65 | 1.73 | 1.81 | 1.89 | 1.96 | 2.04 |
| 17.25 | 0.39 | 0.48 | 0.58 | 0.67 | 0.76 | 0.85 | 0.94 | 1.03 | 1.11 | 1.20 | 1.29 | 1.37 | 1.45 | 1.54 | 1.62 | 1.70 | 1.78 | 1.86 | 1.94 | 2.02 | 2.09 |
| 17.50 | 0.40 | 0.50 | 0.59 | 0.69 | 0.78 | 0.87 | 0.97 | 1.06 | 1.15 | 1.23 | 1.32 | 1.41 | 1.50 | 1.58 | 1.66 | 1.75 | 1.83 | 1.91 | 1.99 | 2.07 | 2.15 |
| 17.75 | 0.41 | 0.51 | 0.61 | 0.71 | 0.80 | 0.90 | 0.99 | 1.09 | 1.18 | 1.27 | 1.36 | 1.45 | 1.54 | 1.62 | 1.71 | 1.80 | 1.88 | 1.96 | 2.05 | 2.13 | 2.21 |
| 18.00 | 0.42 | 0.52 | 0.63 | 0.73 | 0.83 | 0.92 | 1.02 | 1.12 | 1.21 | 1.30 | 1.40 | 1.49 | 1.58 | 1.67 | 1.76 | 1.84 | 1.93 | 2.02 | 2.10 | 2.18 | 2.27 |
| 18.25 | 0.43 | 0.54 | 0.64 | 0.75 | 0.85 | 0.95 | 1.05 | 1.15 | 1.24 | 1.34 | 1.43 | 1.53 | 1.62 | 1.71 | 1.80 | 1.89 | 1.98 | 2.07 | 2.16 | 2.24 | 2.33 |
| 18.50 | 0.45 | 0.55 | 0.66 | 0.77 | 0.87 | 0.97 | 1.08 | 1.18 | 1.28 | 1.37 | 1.47 | 1.57 | 1.66 | 1.76 | 1.85 | 1.94 | 2.03 | 2.12 | 2.21 | 2.30 | 2.39 |
| 18.75 | 0.46 | 0.57 | 0.68 | 0.79 | 0.89 | 1.00 | 1.10 | 1.21 | 1.31 | 1.41 | 1.51 | 1.61 | 1.71 | 1.80 | 1.90 | 1.99 | 2.09 | 2.18 | 2.27 | 2.36 | 2.45 |
| 19.00 | 0.47 | 0.58 | 0.70 | 0.81 | 0.92 | 1.03 | 1.13 | 1.24 | 1.34 | 1.45 | 1.55 | 1.65 | 1.75 | 1.85 | 1.95 | 2.04 | 2.14 | 2.23 | 2.33 | 2.42 | 2.51 |
| 19.25 | 0.48 | 0.60 | 0.71 | 0.83 | 0.94 | 1.05 | 1.16 | 1.27 | 1.38 | 1.48 | 1.59 | 1.69 | 1.79 | 1.90 | 1.99 | 2.09 | 2.19 | 2.29 | 2.38 | 2.48 | 2.57 |
| 19.50 | 0.49 | 0.61 | 0.73 | 0.85 | 0.96 | 1.08 | 1.19 | 1.30 | 1.41 | 1.52 | 1.63 | 1.73 | 1.84 | 1.94 | 2.04 | 2.15 | 2.25 | 2.34 | 2.44 | 2.54 | 2.63 |
| 19.75 | 0.51 | 0.63 | 0.75 | 0.87 | 0.99 | 1.11 | 1.22 | 1.33 | 1.45 | 1.56 | 1.67 | 1.78 | 1.88 | 1.99 | 2.09 | 2.20 | 2.30 | 2.40 | 2.50 | 2.60 | 2.70 |
| 20.00 | 0.52 | 0.65 | 0.77 | 0.89 | 1.01 | 1.13 | 1.25 | 1.37 | 1.48 | 1.60 | 1.71 | 1.82 | 1.93 | 2.04 | 2.14 | 2.25 | 2.36 | 2.46 | 2.56 | 2.66 | 2.76 |
| 20.25 | 0.53 | 0.66 | 0.79 | 0.91 | 1.04 | 1.16 | 1.28 | 1.40 | 1.52 | 1.64 | 1.75 | 1.86 | 1.98 | 2.09 | 2.20 | 2.30 | 2.41 | 2.52 | 2.62 | 2.72 | 2.83 |
| 20.50 | 0.55 | 0.68 | 0.81 | 0.94 | 1.06 | 1.19 | 1.31 | 1.43 | 1.56 | 1.67 | 1.79 | 1.91 | 2.02 | 2.14 | 2.25 | 2.36 | 2.47 | 2.57 | 2.68 | 2.79 | 2.89 |
| 20.75 | 0.56 | 0.69 | 0.83 | 0.96 | 1.09 | 1.22 | 1.34 | 1.47 | 1.59 | 1.71 | 1.83 | 1.95 | 2.07 | 2.19 | 2.30 | 2.41 | 2.52 | 2.63 | 2.74 | 2.85 | 2.96 |
| 21.00 | 0.57 | 0.71 | 0.85 | 0.98 | 1.11 | 1.25 | 1.38 | 1.50 | 1.63 | 1.75 | 1.88 | 2.00 | 2.12 | 2.24 | 2.35 | 2.47 | 2.58 | 2.69 | 2.80 | 2.91 | 3.02 |
| 21.25 | 0.59 | 0.73 | 0.87 | 1.00 | 1.14 | 1.27 | 1.41 | 1.54 | 1.67 | 1.79 | 1.92 | 2.04 | 2.17 | 2.29 | 2.41 | 2.52 | 2.64 | 2.75 | 2.87 | 2.98 | 3.09 |
| 21.50 | 0.60 | 0.74 | 0.89 | 1.03 | 1.17 | 1.30 | 1.44 | 1.57 | 1.70 | 1.83 | 1.96 | 2.09 | 2.21 | 2.34 | 2.46 | 2.58 | 2.70 | 2.81 | 2.93 | 3.05 | 3.16 |
| 21.75 | 0.61 | 0.76 | 0.91 | 1.05 | 1.19 | 1.33 | 1.47 | 1.61 | 1.74 | 1.88 | 2.01 | 2.14 | 2.26 | 2.39 | 2.51 | 2.64 | 2.76 | 2.88 | 2.99 | 3.11 | 3.23 |
| 22.00 | 0.63 | 0.78 | 0.93 | 1.08 | 1.22 | 1.36 | 1.50 | 1.64 | 1.78 | 1.92 | 2.05 | 2.18 | 2.31 | 2.44 | 2.57 | 2.69 | 2.82 | 2.94 | 3.06 | 3.18 | 3.30 |
| 22.25 | 0.64 | 0.80 | 0.95 | 1.10 | 1.25 | 1.39 | 1.54 | 1.68 | 1.82 | 1.96 | 2.09 | 2.23 | 2.36 | 2.49 | 2.62 | 2.75 | 2.88 | 3.00 | 3.12 | 3.25 | 3.36 |
| 22.50 | 0.66 | 0.81 | 0.97 | 1.12 | 1.27 | 1.42 | 1.57 | 1.72 | 1.86 | 2.00 | 2.14 | 2.28 | 2.41 | 2.55 | 2.68 | 2.81 | 2.94 | 3.06 | 3.19 | 3.31 | 3.44 |
| 22.75 | 0.67 | 0.83 | 0.99 | 1.15 | 1.30 | 1.45 | 1.61 | 1.75 | 1.90 | 2.04 | 2.19 | 2.33 | 2.46 | 2.60 | 2.73 | 2.87 | 3.00 | 3.13 | 3.26 | 3.38 | 3.51 |
| 23.00 | 0.69 | 0.85 | 1.01 | 1.17 | 1.33 | 1.49 | 1.64 | 1.79 | 1.94 | 2.09 | 2.23 | 2.37 | 2.52 | 2.65 | 2.79 | 2.93 | 3.06 | 3.19 | 3.32 | 3.45 | 3.58 |
| 23.25 | 0.70 | 0.87 | 1.03 | 1.20 | 1.36 | 1.52 | 1.67 | 1.83 | 1.98 | 2.13 | 2.28 | 2.42 | 2.57 | 2.71 | 2.85 | 2.99 | 3.12 | 3.26 | 3.39 | 3.52 | 3.65 |
| 23.50 | 0.71 | 0.89 | 1.06 | 1.22 | 1.39 | 1.55 | 1.71 | 1.87 | 2.02 | 2.17 | 2.32 | 2.47 | 2.62 | 2.76 | 2.91 | 3.05 | 3.19 | 3.32 | 3.46 | 3.59 | 3.72 |
| 23.75 | 0.73 | 0.91 | 1.08 | 1.25 | 1.42 | 1.58 | 1.74 | 1.90 | 2.06 | 2.22 | 2.37 | 2.52 | 2.67 | 2.82 | 2.96 | 3.11 | 3.25 | 3.39 | 3.53 | 3.66 | 3.80 |
| 24.00 | 0.74 | 0.92 | 1.10 | 1.27 | 1.44 | 1.61 | 1.78 | 1.94 | 2.10 | 2.26 | 2.42 | 2.57 | 2.73 | 2.88 | 3.02 | 3.17 | 3.31 | 3.46 | 3.59 | 3.73 | 3.87 |
| 24.25 | 0.76 | 0.94 | 1.12 | 1.30 | 1.47 | 1.65 | 1.82 | 1.98 | 2.15 | 2.31 | 2.47 | 2.62 | 2.78 | 2.93 | 3.08 | 3.23 | 3.38 | 3.52 | 3.66 | 3.80 | 3.94 |
| 24.50 | 0.78 | 0.96 | 1.15 | 1.33 | 1.50 | 1.68 | 1.85 | 2.02 | 2.19 | 2.35 | 2.52 | 2.68 | 2.83 | 2.99 | 3.14 | 3.29 | 3.44 | 3.59 | 3.73 | 3.88 | 4.02 |
| 24.75 | 0.79 | 0.98 | 1.17 | 1.35 | 1.53 | 1.71 | 1.89 | 2.06 | 2.23 | 2.40 | 2.56 | 2.73 | 2.89 | 3.05 | 3.20 | 3.36 | 3.51 | 3.66 | 3.81 | 3.95 | 4.09 |
| 25.00 | 0.81 | 1.00 | 1.19 | 1.38 | 1.56 | 1.75 | 1.92 | 2.10 | 2.27 | 2.45 | 2.61 | 2.78 | 2.94 | 3.10 | 3.26 | 3.42 | 3.57 | 3.73 | 3.88 | 4.02 | 4.17 |

## Back surface allowance

If it is the concave surface which is to be finished to prescription, the true front surface power $F_1$ of the semi-finished blank must be reliably known or checked with a precision spherometer. The formula for the vertex power allowance now becomes

$$\text{VPA} = \frac{tF_1^z}{1000\,n - tF_1}$$

For example, given $F_1$ = +7.86 D, $t$ = 4.0 mm and $n$ = 1.500, the allowance would be 0.17 D. This is the amount by which the nominal power of the back surface (assumed to be concave) should be *increased*, for example, from −3.00 to −3.17 D.

# Sags of lens surfaces

The derivation of the spherometer formula was given in Chapter 8.

$$s = r - \sqrt{r^2 - y^2}$$

*Tables* 3 and 4 have been calculated for refractive indices of 1.523 and 1.498 respectively. For other index materials, apply the sag formula or multiply the actual surface power $F$ by the fraction

$$(n - 1)/(n' - 1)$$

For example, a +10.00 D surface on 1.700 ($n' = 1.700$) would be reckoned as

$$10.00 \times (0.523/0.700) = +7.47 \text{ D}$$

This is the surface power which would be taken when using the table (*Table 3*).

**Table 3** Sags of lens surfaces at various diameters ($n = 1.523$)

| Surface power (D) | Lens diameter (mm) | | | | | | | | | | | | | | | |
|---|---|---|---|---|---|---|---|---|---|---|---|---|---|---|---|---|
| | 50 | 52 | 54 | 56 | 58 | 60 | 62 | 64 | 66 | 68 | 70 | 72 | 74 | 76 | 78 | 80 |
| 0.25 | 0.15 | 0.16 | 0.17 | 0.19 | 0.20 | 0.22 | 0.23 | 0.24 | 0.26 | 0.28 | 0.29 | 0.31 | 0.33 | 0.35 | 0.36 | 0.38 |
| 0.50 | 0.30 | 0.32 | 0.35 | 0.37 | 0.40 | 0.43 | 0.46 | 0.49 | 0.52 | 0.55 | 0.59 | 0.62 | 0.65 | 0.69 | 0.73 | 0.77 |
| 0.75 | 0.45 | 0.48 | 0.52 | 0.56 | 0.60 | 0.65 | 0.69 | 0.73 | 0.78 | 0.83 | 0.88 | 0.93 | 0.98 | 1.04 | 1.09 | 1.15 |
| 1.00 | 0.60 | 0.65 | 0.70 | 0.75 | 0.80 | 0.86 | 0.92 | 0.98 | 1.04 | 1.11 | 1.17 | 1.24 | 1.31 | 1.38 | 1.46 | 1.53 |
| 1.25 | 0.75 | 0.81 | 0.87 | 0.94 | 1.01 | 1.08 | 1.15 | 1.23 | 1.30 | 1.38 | 1.47 | 1.55 | 1.64 | 1.73 | 1.82 | 1.92 |
| 1.50 | 0.90 | 0.97 | 1.05 | 1.13 | 1.21 | 1.29 | 1.38 | 1.47 | 1.57 | 1.66 | 1.76 | 1.86 | 1.97 | 2.08 | 2.19 | 2.30 |
| 1.75 | 1.05 | 1.13 | 1.22 | 1.31 | 1.41 | 1.51 | 1.61 | 1.72 | 1.83 | 1.94 | 2.06 | 2.18 | 2.30 | 2.43 | 2.56 | 2.69 |
| 2.00 | 1.20 | 1.30 | 1.40 | 1.50 | 1.61 | 1.73 | 1.84 | 1.97 | 2.09 | 2.22 | 2.35 | 2.49 | 2.63 | 2.78 | 2.92 | 3.08 |
| 2.25 | 1.35 | 1.46 | 1.57 | 1.69 | 1.82 | 1.94 | 2.08 | 2.21 | 2.35 | 2.50 | 2.65 | 2.80 | 2.96 | 3.13 | 3.30 | 3.47 |
| 2.50 | 1.50 | 1.62 | 1.75 | 1.88 | 2.02 | 2.16 | 2.31 | 2.46 | 2.62 | 2.78 | 2.95 | 3.12 | 3.30 | 3.48 | 3.67 | 3.86 |
| 2.75 | 1.65 | 1.79 | 1.93 | 2.07 | 2.22 | 2.38 | 2.54 | 2.71 | 2.88 | 3.06 | 3.25 | 3.44 | 3.63 | 3.84 | 4.04 | 4.25 |
| 3.00 | 1.80 | 1.95 | 2.10 | 2.26 | 2.43 | 2.60 | 2.78 | 2.96 | 3.15 | 3.35 | 3.55 | 3.76 | 3.97 | 4.19 | 4.42 | 4.65 |
| 3.25 | 1.95 | 2.11 | 2.28 | 2.45 | 2.63 | 2.82 | 3.01 | 3.21 | 3.42 | 3.63 | 3.85 | 4.08 | 4.31 | 4.55 | 4.80 | 5.05 |
| 3.50 | 2.11 | 2.28 | 2.46 | 2.65 | 2.84 | 3.04 | 3.25 | 3.47 | 3.69 | 3.92 | 4.16 | 4.40 | 4.65 | 4.91 | 5.18 | 5.45 |
| 3.75 | 2.26 | 2.44 | 2.64 | 2.84 | 3.05 | 3.26 | 3.49 | 3.72 | 3.96 | 4.21 | 4.46 | 4.73 | 5.00 | 5.28 | 5.56 | 5.86 |
| 4.00 | 2.41 | 2.61 | 2.82 | 3.03 | 3.26 | 3.49 | 3.73 | 3.98 | 4.23 | 4.50 | 4.77 | 5.05 | 5.34 | 5.64 | 5.95 | 6.27 |
| 4.25 | 2.57 | 2.78 | 3.00 | 3.23 | 3.47 | 3.71 | 3.97 | 4.23 | 4.51 | 4.79 | 5.08 | 5.38 | 5.69 | 6.01 | 6.34 | 6.68 |
| 4.50 | 2.72 | 2.95 | 3.18 | 3.42 | 3.68 | 3.94 | 4.21 | 4.49 | 4.78 | 5.08 | 5.40 | 5.72 | 6.05 | 6.39 | 6.74 | 7.10 |
| 4.75 | 2.88 | 3.11 | 3.36 | 3.62 | 3.89 | 4.17 | 4.45 | 4.75 | 5.06 | 5.38 | 5.71 | 6.05 | 6.40 | 6.77 | 7.14 | 7.52 |
| 5.00 | 3.03 | 3.28 | 3.54 | 3.82 | 4.10 | 4.39 | 4.70 | 5.02 | 5.34 | 5.68 | 6.03 | 6.39 | 6.76 | 7.15 | 7.54 | 7.95 |
| 5.25 | 3.19 | 3.45 | 3.73 | 4.02 | 4.31 | 4.62 | 4.95 | 5.28 | 5.62 | 5.98 | 6.35 | 6.73 | 7.13 | 7.53 | 7.95 | 8.38 |
| 5.50 | 3.35 | 3.62 | 3.91 | 4.22 | 4.53 | 4.86 | 5.19 | 5.55 | 5.91 | 6.29 | 6.68 | 7.08 | 7.49 | 7.92 | 8.37 | 8.82 |
| 5.75 | 3.50 | 3.80 | 4.10 | 4.42 | 4.75 | 5.09 | 5.45 | 5.81 | 6.20 | 6.59 | 7.00 | 7.43 | 7.87 | 8.32 | 8.79 | 9.27 |
| 6.00 | 3.66 | 3.97 | 4.29 | 4.62 | 4.97 | 5.33 | 5.70 | 6.09 | 6.49 | 6.90 | 7.34 | 7.78 | 8.24 | 8.72 | 9.21 | 9.72 |
| 6.25 | 3.82 | 4.14 | 4.48 | 4.82 | 5.19 | 5.56 | 5.95 | 6.36 | 6.78 | 7.22 | 7.67 | 8.14 | 8.62 | 9.13 | 9.64 | 10.18 |
| 6.50 | 3.98 | 4.32 | 4.67 | 5.03 | 5.41 | 5.80 | 6.21 | 6.64 | 7.08 | 7.54 | 8.01 | 8.50 | 9.01 | 9.54 | 10.08 | 10.65 |
| 6.75 | 4.14 | 4.49 | 4.86 | 5.24 | 5.63 | 6.04 | 6.47 | 6.92 | 7.38 | 7.86 | 8.36 | 8.87 | 9.41 | 9.96 | 10.53 | 11.12 |
| 7.00 | 4.31 | 4.67 | 5.05 | 5.45 | 5.86 | 6.29 | 6.73 | 7.20 | 7.68 | 8.18 | 8.71 | 9.25 | 9.80 | 10.39 | 10.99 | 11.61 |
| 7.25 | 4.47 | 4.85 | 5.24 | 5.66 | 6.09 | 6.53 | 7.00 | 7.49 | 7.99 | 8.51 | 9.06 | 9.62 | 10.21 | 10.82 | 11.45 | 12.11 |

| | | | | | | | | | | | | | | | | |
|---|---|---|---|---|---|---|---|---|---|---|---|---|---|---|---|---|
| 7.50 | 4.64 | 5.03 | 5.44 | 5.87 | 6.32 | 6.78 | 7.27 | 7.78 | 8.30 | 8.85 | 9.42 | 10.01 | 10.63 | 11.26 | 11.93 | 12.61 |
| 7.75 | 4.80 | 5.21 | 5.64 | 6.08 | 6.55 | 7.03 | 7.54 | 8.07 | 8.62 | 9.19 | 9.79 | 10.40 | 11.05 | 11.72 | 12.41 | 13.13 |
| 8.00 | 4.97 | 5.39 | 5.84 | 6.30 | 6.78 | 7.29 | 7.82 | 8.37 | 8.94 | 9.54 | 10.16 | 10.80 | 11.48 | 12.18 | 12.91 | 13.67 |
| 8.25 | 5.14 | 5.58 | 6.04 | 6.52 | 7.02 | 7.55 | 8.10 | 8.67 | 9.27 | 9.89 | 10.54 | 11.21 | 11.92 | 12.65 | 13.42 | 14.21 |
| 8.50 | 5.31 | 5.76 | 6.24 | 6.74 | 7.26 | 7.81 | 8.38 | 8.98 | 9.60 | 10.25 | 10.92 | 11.63 | 12.37 | 13.14 | 13.94 | 14.78 |
| 8.75 | 5.48 | 5.95 | 6.45 | 6.96 | 7.51 | 8.07 | 8.67 | 9.29 | 9.94 | 10.61 | 11.32 | 12.06 | 12.83 | 13.63 | 14.48 | 15.36 |
| 9.00 | 5.65 | 6.14 | 6.65 | 7.19 | 7.75 | 8.34 | 8.96 | 9.60 | 10.28 | 10.98 | 11.72 | 12.49 | 13.30 | 14.15 | 15.03 | 15.96 |
| 9.25 | 5.83 | 6.33 | 6.86 | 7.42 | 8.00 | 8.62 | 9.26 | 9.93 | 10.63 | 11.36 | 12.14 | 12.94 | 13.79 | 14.67 | 15.60 | 16.58 |
| 9.50 | 6.00 | 6.53 | 7.08 | 7.65 | 8.26 | 8.89 | 9.56 | 10.26 | 10.99 | 11.75 | 12.56 | 13.40 | 14.29 | 15.22 | 16.20 | 17.23 |
| 9.75 | 6.18 | 6.72 | 7.29 | 7.89 | 8.51 | 9.17 | 9.86 | 10.59 | 11.35 | 12.15 | 12.99 | 13.87 | 14.80 | 15.78 | 16.81 | 17.90 |
| 10.00 | 6.36 | 6.92 | 7.51 | 8.13 | 8.78 | 9.46 | 10.18 | 10.93 | 11.73 | 12.56 | 13.44 | 14.36 | 15.34 | 16.37 | 17.45 | 18.61 |
| 10.25 | 6.54 | 7.12 | 7.73 | 8.37 | 9.04 | 9.75 | 10.50 | 11.28 | 12.11 | 12.98 | 13.90 | 14.87 | 15.89 | 16.97 | 18.12 | 19.35 |
| 10.50 | 6.73 | 7.32 | 7.95 | 8.62 | 9.31 | 10.05 | 10.82 | 11.64 | 12.50 | 13.41 | 14.37 | 15.39 | 16.46 | 17.61 | 18.83 | 20.13 |
| 10.75 | 6.91 | 7.53 | 8.18 | 8.87 | 9.59 | 10.35 | 11.16 | 12.01 | 12.90 | 13.85 | 14.86 | 15.93 | 17.06 | 18.27 | 19.57 | 20.96 |
| 11.00 | 7.10 | 7.74 | 8.41 | 9.12 | 9.87 | 10.66 | 11.50 | 12.38 | 13.32 | 14.31 | 15.37 | 16.49 | 17.69 | 18.97 | 20.35 | 21.84 |
| 11.25 | 7.29 | 7.95 | 8.64 | 9.38 | 10.15 | 10.98 | 11.84 | 12.77 | 13.74 | 14.78 | 15.89 | 17.07 | 18.34 | 19.71 | 21.19 | 22.80 |
| 11.50 | 7.49 | 8.17 | 8.88 | 9.64 | 10.45 | 11.30 | 12.20 | 13.16 | 14.18 | 15.27 | 16.44 | 17.69 | 19.03 | 20.49 | 22.08 | 23.84 |
| 11.75 | 7.68 | 8.38 | 9.12 | 9.91 | 10.74 | 11.63 | 12.57 | 13.57 | 14.64 | 15.78 | 17.01 | 18.33 | 19.77 | 21.33 | 23.06 | 24.99 |
| 12.00 | 7.88 | 8.60 | 9.37 | 10.18 | 11.05 | 11.97 | 12.95 | 13.99 | 15.11 | 16.32 | 17.61 | 19.02 | 20.55 | 22.24 | 24.13 | 26.28 |
| 12.25 | 8.09 | 8.83 | 9.62 | 10.46 | 11.36 | 12.32 | 13.34 | 14.43 | 15.61 | 16.87 | 18.24 | 19.74 | 21.39 | 23.23 | 25.32 | 27.77 |
| 12.50 | 8.29 | 9.06 | 9.88 | 10.75 | 11.68 | 12.68 | 13.74 | 14.88 | 16.12 | 17.46 | 18.91 | 20.52 | 22.31 | 24.33 | 26.69 | 29.57 |
| 12.75 | 8.50 | 9.29 | 10.14 | 11.04 | 12.01 | 13.04 | 14.16 | 15.36 | 16.66 | 18.07 | 19.63 | 21.36 | 23.31 | 25.57 | 28.31 | 31.93 |
| 13.00 | 8.71 | 9.53 | 10.41 | 11.34 | 12.35 | 13.43 | 14.59 | 15.85 | 17.22 | 18.72 | 20.39 | 22.27 | 24.43 | 27.02 | 30.36 | 35.93 |
| 13.25 | 8.93 | 9.77 | 10.68 | 11.65 | 12.69 | 13.82 | 15.04 | 16.36 | 17.81 | 19.42 | 21.22 | 23.28 | 25.72 | 28.79 | 33.39 | |
| 13.50 | 9.15 | 10.02 | 10.96 | 11.97 | 13.05 | 14.23 | 15.51 | 16.90 | 18.45 | 20.17 | 22.13 | 24.43 | 27.26 | 31.20 | | |
| 13.75 | 9.37 | 10.27 | 11.25 | 12.29 | 13.42 | 14.65 | 16.00 | 17.48 | 19.12 | 20.98 | 23.14 | 25.76 | 29.22 | 36.37 | | |
| 14.00 | 9.60 | 10.53 | 11.54 | 12.63 | 13.81 | 15.10 | 16.51 | 18.08 | 19.85 | 21.88 | 24.30 | 27.38 | 32.20 | | | |
| 14.25 | 9.83 | 10.80 | 11.84 | 12.97 | 14.21 | 15.56 | 17.05 | 18.73 | 20.64 | 22.88 | 25.66 | 29.56 | | | | |
| 14.50 | 10.07 | 11.07 | 12.15 | 13.33 | 14.62 | 16.04 | 17.63 | 19.43 | 21.51 | 24.03 | 27.35 | 33.84 | | | | |
| 14.75 | 10.31 | 11.35 | 12.47 | 13.70 | 15.06 | 16.56 | 18.25 | 20.19 | 22.49 | 25.40 | 29.78 | | | | | |
| 15.00 | 10.56 | 11.64 | 12.81 | 14.09 | 15.51 | 17.10 | 18.91 | 21.02 | 23.61 | 27.14 | | | | | | |
| 15.25 | 10.82 | 11.93 | 13.15 | 14.49 | 15.99 | 17.68 | 19.63 | 21.96 | 24.96 | 29.81 | | | | | | |
| 15.50 | 11.08 | 12.24 | 13.51 | 14.91 | 16.49 | 18.30 | 20.42 | 23.04 | 26.71 | | | | | | | |
| 15.75 | 11.35 | 12.55 | 13.88 | 15.36 | 17.03 | 18.97 | 21.30 | 24.34 | 29.51 | | | | | | | |

*Continued*

**Table 3** *Continued*

| Surface power (D) | Lens diameter (mm) | | | | | | | | | | | | | | | |
|---|---|---|---|---|---|---|---|---|---|---|---|---|---|---|---|---|
| | 50 | 52 | 54 | 56 | 58 | 60 | 62 | 64 | 66 | 68 | 70 | 72 | 74 | 76 | 78 | 80 |
| 16.00 | 11.63 | 12.88 | 14.26 | 15.82 | 17.61 | 19.71 | 22.32 | 26.02 | | | | | | | | |
| 16.25 | 11.92 | 13.21 | 14.67 | 16.31 | 18.23 | 20.53 | 23.53 | 28.74 | | | | | | | | |
| 16.50 | 12.21 | 13.57 | 15.09 | 16.84 | 18.90 | 21.46 | 25.09 | | | | | | | | | |
| 16.75 | 12.52 | 13.93 | 15.54 | 17.41 | 19.65 | 22.57 | 27.49 | | | | | | | | | |
| 17.00 | 12.84 | 14.32 | 16.02 | 18.02 | 20.49 | 23.95 | | | | | | | | | | |
| 17.25 | 13.17 | 14.72 | 16.53 | 18.69 | 21.47 | 25.93 | | | | | | | | | | |
| 17.50 | 13.51 | 15.15 | 17.07 | 19.44 | 22.66 | | | | | | | | | | | |
| 17.75 | 13.87 | 15.60 | 17.67 | 20.29 | 24.25 | | | | | | | | | | | |
| 18.00 | 14.25 | 16.09 | 18.32 | 21.30 | 27.26 | | | | | | | | | | | |
| 18.25 | 14.65 | 16.61 | 19.05 | 22.55 | | | | | | | | | | | | |
| 18.50 | 15.07 | 17.17 | 19.89 | 24.37 | | | | | | | | | | | | |
| 18.75 | 15.52 | 17.79 | 20.89 | | | | | | | | | | | | | |
| 19.00 | 16.01 | 18.49 | 22.17 | | | | | | | | | | | | | |
| 19.25 | 16.53 | 19.29 | 24.14 | | | | | | | | | | | | | |
| 19.50 | 17.11 | 20.24 | | | | | | | | | | | | | | |
| 19.75 | 17.75 | 21.46 | | | | | | | | | | | | | | |
| 20.00 | 18.48 | 23.35 | | | | | | | | | | | | | | |
| 20.25 | 19.34 | | | | | | | | | | | | | | | |
| 20.50 | 20.43 | | | | | | | | | | | | | | | |
| 20.75 | 22.00 | | | | | | | | | | | | | | | |
| 21.00 | | | | | | | | | | | | | | | | |

**Table 4** Sags of lens surfaces at various diameters ($n = 1.498$)

| Surface power (D) | Lens diameter (mm) | | | | | | | | | | | | | | | |
|---|---|---|---|---|---|---|---|---|---|---|---|---|---|---|---|---|
| | 50 | 52 | 54 | 56 | 58 | 60 | 62 | 64 | 66 | 68 | 70 | 72 | 74 | 76 | 78 | 80 |
| 0.25 | 0.16 | 0.17 | 0.18 | 0.20 | 0.21 | 0.23 | 0.24 | 0.26 | 0.27 | 0.29 | 0.31 | 0.33 | 0.34 | 0.36 | 0.38 | 0.40 |
| 0.50 | 0.31 | 0.34 | 0.37 | 0.39 | 0.42 | 0.45 | 0.48 | 0.51 | 0.55 | 0.58 | 0.61 | 0.65 | 0.69 | 0.72 | 0.76 | 0.80 |
| 0.75 | 0.47 | 0.51 | 0.55 | 0.59 | 0.63 | 0.68 | 0.72 | 0.77 | 0.82 | 0.87 | 0.92 | 0.98 | 1.03 | 1.09 | 1.15 | 1.20 |
| 1.00 | 0.63 | 0.68 | 0.73 | 0.79 | 0.84 | 0.90 | 0.96 | 1.03 | 1.09 | 1.16 | 1.23 | 1.30 | 1.38 | 1.45 | 1.53 | 1.61 |
| 1.25 | 0.78 | 0.85 | 0.92 | 0.98 | 1.06 | 1.13 | 1.21 | 1.29 | 1.37 | 1.45 | 1.54 | 1.63 | 1.72 | 1.81 | 1.91 | 2.01 |
| 1.50 | 0.94 | 1.02 | 1.10 | 1.18 | 1.27 | 1.36 | 1.45 | 1.54 | 1.64 | 1.74 | 1.85 | 1.96 | 2.07 | 2.18 | 2.30 | 2.42 |
| 1.75 | 1.10 | 1.19 | 1.28 | 1.38 | 1.48 | 1.58 | 1.69 | 1.80 | 1.92 | 2.04 | 2.16 | 2.28 | 2.41 | 2.55 | 2.68 | 2.82 |
| 2.00 | 1.26 | 1.36 | 1.47 | 1.58 | 1.69 | 1.81 | 1.94 | 2.06 | 2.19 | 2.33 | 2.47 | 2.61 | 2.76 | 2.91 | 3.07 | 3.23 |
| 2.25 | 1.42 | 1.53 | 1.65 | 1.78 | 1.91 | 2.04 | 2.18 | 2.32 | 2.47 | 2.62 | 2.78 | 2.94 | 3.11 | 3.28 | 3.46 | 3.64 |
| 2.50 | 1.57 | 1.70 | 1.84 | 1.98 | 2.12 | 2.27 | 2.42 | 2.58 | 2.75 | 2.92 | 3.10 | 3.28 | 3.46 | 3.65 | 3.85 | 4.05 |
| 2.75 | 1.73 | 1.87 | 2.02 | 2.18 | 2.33 | 2.50 | 2.67 | 2.85 | 3.03 | 3.22 | 3.41 | 3.61 | 3.82 | 4.03 | 4.25 | 4.47 |
| 3.00 | 1.89 | 2.05 | 2.21 | 2.38 | 2.55 | 2.73 | 2.92 | 3.11 | 3.31 | 3.52 | 3.73 | 3.95 | 4.17 | 4.40 | 4.64 | 4.89 |
| 3.25 | 2.05 | 2.22 | 2.40 | 2.58 | 2.77 | 2.96 | 3.17 | 3.38 | 3.59 | 3.82 | 4.05 | 4.28 | 4.53 | 4.78 | 5.04 | 5.31 |
| 3.50 | 2.21 | 2.39 | 2.58 | 2.78 | 2.98 | 3.20 | 3.41 | 3.64 | 3.88 | 4.12 | 4.37 | 4.62 | 4.89 | 5.16 | 5.44 | 5.73 |
| 3.75 | 2.37 | 2.57 | 2.77 | 2.98 | 3.20 | 3.43 | 3.67 | 3.91 | 4.16 | 4.42 | 4.69 | 4.97 | 5.25 | 5.55 | 5.85 | 6.16 |
| 4.00 | 2.53 | 2.74 | 2.96 | 3.19 | 3.42 | 3.66 | 3.92 | 4.18 | 4.45 | 4.73 | 5.02 | 5.31 | 5.62 | 5.93 | 6.26 | 6.59 |
| 4.25 | 2.70 | 2.92 | 3.15 | 3.39 | 3.64 | 3.90 | 4.17 | 4.45 | 4.74 | 5.04 | 5.34 | 5.66 | 5.99 | 6.33 | 6.67 | 7.03 |
| 4.50 | 2.86 | 3.09 | 3.34 | 3.60 | 3.86 | 4.14 | 4.43 | 4.72 | 5.03 | 5.35 | 5.67 | 6.01 | 6.36 | 6.72 | 7.09 | 7.47 |
| 4.75 | 3.02 | 3.27 | 3.53 | 3.80 | 4.09 | 4.38 | 4.68 | 5.00 | 5.32 | 5.66 | 6.01 | 6.37 | 6.74 | 7.12 | 7.52 | 7.92 |
| 5.00 | 3.19 | 3.45 | 3.73 | 4.01 | 4.31 | 4.62 | 4.94 | 5.27 | 5.62 | 5.98 | 6.35 | 6.73 | 7.12 | 7.53 | 7.94 | 8.38 |
| 5.25 | 3.35 | 3.63 | 3.92 | 4.22 | 4.54 | 4.86 | 5.20 | 5.55 | 5.92 | 6.30 | 6.69 | 7.09 | 7.51 | 7.94 | 8.38 | 8.84 |
| 5.50 | 3.52 | 3.81 | 4.11 | 4.43 | 4.76 | 5.11 | 5.47 | 5.84 | 6.22 | 6.62 | 7.03 | 7.46 | 7.90 | 8.35 | 8.82 | 9.30 |
| 5.75 | 3.68 | 3.99 | 4.31 | 4.65 | 4.99 | 5.36 | 5.73 | 6.12 | 6.53 | 6.95 | 7.38 | 7.83 | 8.29 | 8.77 | 9.27 | 9.78 |
| 6.00 | 3.85 | 4.17 | 4.51 | 4.86 | 5.23 | 5.61 | 6.00 | 6.41 | 6.83 | 7.28 | 7.73 | 8.20 | 8.69 | 9.20 | 9.72 | 10.26 |
| 6.25 | 4.02 | 4.36 | 4.71 | 5.08 | 5.46 | 5.86 | 6.27 | 6.70 | 7.15 | 7.61 | 8.09 | 8.59 | 9.10 | 9.63 | 10.19 | 10.76 |
| 6.50 | 4.19 | 4.54 | 4.91 | 5.29 | 5.69 | 6.11 | 6.54 | 7.00 | 7.46 | 7.95 | 8.45 | 8.97 | 9.52 | 10.08 | 10.66 | 11.26 |
| 6.75 | 4.36 | 4.73 | 5.11 | 5.51 | 5.93 | 6.37 | 6.82 | 7.29 | 7.78 | 8.29 | 8.82 | 9.37 | 9.94 | 10.53 | 11.14 | 11.77 |

*Continued*

**Table 4** Continued

|  | Lens diameter (mm) | | | | | | | | | | | | | | | |
|---|---|---|---|---|---|---|---|---|---|---|---|---|---|---|---|---|
| Surface power (D) | 50 | 52 | 54 | 56 | 58 | 60 | 62 | 64 | 66 | 68 | 70 | 72 | 74 | 76 | 78 | 80 |
| 7.00 | 4.53 | 4.92 | 5.32 | 5.74 | 6.17 | 6.63 | 7.10 | 7.59 | 8.11 | 8.64 | 9.19 | 9.77 | 10.37 | 10.99 | 11.63 | 12.30 |
| 7.25 | 4.71 | 5.11 | 5.52 | 5.96 | 6.41 | 6.89 | 7.38 | 7.90 | 8.44 | 8.99 | 9.57 | 10.18 | 10.80 | 11.45 | 12.13 | 12.83 |
| 7.50 | 4.88 | 5.30 | 5.73 | 6.19 | 6.66 | 7.16 | 7.67 | 8.21 | 8.77 | 9.35 | 9.96 | 10.59 | 11.25 | 11.93 | 12.64 | 13.38 |
| 7.75 | 5.06 | 5.49 | 5.94 | 6.41 | 6.91 | 7.42 | 7.96 | 8.52 | 9.11 | 9.72 | 10.36 | 11.02 | 11.71 | 12.42 | 13.17 | 13.95 |
| 8.00 | 5.23 | 5.68 | 6.15 | 6.65 | 7.16 | 7.70 | 8.26 | 8.84 | 9.46 | 10.09 | 10.76 | 11.45 | 12.17 | 12.93 | 13.71 | 14.53 |
| 8.25 | 5.41 | 5.88 | 6.37 | 6.88 | 7.41 | 7.97 | 8.56 | 9.17 | 9.81 | 10.47 | 11.17 | 11.89 | 12.65 | 13.44 | 14.27 | 15.14 |
| 8.50 | 5.60 | 6.08 | 6.58 | 7.12 | 7.67 | 8.25 | 8.86 | 9.50 | 10.17 | 10.86 | 11.59 | 12.35 | 13.14 | 13.98 | 14.85 | 15.76 |
| 8.75 | 5.78 | 6.28 | 6.80 | 7.36 | 7.93 | 8.54 | 9.17 | 9.84 | 10.53 | 11.26 | 12.02 | 12.82 | 13.65 | 14.52 | 15.44 | 16.40 |
| 9.00 | 5.96 | 6.48 | 7.03 | 7.60 | 8.20 | 8.83 | 9.49 | 10.18 | 10.90 | 11.66 | 12.46 | 13.29 | 14.17 | 15.09 | 16.06 | 17.08 |
| 9.25 | 6.15 | 6.69 | 7.25 | 7.84 | 8.47 | 9.12 | 9.81 | 10.53 | 11.29 | 12.08 | 12.91 | 13.79 | 14.71 | 15.68 | 16.70 | 17.78 |
| 9.50 | 6.34 | 6.89 | 7.48 | 8.09 | 8.74 | 9.42 | 10.14 | 10.89 | 11.68 | 12.51 | 13.38 | 14.30 | 15.26 | 16.29 | 17.37 | 18.51 |
| 9.75 | 6.53 | 7.10 | 7.71 | 8.35 | 9.02 | 9.73 | 10.47 | 11.25 | 12.08 | 12.94 | 13.86 | 14.82 | 15.84 | 16.92 | 18.07 | 19.28 |
| 10.00 | 6.72 | 7.32 | 7.95 | 8.61 | 9.30 | 10.04 | 10.81 | 11.63 | 12.49 | 13.39 | 14.35 | 15.37 | 16.44 | 17.59 | 18.80 | 20.10 |
| 10.25 | 6.92 | 7.53 | 8.18 | 8.87 | 9.59 | 10.36 | 11.16 | 12.01 | 12.91 | 13.86 | 14.87 | 15.93 | 17.07 | 18.28 | 19.58 | 20.97 |
| 10.50 | 7.12 | 7.75 | 8.43 | 9.14 | 9.89 | 10.68 | 11.52 | 12.40 | 13.34 | 14.34 | 15.40 | 16.52 | 17.73 | 19.02 | 20.40 | 21.90 |
| 10.75 | 7.32 | 7.97 | 8.67 | 9.41 | 10.19 | 11.01 | 11.88 | 12.81 | 13.79 | 14.84 | 15.95 | 17.14 | 18.42 | 19.79 | 21.28 | 22.91 |
| 11.00 | 7.52 | 8.20 | 8.92 | 9.68 | 10.49 | 11.35 | 12.26 | 13.23 | 14.26 | 15.36 | 16.53 | 17.79 | 19.15 | 20.63 | 22.24 | 24.02 |
| 11.25 | 7.73 | 8.43 | 9.18 | 9.97 | 10.81 | 11.70 | 12.65 | 13.66 | 14.74 | 15.90 | 17.14 | 18.48 | 19.93 | 21.52 | 23.28 | 25.25 |
| 11.50 | 7.94 | 8.66 | 9.44 | 10.26 | 11.13 | 12.06 | 13.05 | 14.11 | 15.24 | 16.46 | 17.77 | 19.20 | 20.76 | 22.49 | 24.43 | 26.64 |
| 11.75 | 8.15 | 8.90 | 9.70 | 10.55 | 11.46 | 12.43 | 13.46 | 14.57 | 15.76 | 17.05 | 18.45 | 19.98 | 21.67 | 23.56 | 25.72 | 28.29 |
| 12.00 | 8.36 | 9.14 | 9.97 | 10.85 | 11.80 | 12.81 | 13.89 | 15.05 | 16.31 | 17.67 | 19.17 | 20.72 | 22.65 | 24.76 | 27.23 | 30.33 |
| 12.25 | 8.58 | 9.39 | 10.25 | 11.16 | 12.15 | 13.20 | 14.33 | 15.55 | 16.88 | 18.33 | 19.93 | 21.72 | 23.75 | 26.13 | 29.08 | 33.21 |
| 12.50 | 8.81 | 9.64 | 10.53 | 11.48 | 12.50 | 13.60 | 14.79 | 16.08 | 17.49 | 19.04 | 20.76 | 22.72 | 25.00 | 27.78 | 31.55 |  |
| 12.75 | 9.04 | 9.90 | 10.82 | 11.81 | 12.87 | 14.03 | 15.27 | 16.63 | 18.13 | 19.79 | 21.67 | 23.84 | 26.46 | 29.90 | 36.33 |  |
| 13.00 | 9.27 | 10.16 | 11.12 | 12.15 | 13.26 | 14.46 | 15.78 | 17.22 | 18.82 | 20.61 | 22.68 | 25.14 | 28.28 | 33.21 |  |  |
| 13.25 | 9.51 | 10.43 | 11.42 | 12.49 | 13.65 | 14.92 | 16.30 | 17.84 | 19.55 | 21.51 | 23.82 | 26.69 | 30.81 |  |  |  |

| | | | | | | | | | | | | |
|---|---|---|---|---|---|---|---|---|---|---|---|---|
| 13.50 | 9.75 | 10.71 | 11.74 | 12.85 | 14.07 | 15.40 | 16.86 | 18.50 | 20.36 | 22.52 | 25.16 | 28.71 |
| 13.75 | 10.00 | 10.99 | 12.06 | 13.22 | 14.50 | 15.90 | 17.46 | 19.21 | 21.24 | 23.67 | 26.80 | 31.97 |
| 14.00 | 10.25 | 11.28 | 12.39 | 13.61 | 14.95 | 16.43 | 18.09 | 19.99 | 22.23 | 25.03 | 29.06 | |
| 14.25 | 10.51 | 11.58 | 12.74 | 14.01 | 15.42 | 16.99 | 18.77 | 20.85 | 23.37 | 26.75 | | |
| 14.50 | 10.78 | 11.89 | 13.10 | 14.43 | 15.91 | 17.59 | 19.52 | 21.81 | 24.74 | 29.29 | | |
| 14.75 | 11.05 | 12.20 | 13.47 | 14.87 | 16.44 | 18.23 | 20.34 | 22.92 | 26.50 | | | |
| 15.00 | 11.34 | 12.53 | 13.86 | 15.33 | 17.00 | 18.93 | 21.26 | 24.26 | 29.30 | | | |
| 15.25 | 11.63 | 12.88 | 14.26 | 15.82 | 17.60 | 19.71 | 22.32 | 26.01 | | | | |
| 15.50 | 11.93 | 13.23 | 14.69 | 16.34 | 18.26 | 20.57 | 23.60 | 28.94 | | | | |
| 15.75 | 12.24 | 13.60 | 15.13 | 16.89 | 18.97 | 21.56 | 25.27 | | | | | |
| 16.00 | 12.56 | 13.99 | 15.61 | 17.49 | 19.77 | 22.75 | 28.04 | | | | | |
| 16.25 | 12.90 | 14.40 | 16.11 | 18.14 | 20.67 | 24.27 | | | | | | |
| 16.50 | 13.25 | 14.82 | 16.66 | 18.86 | 21.74 | 26.64 | | | | | | |
| 16.75 | 13.61 | 15.28 | 17.24 | 19.68 | 23.07 | | | | | | | |
| 17.00 | 14.00 | 15.76 | 17.88 | 20.61 | 24.98 | | | | | | | |
| 17.25 | 14.40 | 16.28 | 18.60 | 21.75 | | | | | | | | |
| 17.50 | 14.83 | 16.85 | 19.41 | 23.25 | | | | | | | | |
| 17.75 | 15.29 | 17.47 | 20.36 | 25.91 | | | | | | | | |
| 18.00 | 15.78 | 18.16 | 21.53 | | | | | | | | | |
| 18.25 | 16.31 | 18.94 | 23.18 | | | | | | | | | |
| 18.50 | 16.89 | 19.87 | | | | | | | | | | |
| 18.75 | 17.54 | 21.03 | | | | | | | | | | |
| 19.00 | 18.28 | 22.72 | | | | | | | | | | |
| 19.25 | 19.14 | | | | | | | | | | | |
| 19.50 | 20.22 | | | | | | | | | | | |
| 19.75 | 21.76 | | | | | | | | | | | |
| 20.00 | | | | | | | | | | | | |
| 20.25 | | | | | | | | | | | | |
| 20.50 | | | | | | | | | | | | |
| 20.75 | | | | | | | | | | | | |
| 21.00 | | | | | | | | | | | | |

# Powers of cylinders at oblique meridians

In any cylindrical surface, the curvature varies from zero in the axis meridian to a maximum in any meridian perpendicular to the axis. In any oblique meridian making an angle $\theta$ with the axis, the curvature would have some intermediate value. For the purpose of calculating lens thicknesses we could express this curvature as the 'notional' power of the cylinder in the given meridian. If we denote it by $C_\theta$ and the power of the cylinder by $C$, then

$$C_\theta = C \sin^2 \theta$$

Similarly, the notional power of a toroidal surface of base curve $B$ in a meridian at $\theta$ from the base curve meridian can be taken as

$$B + C \sin^2 \theta$$

*Table 5* gives values of $C_\theta$ for cylinder powers up to 6.00 D and for values of $\theta$ at every 5 degree intervals. It shows, for example, that a 2.50 D cylinder with its axis at 65 degrees (or 115 degrees) has a notional power of 2.05 D in the horizontal meridian.

**Table 5** Notional surface power of cylinders in oblique meridians

| Cylinder power (D) | Angle between oblique meridian and cylinder axis | | | | | | | | | | | | | | | | |
|---|---|---|---|---|---|---|---|---|---|---|---|---|---|---|---|---|---|
| | 5° | 10° | 15° | 20° | 25° | 30° | 35° | 40° | 45° | 50° | 55° | 60° | 65° | 70° | 75° | 80° | 85° |
| 0.25 | 0.00 | 0.01 | 0.02 | 0.03 | 0.04 | 0.06 | 0.08 | 0.10 | 0.12 | 0.15 | 0.17 | 0.19 | 0.21 | 0.22 | 0.23 | 0.24 | 0.25 |
| 0.50 | 0.00 | 0.02 | 0.03 | 0.06 | 0.09 | 0.12 | 0.16 | 0.21 | 0.25 | 0.29 | 0.34 | 0.37 | 0.41 | 0.44 | 0.47 | 0.48 | 0.50 |
| 0.75 | 0.01 | 0.02 | 0.05 | 0.09 | 0.13 | 0.19 | 0.25 | 0.31 | 0.37 | 0.44 | 0.50 | 0.56 | 0.62 | 0.66 | 0.70 | 0.73 | 0.74 |
| 1.00 | 0.01 | 0.03 | 0.07 | 0.12 | 0.18 | 0.25 | 0.33 | 0.41 | 0.50 | 0.59 | 0.67 | 0.75 | 0.82 | 0.88 | 0.93 | 0.97 | 0.99 |
| 1.25 | 0.01 | 0.04 | 0.08 | 0.15 | 0.22 | 0.31 | 0.41 | 0.52 | 0.62 | 0.73 | 0.84 | 0.94 | 1.03 | 1.10 | 1.17 | 1.21 | 1.24 |
| 1.50 | 0.01 | 0.05 | 0.10 | 0.18 | 0.27 | 0.37 | 0.49 | 0.62 | 0.75 | 0.88 | 1.01 | 1.12 | 1.23 | 1.32 | 1.40 | 1.45 | 1.49 |
| 1.75 | 0.02 | 0.05 | 0.12 | 0.20 | 0.31 | 0.44 | 0.58 | 0.72 | 0.87 | 1.03 | 1.17 | 1.31 | 1.44 | 1.55 | 1.63 | 1.70 | 1.73 |
| 2.00 | 0.02 | 0.06 | 0.13 | 0.23 | 0.36 | 0.50 | 0.66 | 0.83 | 1.00 | 1.17 | 1.34 | 1.50 | 1.64 | 1.77 | 1.87 | 1.94 | 1.98 |
| 2.25 | 0.02 | 0.07 | 0.15 | 0.26 | 0.40 | 0.56 | 0.74 | 0.93 | 1.12 | 1.32 | 1.51 | 1.69 | 1.85 | 1.99 | 2.10 | 2.18 | 2.23 |
| 2.50 | 0.02 | 0.08 | 0.17 | 0.29 | 0.45 | 0.62 | 0.82 | 1.03 | 1.25 | 1.47 | 1.68 | 1.87 | 2.05 | 2.21 | 2.33 | 2.42 | 2.48 |
| 2.75 | 0.02 | 0.08 | 0.18 | 0.32 | 0.49 | 0.69 | 0.90 | 1.14 | 1.37 | 1.61 | 1.85 | 2.06 | 2.26 | 2.43 | 2.57 | 2.67 | 2.73 |
| 3.00 | 0.02 | 0.09 | 0.20 | 0.35 | 0.54 | 0.75 | 0.99 | 1.24 | 1.50 | 1.76 | 2.01 | 2.25 | 2.46 | 2.65 | 2.80 | 2.91 | 2.98 |
| 3.25 | 0.02 | 0.10 | 0.22 | 0.38 | 0.58 | 0.81 | 1.07 | 1.34 | 1.62 | 1.91 | 2.18 | 2.44 | 2.67 | 2.87 | 3.03 | 3.15 | 3.23 |
| 3.50 | 0.03 | 0.11 | 0.23 | 0.41 | 0.63 | 0.87 | 1.15 | 1.45 | 1.75 | 2.05 | 2.35 | 2.62 | 2.87 | 3.09 | 3.27 | 3.39 | 3.47 |
| 3.75 | 0.03 | 0.11 | 0.25 | 0.44 | 0.67 | 0.94 | 1.23 | 1.55 | 1.87 | 2.20 | 2.52 | 2.81 | 3.08 | 3.31 | 3.50 | 3.64 | 3.72 |
| 4.00 | 0.03 | 0.12 | 0.27 | 0.47 | 0.71 | 1.00 | 1.32 | 1.65 | 2.00 | 2.35 | 2.68 | 3.00 | 3.29 | 3.53 | 3.73 | 3.88 | 3.97 |
| 4.25 | 0.03 | 0.13 | 0.28 | 0.50 | 0.76 | 1.06 | 1.40 | 1.76 | 2.12 | 2.49 | 2.85 | 3.19 | 3.49 | 3.75 | 3.97 | 4.12 | 4.22 |
| 4.50 | 0.03 | 0.14 | 0.30 | 0.53 | 0.80 | 1.12 | 1.48 | 1.86 | 2.25 | 2.64 | 3.02 | 3.37 | 3.70 | 3.97 | 4.20 | 4.36 | 4.47 |
| 4.75 | 0.03 | 0.14 | 0.32 | 0.56 | 0.85 | 1.19 | 1.56 | 1.96 | 2.37 | 2.79 | 3.19 | 3.56 | 3.90 | 4.19 | 4.43 | 4.61 | 4.72 |
| 5.00 | 0.04 | 0.15 | 0.33 | 0.58 | 0.89 | 1.25 | 1.65 | 2.07 | 2.50 | 2.93 | 3.35 | 3.75 | 4.11 | 4.42 | 4.67 | 4.85 | 4.96 |
| 5.25 | 0.04 | 0.16 | 0.35 | 0.61 | 0.94 | 1.31 | 1.73 | 2.17 | 2.62 | 3.08 | 3.52 | 3.94 | 4.31 | 4.64 | 4.90 | 5.09 | 5.21 |
| 5.50 | 0.04 | 0.17 | 0.37 | 0.64 | 0.98 | 1.37 | 1.81 | 2.27 | 2.75 | 3.23 | 3.69 | 4.12 | 4.52 | 4.86 | 5.13 | 5.33 | 5.46 |
| 5.75 | 0.04 | 0.17 | 0.39 | 0.67 | 1.03 | 1.44 | 1.89 | 2.38 | 2.87 | 3.37 | 3.86 | 4.31 | 4.72 | 5.08 | 5.36 | 5.58 | 5.71 |
| 6.00 | 0.05 | 0.18 | 0.40 | 0.70 | 1.07 | 1.50 | 1.97 | 2.48 | 3.00 | 3.52 | 4.03 | 4.50 | 4.93 | 5.30 | 5.60 | 5.82 | 5.95 |

# Decentrations and prismatic effects

## Spherical lenses

*Table 6* gives the prismatic effect due to decentration of a spherical lens by a given amount in millimetres. It can also be used in reverse, by scanning along the appropriate line and interpolating when necessary, to find the decentration needed to produce a prescribed prismatic effect. For example, the decentration needed to obtain $1.0^\triangle$ with a 3.75 D lens is found to be 2.7 mm to the nearest 0.1 mm.

### General mathematical solution

The following outlines a general mathematical solution to problems concerning decentration and prisms, as an alternative to graphical methods. Provided that the various sign conventions described are strictly observed, no difficulties should arise in calculation.

### *Position of a specified point*

The position of any point P on a lens is defined by its horizontal distance $x$ from a vertical line through the optical centre (O) of the lens and its vertical distance $y$ from a horizontal line through O. The coordinates $x$ and $y$ are subject to a special sign convention as follows:

> P inwards from O      : $x$ positive
> P outwards from O   : $x$ negative
> P upwards from O    : $y$ positive
> P downwards from O : $y$ negative

Note that $x$ and $y$ are invariably to be given in *centimetres*.

### *Prism components and bast settings*

The horizontal component of the prismatic effects is denoted by $H$ and the vertical component by $V$, subject to the following convention:

> Base in       : $H$ negative
> Base out    : $H$ positive
> Base up     : $V$ negative
> Base down : $V$ positive

**Table 6** Spherical lenses: prismatic effect (in Δ) of decentration

| Lens power | Decentration (mm) | | | | | | | | | | | |
|---|---|---|---|---|---|---|---|---|---|---|---|---|
| | 0.5 | 1.0 | 1.5 | 2.0 | 2.5 | 3.0 | 3.5 | 4.0 | 4.5 | 5.0 | 5.5 | 6.0 |
| 0.25 | 0.01 | 0.03 | 0.04 | 0.05 | 0.06 | 0.08 | 0.09 | 0.10 | 0.11 | 0.13 | 0.14 | 0.15 |
| 0.50 | 0.03 | 0.05 | 0.08 | 0.10 | 0.13 | 0.15 | 0.18 | 0.20 | 0.23 | 0.25 | 0.28 | 0.30 |
| 0.75 | 0.04 | 0.08 | 0.11 | 0.15 | 0.19 | 0.23 | 0.26 | 0.30 | 0.34 | 0.38 | 0.41 | 0.45 |
| 1.00 | 0.05 | 0.10 | 0.15 | 0.20 | 0.25 | 0.30 | 0.35 | 0.40 | 0.45 | 0.50 | 0.55 | 0.60 |
| 1.25 | 0.06 | 0.13 | 0.19 | 0.25 | 0.31 | 0.38 | 0.44 | 0.50 | 0.56 | 0.63 | 0.69 | 0.75 |
| 1.50 | 0.08 | 0.15 | 0.23 | 0.30 | 0.38 | 0.45 | 0.53 | 0.60 | 0.68 | 0.75 | 0.83 | 0.90 |
| 1.75 | 0.09 | 0.18 | 0.26 | 0.35 | 0.44 | 0.53 | 0.61 | 0.70 | 0.79 | 0.88 | 0.96 | 1.05 |
| 2.00 | 0.10 | 0.20 | 0.30 | 0.40 | 0.50 | 0.60 | 0.70 | 0.80 | 0.90 | 1.00 | 1.10 | 1.20 |
| 2.25 | 0.11 | 0.23 | 0.34 | 0.45 | 0.56 | 0.68 | 0.79 | 0.90 | 1.01 | 1.13 | 1.24 | 1.35 |
| 2.50 | 0.13 | 0.25 | 0.38 | 0.50 | 0.63 | 0.75 | 0.88 | 1.00 | 1.13 | 1.25 | 1.38 | 1.50 |
| 2.75 | 0.14 | 0.28 | 0.41 | 0.55 | 0.69 | 0.83 | 0.96 | 1.10 | 1.24 | 1.38 | 1.51 | 1.65 |
| 3.00 | 0.15 | 0.30 | 0.45 | 0.60 | 0.75 | 0.90 | 1.05 | 1.20 | 1.35 | 1.50 | 1.65 | 1.80 |
| 3.25 | 0.16 | 0.33 | 0.49 | 0.65 | 0.81 | 0.98 | 1.14 | 1.30 | 1.46 | 1.63 | 1.79 | 1.95 |
| 3.50 | 0.18 | 0.35 | 0.53 | 0.70 | 0.88 | 1.05 | 1.23 | 1.40 | 1.58 | 1.75 | 1.93 | 2.10 |
| 3.75 | 0.19 | 0.38 | 0.56 | 0.75 | 0.94 | 1.13 | 1.31 | 1.50 | 1.69 | 1.88 | 2.06 | 2.25 |
| 4.00 | 0.20 | 0.40 | 0.60 | 0.80 | 1.00 | 1.20 | 1.40 | 1.60 | 1.80 | 2.00 | 2.20 | 2.40 |
| 4.50 | 0.23 | 0.45 | 0.68 | 0.90 | 1.13 | 1.35 | 1.58 | 1.80 | 2.03 | 2.25 | 2.48 | 2.70 |
| 5.00 | 0.25 | 0.50 | 0.75 | 1.00 | 1.25 | 1.50 | 1.75 | 2.00 | 2.25 | 2.50 | 2.75 | 3.00 |
| 5.50 | 0.28 | 0.55 | 0.83 | 1.10 | 1.38 | 1.65 | 1.93 | 2.20 | 2.48 | 2.75 | 3.03 | 3.30 |
| 6.00 | 0.30 | 0.60 | 0.90 | 1.20 | 1.50 | 1.80 | 2.10 | 2.40⁻ | 2.70 | 3.00 | 3.30 | 3.60 |
| 6.50 | 0.33 | 0.65 | 0.98 | 1.30 | 1.63 | 1.95 | 2.28 | 2.60 | 2.93 | 3.25 | 3.58 | 3.90 |
| 7.00 | 0.35 | 0.70 | 1.05 | 1.40 | 1.75 | 2.10 | 2.45 | 2.80 | 3.15 | 3.50 | 3.85 | 4.20 |
| 7.50 | 0.38 | 0.75 | 1.13 | 1.50 | 1.88 | 2.25 | 2.63 | 3.00 | 3.38 | 3.75 | 4.13 | 4.50 |
| 8.00 | 0.40 | 0.80 | 1.20 | 1.60 | 2.00 | 2.40 | 2.80 | 3.20 | 3.60 | 4.00 | 4.40 | 4.80 |
| 8.50 | 0.43 | 0.85 | 1.28 | 1.70 | 2.13 | 2.55 | 2.98 | 3.40 | 3.83 | 4.25 | 4.68 | 5.10 |
| 9.00 | 0.45 | 0.90 | 1.35 | 1.80 | 2.25 | 2.70 | 3.15 | 3.60 | 4.05 | 4.50 | 4.95 | 5.40 |
| 9.50 | 0.48 | 0.95 | 1.43 | 1.90 | 2.38 | 2.85 | 3.33 | 3.80 | 4.28 | 4.75 | 5.23 | 5.70 |
| 10.00 | 0.50 | 1.00 | 1.50 | 2.00 | 2.50 | 3.00 | 3.50 | 4.00 | 4.50 | 5.00 | 5.50 | 6.00 |
| 10.50 | 0.53 | 1.05 | 1.58 | 2.10 | 2.63 | 3.15 | 3.68 | 4.20 | 4.73 | 5.25 | 5.78 | 6.30 |
| 11.00 | 0.55 | 1.10 | 1.65 | 2.20 | 2.75 | 3.30 | 3.85 | 4.40 | 4.95 | 5.50 | 6.05 | 6.60 |
| 11.50 | 0.58 | 1.15 | 1.73 | 2.30 | 2.88 | 3.45 | 4.03 | 4.60 | 5.18 | 5.75 | 6.33 | 6.90 |
| 12.00 | 0.60 | 1.20 | 1.80 | 2.40 | 3.00 | 3.60 | 4.20 | 4.80 | 5.40 | 6.00 | 6.60 | 7.20 |
| 12.50 | 0.63 | 1.25 | 1.88 | 2.50 | 3.13 | 3.75 | 4.38 | 5.00 | 5.63 | 6.25 | 6.88 | 7.50 |
| 13.00 | 0.65 | 1.30 | 1.95 | 2.60 | 3.25 | 3.90 | 4.55 | 5.20 | 5.85 | 6.50 | 7.15 | 7.80 |
| 13.50 | 0.68 | 1.35 | 2.03 | 2.70 | 3.38 | 4.05 | 4.73 | 5.40 | 6.08 | 6.75 | 7.43 | 8.10 |
| 14.00 | 0.70 | 1.40 | 2.10 | 2.80 | 3.50 | 4.20 | 4.90 | 5.60 | 6.30 | 7.00 | 7.70 | 8.40 |
| 14.50 | 0.73 | 1.45 | 2.18 | 2.90 | 3.63 | 4.35 | 5.08 | 5.80 | 6.53 | 7.25 | 7.98 | 8.70 |
| 15.00 | 0.75 | 1.50 | 2.25 | 3.00 | 3.75 | 4.50 | 5.25 | 6.00 | 6.75 | 7.50 | 8.25 | 9.00 |
| 15.50 | 0.78 | 1.55 | 2.33 | 3.10 | 3.88 | 4.65 | 5.43 | 6.20 | 6.98 | 7.75 | 8.53 | 9.30 |
| 16.00 | 0.80 | 1.60 | 2.40 | 3.20 | 4.00 | 4.80 | 5.60 | 6.40 | 7.20 | 8.00 | 8.80 | 9.60 |
| 16.50 | 0.83 | 1.65 | 2.48 | 3.30 | 4.13 | 4.95 | 5.78 | 6.60 | 7.43 | 8.25 | 9.08 | 9.90 |
| 17.00 | 0.85 | 1.70 | 2.55 | 3.40 | 4.25 | 5.10 | 5.95 | 6.80 | 7.65 | 8.50 | 9.35 | 10.20 |
| 17.50 | 0.88 | 1.75 | 2.63 | 3.50 | 4.38 | 5.25 | 6.13 | 7.00 | 7.88 | 8.75 | 9.63 | 10.50 |
| 18.00 | 0.90 | 1.80 | 2.70 | 3.60 | 4.50 | 5.40 | 6.30 | 7.20 | 8.10 | 9.00 | 9.90 | 10.80 |
| 18.50 | 0.93 | 1.85 | 2.78 | 3.70 | 4.63 | 5.55 | 6.48 | 7.40 | 8.33 | 9.25 | 10.18 | 11.10 |
| 19.00 | 0.95 | 1.90 | 2.85 | 3.80 | 4.75 | 5.70 | 6.65 | 7.60 | 8.55 | 9.50 | 10.45 | 11.40 |
| 19.50 | 0.98 | 1.95 | 2.93 | 3.90 | 4.88 | 5.85 | 6.83 | 7.80 | 8.78 | 9.75 | 10.73 | 11.70 |
| 20.00 | 1.00 | 2.00 | 3.00 | 4.00 | 5.00 | 6.00 | 7.00 | 8.00 | 9.00 | 10.00 | 11.00 | 12.00 |

## Axis direction

The cylinder axis direction is denoted by $\phi$, always considered positive and expressed as follows:

R eye : $\phi$ is 180 degrees minus the axis direction in standard notation

L eye : $\phi$ is the axis direction in standard notation.

## Coefficients

The first step is to calculate the value of the coefficients $A$, $B$ and $D$ from the following expressions:

$$A = S + C \sin^2 \phi$$
$$B = C \sin \phi \cos \phi$$
$$D = S + C \cos^2 \phi$$

in which $S$ is the spherical power and $C$ the cylindrical power of the lens.

## To find the prismatic effect at a specified point p

$$H = Ax + By$$
$$V = Bx + Dy$$

*Example:* Find the prismatic effect at a point 8 mm below and 2 mm inwards from the optical centre of the lens

L +3.75 DS +2.50 DC ax. 50°

The working details are

$$S = +3.75 \qquad x = 0.2$$
$$C = +2.50 \qquad y = -0.8$$
$$\phi = 50°$$

from which the values of the coefficients are found to be

$$A = 5.217$$
$$B = 1.231$$

and

$$D = 4.783$$

Finally

$$H = 5.217 \times 0.2 + 1.231 \times (-0.8) = 0.0586$$
$$= 0.06^\Delta \text{ base out}$$

and

$$V = 1.231 \times 0.2 + 4.783 \times (-0.8) = -3.5802$$
$$= 3.58^\Delta \text{ base up}$$

*To find the decentration required to produce a given prismatic effect*

The horizontal component $h$ and vertical component $v$ of the required decentration are found from

$$h = \frac{-DH + BV}{S(S + C)}$$

$$v = \frac{BH - AV}{S(S + C)}$$

Note that $h$ and $v$ are subject to the same sign convention as $x$ and $y$.

*Example:* Find the decentration needed to produce the prescribed prismatic effect, the lens being

R –2.00 DS –1.00 DC ax. 60°
1Δ base up 2Δ base in

The working details are

$S = -2.00$          $H = -2$
$C = -1.00$          $V = +1$
$\phi = (180 - 60) = 120°$

from which the values of the coefficients are found to be

$A = -2.75$
$B = 0.433$

and

$D = -2.25$

Finally

$$h = \frac{2.25 \times (-2) + 0.433 \times (-1)}{-2.00 \times (-3.00)}$$

$$= -0.822 \, \text{cm}$$

$$= 8.2 \, \text{mm out}$$

$$v = \frac{0.433 \times (-2) + 2.75 \times (-1)}{-2.00 \times (-3.00)}$$

$$= -0.603 \, \text{cm}$$

$$= 6.0 \, \text{mm down}$$

# Compensation for change in vertex distance

Whenever lens powers exceed about 5.00 D, attention should be paid to the vertex distance, that is, the separation between the back vertex of the lens and the cornea. This distance should then be measured by the prescriber and noted on the prescription. If the lens subsequently dispensed is fitted at some other vertex distance, the onus is on the dispenser to modify the prescription when necessary, or indicate on the prescription either the two distances (testing and fitting) or the difference between them and whether the lens has moved closer or farther from the eye. This allows some compensation to be made by the prescription house. Otherwise, serious errors may be introduced.

*Table 7* gives the modified power needed to compensate for a change in the vertex distance. If a plus lens is fitted closer to the eye or a minus lens further from the eye, its power must be increased. Conversely, a plus lens fitted further from the eye or a minus lens fitted closer to the eye must have their powers decreased.

In the case of astigmatic prescriptions, each principal meridian must be dealt with separately.

*Example:* An aphakic eye is corrected for distance by

+14.00 DS +1.50 DC

fitted at 15 mm from the cornea. What modified prescription is needed if the vertex distance is decreased to 12 mm?

The two principal powers are +14.00 and +15.50 D, and the lens is to be moved 3 mm closer to the eye. *Table 7* shows that the modified principal powers should be +14.61 D and +16.26 D. Rounding off may require some consideration, as in this case. The possible alternative prescriptions would be

+14.50 DS +1.75 DC

or

+14.75 DS +1.50 DC

In both cases, the stronger principal power would be +16.25 D.

**Table 7** Modified powers to compensate for change in vertex distance

| Plus lens fitted further from eye or minus lens fitted closer to eye | | | | | | | Plus lens fitted closer to eye or minus lens fitted further from eye | | | | | |
|---|---|---|---|---|---|---|---|---|---|---|---|---|
| Change in vertex distance (mm) | | | | | | Original power | Change in vertex distance (mm) | | | | | |
| 6 | 5 | 4 | 3 | 2 | 1 | | 1 | 2 | 3 | 4 | 5 | 6 |
| 4.38 | 4.40 | 4.42 | 4.44 | 4.46 | 4.48 | **4.50** | 4.52 | 4.54 | 4.56 | 4.58 | 4.60 | 4.62 |
| 4.85 | 4.88 | 4.90 | 4.93 | 4.95 | 4.98 | **5.00** | 5.03 | 5.05 | 5.08 | 5.10 | 5.13 | 5.15 |
| 5.32 | 5.35 | 5.38 | 5.41 | 5.44 | 5.47 | **5.50** | 5.53 | 5.56 | 5.59 | 5.62 | 5.66 | 5.69 |
| 5.79 | 5.83 | 5.86 | 5.89 | 5.93 | 5.96 | **6.00** | 6.04 | 6.07 | 6.11 | 6.15 | 6.19 | 6.22 |
| 6.26 | 6.30 | 6.34 | 6.38 | 6.42 | 6.46 | **6.50** | 6.54 | 6.59 | 6.63 | 6.67 | 6.72 | 6.76 |
| 6.72 | 6.76 | 6.81 | 6.86 | 6.90 | 6.95 | **7.00** | 7.05 | 7.10 | 7.15 | 7.20 | 7.25 | 7.31 |
| 7.18 | 7.23 | 7.28 | 7.33 | 7.39 | 7.44 | **7.50** | 7.56 | 7.61 | 7.67 | 7.73 | 7.79 | 7.85 |
| 7.63 | 7.69 | 7.75 | 7.81 | 7.87 | 7.94 | **8.00** | 8.06 | 8.13 | 8.20 | 8.26 | 8.33 | 8.40 |
| 8.09 | 8.15 | 8.22 | 8.29 | 8.36 | 8.43 | **8.50** | 8.57 | 8.65 | 8.72 | 8.80 | 8.88 | 8.96 |
| 8.54 | 8.61 | 8.69 | 8.76 | 8.84 | 8.92 | **9.00** | 9.08 | 9.17 | 9.25 | 9.34 | 9.42 | 9.51 |
| 8.99 | 9.07 | 9.15 | 9.24 | 9.32 | 9.41 | **9.50** | 9.59 | 9.68 | 9.78 | 9.88 | 9.97 | 10.07 |
| 9.43 | 9.52 | 9.62 | 9.71 | 9.80 | 9.90 | **10.00** | 10.10 | 10.20 | 10.31 | 10.42 | 10.53 | 10.64 |
| 9.88 | 9.98 | 10.08 | 10.18 | 10.28 | 10.39 | **10.50** | 10.61 | 10.73 | 10.84 | 10.96 | 11.08 | 11.21 |
| 10.32 | 10.43 | 10.54 | 10.65 | 10.76 | 10.88 | **11.00** | 11.12 | 11.25 | 11.38 | 11.51 | 11.64 | 11.78 |
| 10.76 | 10.87 | 10.99 | 11.12 | 11.24 | 11.37 | **11.50** | 11.63 | 11.77 | 11.91 | 12.05 | 12.20 | 12.35 |
| 11.19 | 11.32 | 11.45 | 11.58 | 11.72 | 11.86 | **12.00** | 12.15 | 12.30 | 12.45 | 12.61 | 12.77 | 12.93 |
| 11.63 | 11.76 | 11.90 | 12.05 | 12.20 | 12.35 | **12.50** | 12.66 | 12.82 | 12.99 | 13.16 | 13.33 | 13.51 |
| 12.06 | 12.21 | 12.36 | 12.51 | 12.67 | 12.83 | **13.00** | 13.17 | 13.35 | 13.53 | 13.71 | 13.90 | 14.10 |
| 12.49 | 12.65 | 12.81 | 12.97 | 13.15 | 13.32 | **13.50** | 13.68 | 13.87 | 14.07 | 14.27 | 14.48 | 14.69 |
| 12.92 | 13.08 | 13.26 | 13.44 | 13.62 | 13.81 | **14.00** | 14.20 | 14.40 | 14.61 | 14.83 | 15.05 | 15.28 |
| 13.34 | 13.52 | 13.71 | 13.90 | 14.09 | 14.29 | **14.50** | 14.71 | 14.93 | 15.16 | 15.39 | 15.63 | 15.88 |
| 13.76 | 13.95 | 14.15 | 14.35 | 14.56 | 14.78 | **15.00** | 15.23 | 15.46 | 15.71 | 15.96 | 16.22 | 16.48 |
| 14.18 | 14.39 | 14.60 | 14.81 | 15.03 | 15.26 | **15.50** | 15.74 | 16.00 | 16.26 | 16.52 | 16.80 | 17.09 |
| 14.60 | 14.81 | 15.04 | 15.27 | 15.50 | 15.75 | **16.00** | 16.26 | 16.53 | 16.81 | 17.09 | 17.39 | 17.70 |
| 15.01 | 15.24 | 15.48 | 15.72 | 15.97 | 16.23 | **16.50** | 16.78 | 17.06 | 17.36 | 17.67 | 17.98 | 18.31 |
| 15.43 | 15.67 | 15.92 | 16.18 | 16.44 | 16.72 | **17.00** | 17.29 | 17.60 | 17.91 | 18.24 | 18.58 | 18.93 |
| 15.84 | 16.09 | 16.36 | 16.63 | 16.91 | 17.20 | **17.50** | 17.81 | 18.13 | 18.47 | 18.82 | 19.18 | 19.55 |
| 16.25 | 16.51 | 16.79 | 17.08 | 17.37 | 17.68 | **18.00** | 18.33 | 18.67 | 19.03 | 19.40 | 19.78 | 20.18 |
| 16.65 | 16.93 | 17.23 | 17.53 | 17.84 | 18.16 | **18.50** | 18.85 | 19.21 | 19.59 | 19.98 | 20.39 | 20.81 |
| 17.06 | 17.35 | 17.66 | 17.98 | 18.30 | 18.65 | **19.00** | 19.37 | 19.75 | 20.15 | 20.56 | 20.99 | 21.44 |
| 17.46 | 17.77 | 18.09 | 18.42 | 18.77 | 19.13 | **19.50** | 19.89 | 20.29 | 20.71 | 21.15 | 21.61 | 22.08 |
| 17.86 | 18.18 | 18.52 | 18.87 | 19.23 | 19.61 | **20.00** | 20.41 | 20.83 | 21.28 | 21.74 | 22.22 | 22.73 |
| 18.25 | 18.59 | 18.95 | 19.31 | 19.69 | 20.09 | **20.50** | 20.93 | 21.38 | 21.84 | 22.33 | 22.84 | 23.38 |
| 18.65 | 19.00 | 19.37 | 19.76 | 20.15 | 20.57 | **21.00** | 21.45 | 21.92 | 22.41 | 22.93 | 23.46 | 24.03 |
| 19.04 | 19.41 | 19.80 | 20.20 | 20.61 | 21.05 | **21.50** | 21.97 | 22.47 | 22.98 | 23.52 | 24.09 | 24.68 |
| 19.43 | 19.82 | 20.22 | 20.64 | 21.07 | 21.53 | **22.00** | 22.49 | 23.01 | 23.55 | 24.12 | 24.72 | 25.35 |
| 20.21 | 20.63 | 21.06 | 21.52 | 21.99 | 22.48 | **23.00** | 23.54 | 24.11 | 24.70 | 25.33 | 25.99 | 26.68 |
| 20.98 | 21.43 | 21.90 | 22.39 | 22.90 | 23.44 | **24.00** | 24.59 | 25.21 | 25.86 | 26.55 | 27.27 | 28.04 |
| 21.74 | 22.22 | 22.73 | 23.26 | 23.81 | 24.39 | **25.00** | 25.64 | 26.32 | 27.03 | 27.78 | 28.57 | 29.41 |
| 22.49 | 23.01 | 23.55 | 24.12 | 24.71 | 25.34 | **26.00** | 26.69 | 27.43 | 28.20 | 29.02 | 29.89 | 30.81 |
| 23.24 | 23.79 | 24.37 | 24.98 | 25.62 | 26.29 | **27.00** | 27.75 | 28.54 | 29.38 | 30.27 | 31.21 | 32.22 |
| 23.97 | 24.56 | 25.18 | 25.83 | 26.52 | 27.24 | **28.00** | 28.81 | 29.66 | 30.57 | 31.53 | 32.56 | 33.65 |
| 24.70 | 25.33 | 25.99 | 26.68 | 27.41 | 28.18 | **29.00** | 29.87 | 30.79 | 31.76 | 32.81 | 33.92 | 35.11 |
| 25.42 | 26.09 | 26.79 | 27.52 | 28.30 | 29.13 | **30.00** | 30.93 | 31.92 | 32.97 | 34.09 | 35.29 | 36.59 |

# Flow chart for a prescription house

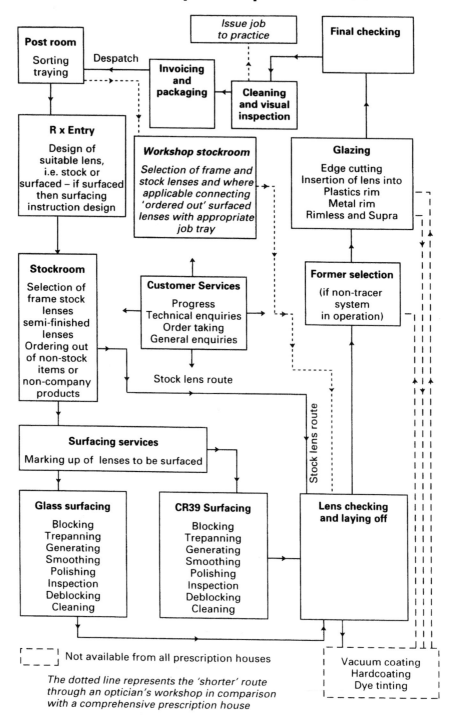

Issue job to practice

Final checking

**Post room**

Sorting traying

Despatch

**Invoicing and packaging**

**Cleaning and visual inspection**

**R x Entry**

Design of suitable lens, i.e. stock or surfaced – if surfaced then surfacing instruction design

**Workshop stockroom**

*Selection of frame and stock lenses and where applicable connecting 'ordered out' surfaced lenses with appropriate job tray*

**Glazing**

Edge cutting
Insertion of lens into
Plastics rim
Metal rim
Rimless and Supra

**Stockroom**

Selection of frame stock lenses semi-finished lenses
Ordering out of non-stock items or non-company products

**Customer Services**

Progress
Technical enquiries
Order taking
General enquiries

**Former selection**

(if non-tracer system in operation)

Stock lens route

Stock lens route

**Surfacing services**

Marking up of lenses to be surfaced

**Glass surfacing**

Blocking
Trepanning
Generating
Smoothing
Polishing
Inspection
Deblocking
Cleaning

**CR39 Surfacing**

Blocking
Trepanning
Generating
Smoothing
Polishing
Inspection
Deblocking
Cleaning

**Lens checking and laying off**

Not available from all prescription houses

Vacuum coating
Hardcoating
Dye tinting

*The dotted line represents the 'shorter' route through an optician's workshop in comparison with a comprehensive prescription house*

# Index

Abbe number (v-value), 272–3
Aberrations, 116
Abuse marks, 211
Accommodation, 9
Acrylic resin frame materials, 35–6
Addition
  focimeter measurements, 177–8
  fused multifocals, 225–7
  prescription order form, 70
  progressives *see* Progressive lenses
Aluminium frame material, 28
Anisometropia, 227
Anti-reflection (AR) coatings, 18,
  293–6
  application, 295–6
Aphakia, 11, 285
Aphakic lens, 285
Aqueous humour, 8
Aspheric lenses, 117, 280–9
  oblique astigmatism/curvature
    error reduction, 284, 285
Astigmatic lenses, 102–10, 116
  cylindrical surface, 102–3
  neutralisation, 163, 164–6
  principle powers, 104–6
  sphero-cylindrical (spherocyl), 103
  transposition, 107
    rules, 107–10
Astigmatism, 3, 11, 102

Back surface, 76
Back vertex, 76
Bad metal, 208
Base curves, 82–3, 116
Bead marks, 211
Best-form series, 116
Bevelled edges/lenses, 186, 196
Bi-prism (slab-off)
  fused multifocals, 227, 228–31
  resin multifocals, 245, 246, 247

Blanks *see* Semi-finished blanks
Blended (seamless) lenticular lenses,
  286, 287
Blind spot, 8
Blocking (pressure distortion), 211
Blocking procedure, 322–3
Bonded bifocals, 266–7
Bonded equitint lenses, 306–8
Box system, 53, 54, 62
Brace bar, 42
Bridge
  dimensions, 56, 57
  metal frames, 41–2
  plastic frames, 44–6
Bruise check, lens surface, 211
Bubbles in lens material, 208

Carbon fibre frame materials, 37–8
Casting system for lens manufacture,
  332
Cataract, 284–5, 315
CE markings, 19, 21
Cellulose acetate frame materials,
  32–5
Cellulose nitrate frame materials,
  31–2
Cellulose propionate frame materials,
  36
Centration, 129–43
  focimeter measurements, 176
Centration distance, 130–1
Centration point, 137
Centre of curvature, 75, 76
Chemical toughening process, 318–19
Chips, 211
Clip-on, 39
Clipover, 39
Colour of lens, 207
Concave lens surface, 75
Constringence, 272

Consumer legislation, 21
Contour eyeshapes, 66
Convex lens surface, 75
Cornea, 7
Crazing, 208
Cribbing (trepanning), 15, 323
Crimping, 331
Curvature error, 281, 283, 284
Curve variation factor (CVF), 270
Curved lenses, 116–22
  neutralisation, 166
Cutting lenses, 183–5
Cutting wheels, 324, 325
Cycling spectacles, 52
Cylinders, powers at oblique
  meridians, 352–3

Datum system, 53, 54, 55, 61–2
Deblocking, 331
Decentration, 130
  prism effects
    spherical lenses, 137–9, 354–7
    sphero-cylinders, 139–43
Differential prism (vertical
  imbalance), 177
Dig, lens surface, 210
Dioptres, 78–9, 103
Dispensing opticians, 5
Dispersion effects
  fused multifocals, 221
  high index materials, 271–2
Distance edging, 74
Diving mask, 50–1
Dress-clips, 49
Dry cutting, 189, 325
Dye tinting, 297, 300–2

EC Directives, 21
Edge forms, 186–9
Edgers
  automatic, 183–5
  dry cut, 189
  hand, 189
Edging, 180
Effective lens diameter, 63–4
Electro-magnetic spectrum, 269, 270,
  271, 290–1
Engraved frames, 41
Equi-concave lens, 81
Equi-convex lens, 81
Executive (E-style) bifocals, 240–1
Eye structure, 7–9
Eyeglasses, 39

Feathers in lens material, 208
Filters see Tinted lenses
Fining, 18
Fitting see Glazing
Flake, 195
Flat-edged lenses, 186, 196
Flexibridge, 42
Focimeter (lens analyser/lensmeter),
  167–79
  applications, 167–8
  automated readings, 167, 168, 173,
    174
  callibration, 173
  centration, 176
  eyepiece design, 168, 169–71
  laying off, 180–1
  lens power determination, 175–6
  preliminary adjustment, 172–3
  prismatic effects, 176
  progressive lenses checking, 261–2
  projection instruments, 168, 171–2,
    173
  verification, 177–9, 205
Folding spectacles, 49
Frames see Spectacle frames
Franklin (split) lenses, 263–7
  bonded, 265–6
  trifocals, 264–5
Front surface, 76
Front vertex, 76
Fused multifocals, 219–35
  construction, 219–20
  fused blanks, 225
  properties, 221–2
  reading addition, 225–7
  shaped (non-circular) segments,
    222–4
  trifocals, 231, 234–5
  vertical prism compensation,
    227–31, 232, 233

Generating process, 15, 18, 324–7
Geometrical lens shapes, 64–6
Geometrical optics, 4
Glare, 315
Glass lenses
  impact protection, 316–19
  manufacture, 14–15
Glass solid multifocals, 236–43
  basic features, 236–8
  Executive (E-style), 240–1
  prism controlled, 242–3
  seamless (blended), 239
  segment diameters/height, 237–8

trifocals, 243
upcurve, 238–9
vertical prism compensation, 241–2
Glazing, 13, 60–1, 180–204
alterations, 197
edge forms, 186–9
faults/defects, 194–6
laying off, 180–3
lens cutting, 183–5
automatic edgers, 183–5, 190
edging formers, 185–6
hand edgers, 189
metal frames, 191–2
strain testing, 193–4
nylon supra mounts, 192–3
plastic frames, 190–1
setting up, 197
standards, 194, 196–7
tools, 197–203
Gold frames, 23, 24–7
gold plating, 26–7
rolled gold, 24–5
Grey lens surface, 209
Grooved edge, 187
Gun sights, 51

Half eyes, 47, 49
lens shapes, 68
Hardcoating, 308–10
dipping method, 309–10
in-mould method, 310
spin method, 309
vacuum coating, 310
Hearing-aid spectacles, 50
High index materials, 268–74, 314
Abbe number (v-value), 272–3
chromatic aberration, 272
constringence, 272
definitions, 268
dispersive power, 271–2
reflections, 273
thickness saving, 270, 271
High powered lenses, 268–74
full aperture, 268
lenticular lenses, 268
minus, 274–7
plus, 277–9
Hinged-front spectacles, 49
Historical aspects, 3–4, 22
aspheric lenses, 286
progressive lenses, 249–51
Holes, 209
Hypermetropia (long-sightedness), 9
Hypoallergic frame materials, 36, 37

Impact protection, 316–19
glass, 316–19
toughening process, 317
polycarbonate, 319
resin, 319
Implant (intra-ocular lens), 285
Integral tints, 297, 298–9
Intelligent Prism Thinning, 241, 256–7
Interpupillary distance, 130–1
Intra-ocular lens (implant), 285
Iris, 8

Joints
metal frames, 43
plastic frames, 46
position, 40, 41

Kitemark, 21
Kryptok bifocals, 219, 220

Laying off, 180–3
Lens, 13–21
aspheric, 117, 280–9
crystalline of eye, 8
definition, 6
dimensions, 55, 56, 61–2
effective diameter, 63–4
size of unglazed frame, 62–3
faults, 207–11
glass, 14–15
photochromic, 15
lenticular see Lenticular lenses
resin, 15–18
shape difference (lens difference),
62
shapes, 61
classification, 64–8
spherical see Spherical lenses
standards, 18–20
Lens analyser (lensmeter) see
Focimeter
Lens measure, 84–5
Lensmeter (lens analyser) see
Focimeter
Lenticular lenses, 268
blended/seamless, 286, 287
minus, 274–7
plus, 277–9
Long-sightedness (hypermetropia), 9
Lorgnettes, 39, 49
Lorgnon (quizzer), 39–40, 49

Macula, 8
Make-up spectacles, 49
Manufacture of lenses, 13–14
  glass, 14–15
  resin, 15–18
  see also Surfacing
Marking/markup (stampout) for
    surfacing, 322
Medical Devices EC Directive, 21
Memory metal frame material, 29
Meniscus lens, 117
  minus, 82
  plus, 81
Meniscus plano prism, 144
Metal spectacle frames
  bridge, 41–2
  glazing, 191–2
  joints, 43
  materials, 23–9
  nomenclature, 40–4
  rims, 42
  sides, 43, 44
Milled edge, 187–8
Mini-lab, 332
Minibevel, 187
Minus (mushroom) lap, 327
Monocles, 39, 49
Motorcycle goggles, 51
Mounting see Glazing
Mounts, 39
Multifocals
  bonded bifocals, 266–7
  Franklin (split) lenses, 263–7
  fused see Fused multifocals
  glass solid, 236–43
  progressives comparison, 255–6
  resin, 244–7
  semi-finished blanks, 115
Mushroom (minus) lap, 327
Myopia (short-sightedness), 10
Myopic rings, 268

Natural frame materials, 29–30
Neutralisation, 161–6
  astigmatic lenses, 163, 164–6
  curved lenses, 166
  general rules, 163
  scissors movements, 163
  spherical lenses, 164
  transverse movements, 161–2
Nickel silver frame material, 27
Nylon frame materials, 37
Nylon supra mounts, glazing, 192–3

Oblique astigmatism, 281–2, 283
Ophthalmic medical practitioners, 5
Ophthalmic opticians (optometrists), 5
Ophthalmic optics, 4
Ophthalmology, 4
Optic nerve, 8
Optical axis, 75, 76
Optical centre, 76, 129
  displacement effect of prism, 135–7
  focimeter location, 176
  neutralisation test, 162
Optics, 4
Optyl frame material, 36–7
Oval eyeshape, 65
Over-specs, 51

Pad bridge, 40, 41–2, 44, 45
Panoptic shaped segments, 223
Perimetric lens shapes, 66
Periscope lens, 82
Personal Protective Equipment EC
    Directive, 21
Photochromic lenses, 15, 303–6
  fused multifocals, 221
  toughening process, 318
Photorefractive keratectomy, 4
Pilot eyeshape, 67
Pin beveller, 189
Plano-concave lens, 81
Plano-convex lens, 81
Plastic spectacle frames
  glazing, 190–1
  materials, 29, 30–7
  nomenclature, 44–7
Plus (saucer) lap, 327
Polarised lenses, 314–15
Polished edge, 188
Polishing, 15, 17, 330–1
Polishing burn, 209
Polycarbonate lens, 319
  manufacture, 17–18
Power
  cylindrical lens, 103
    at oblique meridians, 352–3
  focimeter measurements, 175–6, 177
    automated readings, 167, 168,
      173, 174
  neutralisation test, 161
  prisms, 147–9
  spherical lens, 78–9
  sphero-cylindrical (spherocyl) lens,
    104–6
Power rings, 268
Prentice's rule, 132, 228

Presbyopia, 10, 248, 249, 263
Prescription, 6
Prescription house, 13
  flow chart, 360
Prescription order form, 69–74
  add for multifocals/progressives, 70
  centration distance, 70–1, 72
  geometrical inset, 72–3
  optical inset, 73
  segment position, 71–2
  Standard Axis Notation, 70
  standards, 69
Pressure distortion, 211
Prism by decentration
  spherical lenses, 137–8
  sphero-cylinders, 139–43
Prism dioptres, 132, 147
Prism thinning
  Executive (E-style) bifocals, 240–1
  progressive lenses, 256–7
Prism/lens combination, 135–7
Prismatic effects
  focimeter measurements, 176
  plano-cylinder, 134–5
  spherical lenses, 131–4
Prisms, ophthalmic, 144–60
  base setting, 150–2
  compounding/resolving, 153–60
  definitions, 144
  deviation, 145
  dividing (splitting), 152–3
  power, 147–9
  thickness difference, 149–50, 151
  units of angle, 145–7
  uses, 145
PRO (pantoscopic round oval)
    eyeshape, 65–6
Progressive addition lenses (PALs) see
    Progressive lenses
Progressive lenses, 248–62
  asymmetrical designs, 253, 254
  design advances, 258–9
  focimeter checking, 261–2
  hard/soft designs, 254–5
  main elements, 248, 249
  Maitenaz design, 251
  markings/engravings, 260, 261
  multifocals comparison, 255–6
  patient adaptation, 248–9
  prism checking point, 261
  prism thinning, 256–7
  semi-finished blanks, 115
  symmetrical designs, 252, 253
  unwanted astigmatic effects, 258
  vocational designs, 257

Ptosis spectacles, 50
Pupil, 7
Pushing in (springing in), 180, 191

Quadra eyeshape, 66
Quality of optical products, 20–1
Quizzer (lorgnon), 39–40, 49

Radius of curvature, 75, 76, 83, 84
Recumbent spectacles, 50
Reflections
  at normal incidence, 292
  causes, 291–2
Refraction, 4–5
Refractive index, 14, 20
  measurement wavelengths, 268–9
  standards, 268
Resin lenses
  hardcoating, 308–10
  impact protection, 319
  manufacture, 15–18
Resin multifocals, 244–7
  high index resins, 247
  segment sizes/shapes, 244, 245
  vertical prism compensation, 245–7
Respiration spectacles, 52
Retina, 8
Reversible spectacles, 52
Rimless fitting, 180, 193
Rimless spectacles, 47, 196
  lens shapes, 67, 68
  strain testing, 193–4
Rims, 42
Round eyeshape, 64–5

Safety chamfers, 188–9, 195
Safety spectacles, 50
  see also Impact protection
Sag
  formula, 87–96
  gauge (high-precision spherometer),
    85–6
  lens surface, 345–51
Saucer (plus) lap, 327
Scalloped edge, 188
Sclera, 8
Scratches, 210
Seamless (blended) bifocals, 239
Seamless (blended) lenticular lenses,
    286, 287
Second principle focus, 77, 132

Semi-finished blanks, 13, 320
  fused, 225
  selection, 321–2
  toric lenses, 115–16
Serengeti lenses, 314
Shadowing, 207
Shadowscope, 207
Shooting spectacles, 51
Short-sightedness (myopia), 10
Sides
  classification, 40, 41
  dimensions, 57, 58
  metal frames, 43, 44
  plastic frames, 47
Silver frame material, 23, 24
Ski spectacles, 51
Slab-off process see Bi-prism
Sleek, 211
Smoothing, 15, 17, 327–30
Snooker spectacles, 49–50
Spark, 195
Spectacle frames
  basic dimensions, 55–8
  carbon fibre, 37–8
  classification, 39–40
  joint positions, 40, 41
  marking, 59
  materials, 22–38
    combination, 40
    desirable properties, 23
  metal, 23–9, 40–4
  nomenclature, 39–52
  nylon, 37
  plastics, 29–37, 40
  rimless spectacles, 47
  sides, 40, 41
  standards, 53–5
  supra spectacles, 47
  vocational, 47–52
Spectral control lenses, 314
Spherical lenses, 75–101, 116
  base curves, 82–3, 96
  definitions, 75–6
  minus (diverging), 77–8, 81, 82
  neutralisation, 164
  plus (converging), 77–8, 81
  power, 78–9
    substance compensation, 97–101
  prism effects, 131–4
    decentration, 137–9
  sag formula, 87–96
  spherometer formula, 83–4
  standard forms, 80–2
  surface power, 80
    lens measure, 84–5

sag gauge (high-precision
    spherometer), 85–6
Sphero-cylindrical lens (spherocyl),
    103
  prism effects in decentration,
    139–43
Spherometer formula, 83–4
Split lenses see Franklin lenses
Springing in (pushing in), 180, 191
SPX frame material, 37
Squash goggles, 51
Stainless steel frame material, 27–8
Stampout (marking/markup) for
    surfacing, 322
Standard Axis Notation, 70
Standards, 18–20
  glazing, 194, 196–7
  prescription order form, 69
  refractive index, 268
  spectacle frame dimensions, 53–5
  toric lens, 112–13
  ultraviolet (UV) absorbers, 312, 313
Starring, 195
Strain, lens, 207
Superopticals, 14
Supra spectacles, 47
Surface coating/tinting, 297, 299–300
Surface power
  lens measure, 84–5
  sag gauge (high-precision
      spherometer), 85–6
Surfacing, 320–33
  blank selection, 321–2
  blocking, 322–3
  cleaning, 331
  deblocking, 331
  generating, 15, 18, 324–7
  instructions, 320–1
  marking, 322
  polishing, 15, 17, 330–1
  smoothing, 15, 17, 327–30
  trepanning/cribbing, 15, 323
Swimming goggles, 51
Synthetic plastic frame materials,
    30–1

Tarnish stains, 208
Telescopic spectacles, 50
Thermal toughening process, 317
Thin toughening process, 317
Tinted lenses, 296–303
  dye tinting, 297, 300–2
  integral tints, 297, 298–9
  regulations/restrictions, 297

surface coating/tinting, 297,
    299–300
transmission data, 302–3
Tinting methods, 297–302
Titanium frame material, 28–9
Toric lenses, 112–15
    curves, 116–22
    semi-finished blanks, 115–16
Toroidal surface, 111, 112
Trepanning (cribbing), 15, 323
Trifocals
    Franklin (split) lenses, 264–5
    fused multifocals, 231, 234–5
    glass solid, 243

Ultifo progressive lenses, 250
Ultraviolet inhibitors, 311–14
    spectral control, 314
    standards, 313
Ultraviolet light components, 312
Ultraviolet sunspecs, 52
Uncut lenses, 13, 60
    prescription order form, 73
Univis shaped segments, 222, 223
Upcurve solid bifocals, 238–9
Upswept eyeshape, 67

Varilux progressive lenses, 251
Veins in lens material, 208
Verification, 205–11
    checklist, 205–7
    focimeter (lens analyser/lensmeter),
        177–9
    lens faults, 207–11
    lens inspection, 206–7
Vertex distance compensation, 358–9
Vertex power allowances, 337–44
Vertical prism compensation
    fused multifocals, 227–31, 232, 233
    glass solid multifocals, 241–2
    resin multifocals, 245–7
Visible spectrum, 269
Vitreous humour, 8
Vocational designs
    frames/mounts, 47–52
    progressive lenses, 257

Wafer laminating system, 333
Water resistant coating, 310–11
Waves, lens surface, 209–10
Welding goggles, 52